A Resource for Nurse Anesthesia Educators

Bernadette Henrichs, CRNA, PhD, CCRN
Judy Thompson, CRNA, MS, APRN

Published by
American Association of Nurse Anesthetists

American Association of Nurse Anesthetists
222 South Prospect Avenue
Park Ridge, IL 60068-4001

Printed in the United States of America

Last digit indicates print number: 10 9 8 7 6 5 4 3

The author(s) and publisher have done everything possible to make this book accurate, up to date, and in accord with accepted standards at the time of publication. The authors, editors, and publisher are not responsible for errors or omissions or for consequences from application of the book, and make no warranty, expressed or implied, in regard to the contents of the book. Any practice described in this book should be applied by the reader in accordance with professional standards of care used in regard to the unique circumstances that may apply in each situation.

Library of Congress has cataloged the first printing as follows:

A resource for nurse anesthesia educators / Judy Thompson and Bernadette Henrichs, editors.
    p. ; cm.
 Includes bibliographical references.
 ISBN 978-0-9700279-6-2 (pbk.)
 1. Nurse anesthetists--Study and teaching. I. Thompson, Judy, 1948- II. Henrichs, Bernadette, 1960- III. American Association of Nurse Anesthetists.
 [DNLM: 1. Nurse Anesthetists--education. 2. Anesthesia--nursing.
 3. Education, Nursing. WY 18 R4325 2009]
  RD80.7.R47 2009
  617.9'6076--dc22
                        2009023000

Dedication

Live as if you were to die tomorrow. Learn as if you were to live forever.

–Mahatma Gandhi

This book is dedicated to all the students and instructors in my life who have made me what I am today.

Bernadette Henrichs, CRNA, PhD, CCRN

This book is dedicated to my mother, Betty Thompson, for all her love, encouragement and inspiration. I am who I am because of you. I also dedicate this book to all the students who graduated from St Raphael's since 1983 that I have had the good fortune to work with and learn from all these years.

Judy Thompson, CRNA, MS, APRN

Contributors

Chuck Biddle, CRNA, PhD
Professor and Staff Anesthetist
Virginia Commonwealth University Medical Center
Richmond, Virginia

Pamela K. Blackwell, JD
Associate Director, Federal Regulatory and Payment Policy
American Association of Nurse Anesthetists
Washington, DC

Vicki Coopmans, CRNA, PhD
Associate Professor
Assistant Director, Nurse Anesthesia Program
Goldfarb School of Nursing at Barnes-Jewish College
Saint Louis, Missouri

Francis Gerbasi, CRNA, PhD
Executive Director
Council on Accreditation of Nurse Anesthesia Educational Programs
American Association of Nurse Anesthetists
Park Ridge, Illinois

Richard E. Haas, CRNA, PhD, PHRN
Program Director
WellSpan Health Nurse Anesthetist Program
York College of Pennsylvania
York, Pennsylvania

William Hartland Jr, CRNA, PhD
Associate Professor, Director of Education
Department of Nurse Anesthesia, School of Allied Health Professions
Virginia Commonwealth University
Richmond, Virginia

Bernadette Henrichs, CRNA, PhD, CCRN
Professor and Director, Nurse Anesthesia Program
Goldfarb School of Nursing at Barnes-Jewish College
Saint Louis, Missouri

Betty J. Horton, CRNA, PhD
Education Consultant
Self-Employed
Tower Hill, Illinois

Anne Marie Hranchook, CRNA, MSN
Assistant Director
Beaumont Graduate Program of Nurse Anesthesia
Oakland University
Rochester, Michigan

Lillia M. Loriz, PhD, ARNP, BC
Director
School of Nursing
University of North Florida
Jacksonville, Florida

Alfred E. Lupien, CRNA, PhD, FAAN
Director and Professor
Graduate Program in Nurse Anesthesia
Mount Marty College
Sioux Falls, South Dakota

Kiran Macha, MBBS, MPH
Clinical Research Coordinator
Nurse Anesthetist Program
School of Nursing
University of North Florida
Jacksonville, Florida

Mary Jeanette Mannino, CRNA, JD
Private Practice
Laguna Niguel, California
Adjunct faculty
Gonzaga University
Spokane, Washington

Maura S. McAuliffe, CRNA, PhD, FAAN
Professor and Program Director
East Carolina University College of Nursing
Nurse Anesthesia Program
Greenville, North Carolina

John P. McDonough, CRNA, EdD, ARNP
Professor and Director, Nurse Anesthetist Program
Associate Director for Graduate Studies
School of Nursing
University of North Florida
Jacksonville, Florida

John J. McFadden, CRNA, PhD
Associate Dean and Chair
Division of Graduate Clinical Sciences
Barry University College of Health Sciences
Miami Shores, Florida

Lisa Mileto, CRNA, MS
Director
Beaumont Graduate Program of Nurse Anesthesia
Oakland University
Rochester, Michigan

Charles A. Reese, CRNA, PhD
Associate Professor, Department of Anesthesiology
Associate Professor, Department of Obstetrics and Gynecology
Medical College of Virginia Physicians
Virginia Commonwealth University Medical Center
Richmond, Virginia

Elizabeth Monti Seibert, CRNA, PhD
Program Administrator
Nurse Anesthesia Program
Otterbein College/Grant Medical Center
Columbus, Ohio

Lisa J. Thiemann, CRNA, MNA
Senior Director, Professional Practice
American Association of Nurse Anesthetists
Park Ridge, Illinois

Judy Thompson, CRNA, MS, APRN
Program Director
Hospital of St Raphael
School of Nurse Anesthesia
New Haven, Connecticut

Lawrence Howard Truver, CRNA, MSNA
Locum Tenens CRNA
Charleston, South Carolina

Sandra K. Tunajek, CRNA, DNP
Former Executive Director, Council for Public Interest in Anesthesia
Director, AANA Wellness Program (2005-2008)
American Association of Nurse Anesthetists
Park Ridge, Illinois

Lynne M. Van Wormer, CRNA, MSN
Clinical Graduate Director
Center for Nurse Anesthesiology
Albany Medical College
Albany, New York

Celeste G. Villanueva, CRNA, MS
Program Director
Samuel Merritt University
Oakland, California

Kathleen Wren, CRNA, PhD
Professor and Chair
Nurse Anesthesia Department
Florida Hospital College of Health Sciences
Orlando, Florida

Timothy Wren, RN, DNP
Professor
Nursing Department
Florida Hospital College of Health Sciences
Orlando, Florida

Foreword

We are delighted to introduce to you *A Resource for Nurse Anesthesia Educators*. This book was compiled for all of you who serve or aspire to serve in the roles of preceptor, educator, or mentor to student nurse anesthetists. In this volume, we have provided informative chapters on many of the major issues related to educating our future colleagues. The authors of these chapters are among the most experienced nurse anesthesia educators in our field today. We hope that this one-of-a-kind volume will encourage nurse anesthetists who have an interest in teaching and inspire experienced educators to be even better teachers.

This book has been in the works for several years. It began as a guide for clinical preceptors, but through our research on the needs of faculty, we chose to broaden our scope to include both didactic and clinical education. We saw the need for a comprehensive and informative book on the theme of "teach us to teach." As nurse anesthetists, we are schooled in the science of anesthesia and its administration, but not necessarily in teaching. As clinicians, we are often called upon to precept our students in the clinical area and to serve as their primary educators. For some of us, the role of teacher comes naturally, but for most of us, it does not. We hope that the knowledge and encouragement of these experienced educators will motivate and educate all of us to do this very important job and to do it well.

The book is divided into 3 sections: the educational process, clinical education, and didactic education. Our goal was to cover many aspects of nurse anesthesia education, such as mentoring our students in research, writing exam questions, performing evaluations, understanding and navigating the Medicare system as it epertains to teaching rules, teaching simulation, and much more.

The future of our profession is in the hands of nurse anesthesia educators, preceptors, and mentors. We all have much to offer our future colleagues. The better prepared we are to do the job right and the more encouragement we can give to the educators of the future, the stronger and more effective we will be.

The Editors

A Resource for Nurse Anesthesia Educators

Table of Contents

SECTION II – Clinical Education

SECTION III – Didactic Education

Section I

The Educational Process

Chapter 1

Socratic Method and Its Use in Teaching Student Nurse Anesthetists

Richard E. Haas, CRNA, PhD, PHRN

Key Points

- The use of Socratic instruction is imperative to determine the depth of knowledge of your students.

- A tone of openness to dialogue and the importance of questioning concepts must be set for Socratic instruction to succeed.

- Good Socratic instructors know that after any question is asked, they must have the necessary background to know a correct answer and evaluate the extent to which the student's response is correct.

- Although Socratic instruction usually is associated with one-to-one clinical instruction, it may be modified easily for use in small groups.

An Open Letter to the Clinical or Didactic Faculty Member

Dear Fellow Teacher:

I know you. You aren't a "facilitator" or a "guide." You are a teacher. You know your profession and know it well. It is your passion as well as your vocation. You take your specialized clinical skills and intuitive abilities and pass them along to the next generation of nurse anesthetists.

Teaching student anesthetists is demanding. For clinical instructors, it is frequently an unpaid "benefit" of your position. Oh, sometimes you get a title (eg, "preceptor," "clinical faculty," or "adjunct lecturer"), free run of the medical library, and a really cool line on your resume, but usually that is it. Socrates, the father of instruction in just about everything, would have been proud of you because he made it a point to *never* take payment for his teaching.[1] Few people in healthcare make as great a contribution to the future successes of our profession as you do.

The general public doesn't know who you are, but we in nurse anesthesia education circles do. We have seen you, there in the trenches. You are watching, teaching, cajoling, praising, and yes, even sometimes growling at the students assigned to you. We have seen you, because we have been there with you.

Well, friends and colleagues, it is time to let the cat out of the bag. There is a way to teach that is enjoyable, fun, exciting, and stimulating for both you and your students. The technique has been around for thousands of years, and I indirectly referred to it earlier. If you think back over your own education, you probably have been exposed to it yourself. It is the Socratic method. Okay, now stop sighing and rolling your eyes! I'm not going to get all philosophical.

Breathe deeply, in and out . . . there, feel better? The Socratic method is actually a straightforward technique that can help you to be a better teacher. Here is the payoff of Socratic instruction: not only will you be an effective teacher, but you'll be a popular teacher as well. Most students, especially the professionals we teach, *love* this technique.[2] They love it in spite of the fact that it makes them work harder than ever; most love it *because* of this fact. One student went so far as to refer to this type of instruction as "good grillin."[1]

The good news is that the Socratic method works much better with small groups and works best with individuals—precisely the way we teach in the operating room. Socrates saw the teacher-student relationship in the "two-on-a-log" model: a student on one end of the log and a teacher on the other.

This type of teaching results in a deep and profound understanding of the material presented. You get to experience the joy every teacher seeks: that of seeing students truly engaged with and succeeding in their studies. So join me as I let you in on the secrets of the Socratic method. You and your students will be glad you did.

Professionally,

Rich

Introduction

This chapter is divided into 3 parts. The first part concerns background and basics, focusing briefly on Socrates himself and the nature of his breakthrough in instruction. It also will show you how to set the tone for your instruction and will provide some concrete suggestions for dealing with small groups. Part 2 discusses the instruction itself: a kind of "how-to-do-it" manual. It also includes some concrete examples of how the Socratic teacher takes "what everyone knows" and guides students through the perilous waters of truth. Part 3 discusses some of the perceived drawbacks of the Socratic method and seeks to alleviate the concerns teachers may have with its use.

Part 1: Socrates for the Uninterested: Who He Was and Why This Works

...for there is far greater peril in buying knowledge than in buying meat and drink...you cannot buy the wares of knowledge and carry them away in another vessel; when you have paid for them you must receive them into your soul and go your way, either greatly harmed or greatly benefited. . . .[3]

– Plato

Who He Was

Ah yes, the voices of the cynics. Who was this Socrates guy anyway, and what could he possibly say to me in the dawn of the 21st century? I mean really, the guy has been dead for 2,300 years; he didn't have the Internet, computers, televisions, phones, or students with 30-second attention spans. Can he possibly be germane to teaching principles of anesthesia? As Socrates might have said, those are excellent questions! In fact, let's begin by doing as Socrates would have done: break this question into its component parts and carefully examine each part.

Who was Socrates? Born in 470 BC, this questioner after truth was the son of a sculptor, Sophroniscus. Socrates lived in the era that immediately followed the retreat of Xerxes and the end of the war against the Persians, in which Socrates was also a foot soldier. His biggest concern was the teaching of virtuous behavior to a civilization of Greeks, whom he felt were beginning the downfall of their existence. Socrates wrote nothing himself[4]; his existence and dialogues depended on his faithful reporters, Plato and Xenophon, among others. In our "publish or perish" age of graduate education, Socrates might never have received tenure.

Plato was Socrates' student, and knew him for roughly 10 years before Socrates was put to death. Students in Socrates' time frequently lived with or near their teachers and spent untold hours in conversations and lessons with them, and simply living together day in and day out. If our own students were to be with us day and night for 10 years, they would have our every statement tattooed in their memories. They also would know every quirk, smirk, smile, and grimace, every gesture and platitude. They would undoubtedly write things about us we'd never write about ourselves. This is what makes Plato a particularly good source of information about how Socrates taught and how we might go about teaching as Socrates did.

Why His Method Works

There is a great deal more to the "who" of Socrates. If you want more details on the life of Socrates, almost any encyclopedia can reveal as much as you would like to read. Let's move on to the "why" part of the question.

Our original question under discussion was the degree to which there is any importance of Socrates' method today. The sophist would answer that Socrates has the same importance now as in the 20th, 19th, 18th century, (and so on). Sophists were the individuals who arranged for Socrates to be put to death. They specialized in twisting arguments through rhetorical flourishes and were paid quite highly. Kreeft[4] identifies them as the forerunners of both lawyers and advertising executives. Since that is the case, we will put Sophistry behind us and get to the heart of the issue.

Socrates was a seeker: a seeker of information, a seeker of truth, and a seeker of virtue. He found answers by asking questions. He also developed word pictures and insights. Socrates was fond of taking a statement made by a classical Greek author such as Homer and then expanding on it. The expansion was based on the application of the statement to some common occurrence in life, and then following the precept of the statement to its logical end.

There are 2 technical terms used to describe this type of learning: the *elenchus* and the *aporia*.[5] *Elenchus* can be thought of in terms of a series of questions, designed to challenge a concept or idea. They are usually thought of as "why" questions: Why does this happen? What is the nature of this phenomenon? What is the underlying goal of this action? These questions should be open-ended. Dichotomous yes or no, true or false questions are less useful in this type of instruction, but they may be helpful in pinning down terms associated with the question. The *aporia* is generally thought of as a state of confusion or consternation: students are required to come to grips with their statements and deal with the logical results of their answers. Although confusion is often thought of as something bad, confusion can be positive when it precipitates further thought on the part of students. As Green and Rose[6] point out, this type of intellectual probing turns education into, ". . . an active process and not a passive spectator sport." This technique of probing questions followed by answers leading to more questions was referred to (far later in history) as the Socratic method. Actually, the Socratic method, as we use it in modern education, came from the former dean of the Harvard Law School, Christopher Columbus Langdell, who began to use it in 1870.[1]

Despite the fact that most of us are not in the habit of teaching law (as Langdell did) or virtue (as Socrates did), the Socratic method can be transformed easily to fit nearly all of the health sciences. Why? It fits because of the nature of the knowledge we possess and require our students to grasp. The student's rote memorization of a simple list of data points is insufficient to care for the patient. Furthermore, as Tucker[7] points out, the Socratic method is particularly effective for instruction in professions that are self-governing. If specific data are the bricks from which concepts are constructed, we quickly note that all bricks and no mortar cause the house to fall down. The mortar is the connection of data points to the broad concepts of patient care. These concepts sound obtuse, but on further thought they become clearer.

Those who have tried to convert the art and science of patient care to an interactive computer program have rapidly found the failings in this technique. A frequent complaint is that the simulation, no matter how good, is not sufficiently complex to mimic the living, breathing patient. Nurse anesthetists must understand complex relationships and the concepts that undergird the clinical decisions they make. A clinical anesthesia example illustrates this.

Let us assume that an anesthetized patient is hypoxic. Increasing tidal volume or the fraction of inspired oxygen may not work to treat this patient's hypoxia. Why not? Because the nurse anesthetist does not know if the patient's hypoxia is due to:

- An absent heart beat
- A kinked endotracheal tube
- A tumor occluding the bottom part of the trachea
- A toxin preventing the attachment of oxygen molecules to the hemoglobin
- Another cause

The complex relationships between cardiovascular function and pulmonary function must be understood before therapy can be initiated. The seeker of knowledge (also known as your student) must have knowledge beyond the simple recall of data. The teacher's ability to discern the level of the student's knowledge and then to build on that level is the strength of Socratic instruction. Socrates showed that one is able to establish the deep understanding of complex relationships. In this manner, the use of Socrates' technique makes you a more efficient, focused, and interesting teacher. Teaching and students, however, do not exist in a vacuum. Rather, they flourish (or perish) within an educational environment designed to support (or kill) academic endeavors.

Part 2: Setting the Tone

Demolishing Ineffective Habits

This is the part of the chapter that no one, including me, particularly relishes. The Oracle at Delphi, someone with whom Socrates was intimately familiar, said that a key aspect of human development was to "know thyself." It is tough to undo the habits that make us inefficient or ineffective teachers. Socratic instruction, however, requires an atmosphere that makes the students answer questions, and allows students to make mistakes. These mistakes, obviously, can never come at the expense of the care rendered to the patient. Patient safety is the primary reason why you, as the clinical instructor, are present. Students, however, will make decisions throughout the case, and your response to these decisions can educate or demolish the student's learning for the day. How do you set the proper tone each day?

The first step is to understand that most students want to learn. Instructors have repositories of specific and esoteric knowledge locked up inside them. One problem for students is that instructors' actions in the operating room have become so second nature that they have difficulty explaining the reason for doing something. This should not be a cause for dismay, because this instinctive response to patient care needs is actually the hallmark of the expert practitioner.[8] Socratic instruction requires that teachers first unlock this data source in their own heads. In other words, as teachers, it is important to go back and rethink why you do what you do. This is more difficult than it first appears; teachers may find they have forgotten why some of the things they do are important to patient care. They simply know that these interventions work. Worse, teachers may occasionally find out that they have no idea why they do what they do. Do not let this discourage you. Socrates frequently said the only thing he knew for sure was that he didn't really know anything.[4]

The second step is to prepare for the period of instruction, whether in the classroom or in the operating room. The Socratic method is easy if you thoroughly understand the topic you are teaching. Poor Socratic instructors, however, err in thinking that it is enough to simply ask question after question. In fact, after the question is asked, you must have the necessary background both to know a correct answer and to evaluate the extent to which the student's response is correct. Your depth of knowledge in your subject is crucial to successful instruction. If some of your knowledge may be dated or you are uncertain, it is important to review the subject matter before your instruction.

The next step is to set a tone of encouragement in the workplace. This may be seen as one of the most difficult hurdles to jump in the area of clinical instruction. The operating room is frequently not the place where such a tone occurs. In far too many operating rooms, everyone is barking at everyone else. With the advent of crew resource management, this antagonistic tone is beginning to change, but there is still much work to be done. Your abilities may not extend to a cultural sea change for an entire department. It is possible, though, to modify and enhance your interactions with the student. You must break the adversarial pattern in your conversations with your student.

Students need to know 2 important things. The first is that they can present even the most ridiculous idea at minimal personal risk. Saying that an idea is ridiculous is fair game; saying that the person is ridiculous is not. You have far more power than your students, (although their perceptions of your power may be exaggerated). Student nurse anesthetists frequently feel as if they are constantly "on the bubble" or that they are 1 mediocre evaluation away from dismissal. Second, students need to know that they are responsible for their answers and knowledge. Although they are in the learner role, their learning cannot be passive; it must be active. The job of the student is to come equipped with basic knowledge, which increases in complexity throughout the course of their studies. The active portion comes when the teacher requires students to use this bank of knowledge and make inferential voyages into the complexities of administering an anesthetic. Rigorous instruction, however, is not hostile instruction. This topic will be expanded upon further in part 3 of this chapter.

Many nurse anesthetists came from educational programs that had 1 or more instructors whose favorite "teaching" technique was to criticize and berate students for every perceived shortcoming. What did they learn from these instructors? They learned how to respond in a fashion that prevented further criticism and berating. In other words, they learned a lot about how not to get yelled at and very little about how to do anesthesia. In educational and testing parlance, this is a classic error in validity. The instructors thought they were teaching anesthesia. In fact, they were teaching how to behave to not incur their wrath. The overwhelming outcome of that behavior has nothing whatsoever to do with anesthesia.

Your desire, as a good Socratic instructor, is to teach all about anesthesia, and the attributes and qualities that make a good nurse anesthetist. Good teaching happens when you ask students open-ended questions and require that students answer. Sometimes you'll have to wait for the answer. Sometimes you can wait (if you are talking with the student during morning report), and sometimes you cannot (you are aggressively resuscitating the patient). Try this experiment. Ask yourself this question, aloud: "How could I use Socratic instruction with my students?"

Wait 30 seconds in silence for a student to answer. This period of time seems long, but it is important that the student answers the question. Do not worry; you will feel more comfortable with this period of silence as you become more experienced with the Socratic method. To sum up, the tone of your instruction is important. Without an open environment, the Socratic method is reduced to students parroting your whims and desires, some of which may not be correct.

The Technique and Some Examples of Its Use

Teaching is the only major occupation of man for which we have not yet developed tools that make an average person capable of competence and performance. In teaching we rely on the "naturals," the ones who somehow know how to teach.[9]

– Peter F. Drucker

What do you think would happen if you, the teacher, were to try to teach the average student nurse anesthetist everything you know about the conduct of an anesthetic on the very first day of clinical rotation? You would not be surprised to see the student collapse in a gibbering mass in the corner of the operating room. The reason for the collapse would be that there was too much information compressed into too short a time. Indeed, some of the information would not relate at all to the case at hand. Students frequently report that the most daunting part of clinical anesthesia education is the difficulty in vigilantly watching multiple data streams that change continually throughout the case. Yet, interestingly enough, clinical instructors make a mistake similar to this each day.

The mistake is a lack of focus by being a mile wide and an inch deep. When you read Plato's interactions of Socrates with his students, you find that Socrates usually carried his discussions and arguments to a far greater depth of understanding than the original question would seem to imply. Depth of understanding was his goal, because students so equipped could take these principles and apply them to many aspects of life.

As you teach future anesthetists, remember how you learned about your science and craft. Richard Feynman,[10] perhaps the greatest theoretical physicist since Newton, advised his students in this fashion: "You start at the beginning and read as far as you can get until you are lost. Then you start at the beginning again and keep working through until you can understand the whole book." Note that Feynman did not say, "Understand the whole book today!" Grasping complex principles and interrelationships takes time (reflected, at least partially, by the fact that nurse anesthesia programs keep increasing in length).

So how did Socrates do it? What was his secret? Samples[11] stresses some of the more important aspects of Socrates' technique. First, Samples tells us that Socrates began from skepticism. In setting a proper tone, however, cynicism must be banished. Skepticism implies that a truth can be known, but cynicism implies that nothing is correct or true, and that instruction is only a way for the teacher to get something back from the student. Socrates, on the other hand, began by refusing to believe, without evidence, the things that "everyone knows." At some institutions in which I have worked, this crazy person called "everyone" seems to know a lot! Perhaps "everyone" works with you as well. You may have heard such things as "Everyone knows thiopental releases histamine." When the student says something like that, the Socratic instructor responds with a question: "Really? How do you know that? Who says that? What is the evidence for your statement?" Sound familiar? It should, because this is the driving precept behind evidence-based practice. Who would have thought Socrates might be involved in that?

Note that the veracity of the student's statement, at this point in your instruction, is immaterial. "But," you reply, "I thought we were searching for truth." Yes, that is the pursuit of both you and your student. The point of the exercise is for you, the teacher, to determine the depth of your student's knowledge and, if possible, give the student the tools to add to this depth. The use of the mystery person "everyone" may reflect the student's discomfiture or lack of knowledge about the given statement. Your skepticism (actual or assumed) drives the first part of this type of teaching. In the practice of anesthesia, assuming nothing is the start of a good, solid plan.

Next, as Samples[11] further describes, Socrates spoke with people. He did not simply pass the time of day engaging in pleasantries; he really wanted to figure out why they knew what they knew. Adult learners want the instructor to engage them.[2] In the operating room, your conversations with the students can go on throughout the day; however, some surgeons need silence more than they need air. In this case, the operating room is not a good place for Socratic dialogue. Finally, Samples tell us Socrates' method is both inductive (applying general knowledge to a specific instance to see if it works each time) and deductive (seeking clues to a thing by determining consequences).[11] All of this sounds very scientific, philosophical, and erudite. The problem is with converting the concept into practice. One of the best initial ways to learn things is to watch others model the technique you are attempting to learn.

Example 1

I would like you to imagine Sam Student, a mid-level student nurse anesthetist having a clinical conversation with his teacher for the day, Izzie Instructor. They are preparing for their first case of the day. Let's listen in on their conversation.

Sam Student (SS): Uh-oh, I just saw our next patient in the holding area and she has red hair—that means trouble!

Izzie Instructor (II): Really? What do you mean by that? (a properly skeptical Socratic response)

SS: Everyone knows redheads have trouble with anesthesia.

II: What do you mean by trouble?

SS: You know (eyes now rolling) . . . *trouble*

II: No, I don't know. Tell me what you mean.

SS: Well, I'm not sure, but somebody told me that everyone knows that they have trouble.

II: So you really aren't certain, based on your readings or journal articles, what does happen when you give a general anesthetic to someone with red hair? Maybe we should take this a bit further. What have you heard about redheaded patients receiving anesthesia?

What just happened in this encounter with a student? The mysterious "everyone," accompanied by his willing assistant "somebody," has told the student an aphorism which, after an uneasy night's sleep, has grown, developed, and reached the status of incontrovertible fact. The instructor knows, however, that hearing someone say something does not necessarily mean that the statement is true. It is up to the instructor to make the student rethink his paradigm. This is the *elenchus*. It has had the decided effect of creating *aporia* within the student. Note that the instructor has not had to rant and rave or impugn the student's intelligence. He is creating an opportunity for the student to gain more knowledge (or dispel faulty hearsay) and then report back. The instructor has ensured that the student does not change techniques or agents based on questionable data; the student is forced to think through the problem and develop an answer.

Example 2

Here is another example. Let's assume you are the staff anesthetist teaching a student in the operating room. You have only 1 student for the entire day. A good idea is for the Socratic teacher to sit down with the student in advance (particularly the new student) and ask the following question: "What 1 thing do you want to learn well today?" You are allowing the student the freedom to select something with which he or she is unfamiliar. Note that if you haven't set the tone, this interaction cannot occur. The student will start to think thoughts such as: "What am I supposed to be saying right now that will keep me from getting into trouble with this staff anesthetist?" That is precisely the question the student ought not to be struggling with during the course of the instruction. The idea of clinical learning is to take new knowledge (or refine and polish what the student already knows and can do) and apply it toward the best possible patient outcome.

The clinical faculty member now has 2 thoughts: (1) What if the student picks something he or she already knows about? (2) How can only 1 thing be made to last the whole day? The answer to the first question is that it is your responsibility as the teacher to see if the student is trying to "game the system." There will be more on that in later sections, so let's answer the second question first.

A key topic can make a whole day of instruction, provided the instructor hones in on the deeper aspects of the topic. Asking questions does this. Moreover, questions always lead to more questions. The best part of teaching anesthesia is that there are occasions during the case in which there is time for the give and take of instruction while still watching the patient. The Socratic method is designed to get to the root of any question or problem.

Here is a dialog between another student (Sally) and her instructor (Isabel).

Isabel Instructor (II): Good morning, Sally. It looks like we are all set up and ready for a big surgical day. What is the 1 area you want to focus on today?
Sally Student (SS): Today I want to focus on how to correctly mask a patient as part of airway management.
II: Great idea; that is a crucial skill in anesthesia. What do you think are the key aspects of masking the patient?
SS: Correctly fitting the mask, using the oral airway, pressure on the bag . . . .
II: Anything else?
SS: uh… (long pause)
II: How about when the technique can be used? For example, which patients are good candidates for mask anesthesia?
SS: Well, they can be used for . . . .

The student, while learning the psychomotor skill associated with using an anesthesia mask, also has to look at complex relationships related to the skill itself. This is 2-for-the-price-of-1 teaching: efficient and effective.

This conversation can occur while actually administering the anesthetic. If, for example, the student is having difficulty maintaining a seal, the Socratic instructor asks: "Why do you think you are having difficulty?" This question is occurring simultaneously with the teacher's correction of the technique. The patient is protected from hypoxia while the instruction goes on. The non-Socratic instructor would tell the student. "Put your fingers here and here and hold this until I tell you to stop."

You may still have to show the student the correct technique, but it should always be accompanied with the "why" explanation (eg, "I use a mask strap because my hands are too small to get around this patient's mandible."). You are taking the student to a depth never anticipated when "to mask a patient better" was suggested as the learning task for the day. The student thought in terms of psychomotor skill acquisition. You, the Socratic teacher, taught that and more.

Making Simple Diagrams Work

Socrates used visual pictures called metaphors to make his audience understand concepts and issues. The audience of ancient Greece was very much a culture of verbal interaction and narrative tradition. Students of today are from the visual and sound-bite tradition: give me a factoid and give it to me now. This cultural aspect is often thought to stand in the way of the Socratic method. Nothing could be further from the truth.

Socratic teachers always have tools at their sides to battle lack of knowledge each time it rears its head: a pencil and a sheet of paper. "The pen is mightier than the sword," said English novelist and dramatist Edward Bulwer-Lytton and, when combined with a piece of scratch paper, it is certainly mightier than most questions. How do you draw anesthesia? Well, you don't, but things such as neurons, synapses, charts, and graphs that describe various aspects of anesthesia are relatively easy to draw. Let's look at some examples.

Assume that a student comes to you and states that she has read an article describing the effect of the α_2-adrenoreceptor agonist clonidine on blood pressure, and that it seems to have an effect on anesthesia. She now wants to know why a blood pressure medicine could make a patient sleepier. You know that stimulation of these receptors decreases neurotransmitter release from the presynaptic neuron, but that explanation seems a little arcane. How could the Socratic instructor describe this more clearly? Try drawing picture of a neuron (Figure 1.1).

It doesn't look exactly like the polished picture from the expensive textbook, but the simple schematic does the job. It is easy to understand. Let's go back to our hypothetical student's question about the α_2-receptor. We've already discussed the

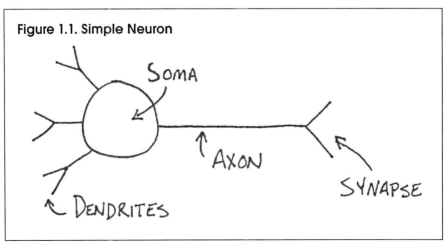

Figure 1.1. Simple Neuron

correct answer; here is the illustration of the phenomenon in an easy format (Figure 1.2).

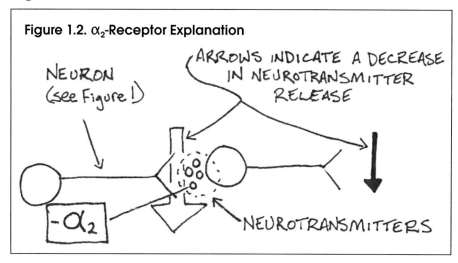

Figure 1.2. α_2-Receptor Explanation

We take the neuron, remove the dendrites, and add a box, some dots, 2 arrows, and a minus sign (inside the α_2 box). We can now see that the release of neurotransmitters (dots) from the presynaptic neuron stimulates the α_2-receptor and provides negative feedback to decrease neurotransmitter release from that same presynaptic neuron. This entire complex discussion was facilitated with lines, dots, arrows, and a box. When combined with your explanation of how things work (along, of course, with your Socratic questions), you have made a difficult process understandable and memorable. Relationships can also be drawn, but here is a strict caveat. The drawing of the relationship reinforces the Socratic instruction, it does not replace it.

Imagine you are explaining the baroreceptor response. An easy way of explaining it would look something like Figure 1.3. The problem here is that it is very easy to forget which arrows go which way, particularly if you are trying to recall this in the heat of anesthesia battles. The clinical teacher knows that the

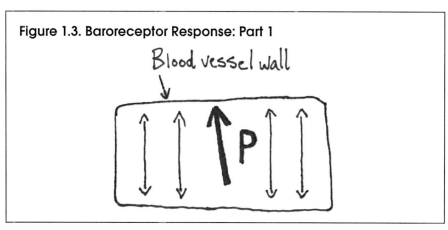

Figure 1.3. Baroreceptor Response: Part 1

(P indicates pressure.)

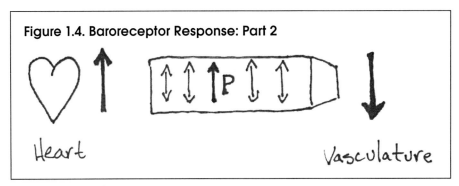

Figure 1.4. Baroreceptor Response: Part 2

Heart

Vasculature

(P indicates pressure.)

baroreceptor is a small sense organ that is sensitive to pressure. As your blood pressure rises, the hydrostatic pressure against the vessels and organs may become too great. The body compensates by decreasing cardiac output (CO). One way of doing this is decreasing heart rate (HR), because CO = HR × stroke volume. The student anesthetist should be familiar with this formula, but providing the preceding formula (or requiring the student to recite it) is simple and efficient. Unfortunately, the harried student will soon forget this quick explanation, which becomes lost in myriad up and down arrows in an ever-increasing list of crucial physiologic relationships.

The Socratic instructor might try something like the following to keep students focused and enhance their understanding of this reflex. Let's begin by assuming the multiple pictures you see in Figures 1.3 through 1.5 are just 1 picture, and that the subsequent diagrams show how objects are added to the original as the discussion goes on. The instructor begins by asking the student a simple and open question. If the pressure inside your blood vessel is too high, can bad things happen to the body and, if so, what bad things?

The student responds (correctly) that vessels could rupture in the brain or elsewhere in the body. The instructor follows up with question 2: What creates high blood pressure? Student answer 2: Cardiac output (heart picture) goes up and/or systemic vascular resistance increases (vessels squeeze down).

The instructor goes on to question 3: "If baroreceptors fire when the blood pressure is high, what do you think their purpose is?" Student response: "To

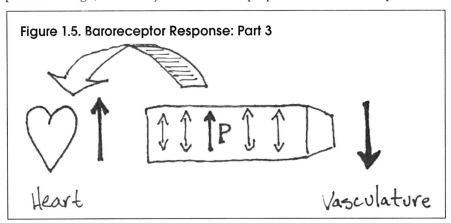

Figure 1.5. Baroreceptor Response: Part 3

Heart

Vasculature

reduce blood pressure." Follow-up question 3A: "Do baroreceptors affect the blood vessels or the heart?" Follow-up answer: They actually affect both, but the primary response is on the heart."

Final point: "If you were the brain, and you wanted to make the body's blood pressure go down, and you couldn't make the vessels bigger, what could you do to the heart?" Final answer: "Make it go slower."

This entire explanation has taken 5 to 10 minutes, but the student has had to work through the problem. The oral and recitation work is accompanied by visual and cognitive work. Pathways are laid down in the brain, and memories are more readily formed than with a 15-second explanation. Furthermore, you can, at later points, require the student to reproduce this drawing, creating a more solid memory pattern upon which to build. In short, hearing something, then reading it, then explaining it, and then reproducing it builds the memories required for the competent CRNA.

Part 3: Concerns Regarding the Socratic Method

By now the discerning teacher is asking the question: "Is there any possible downside to this type of instruction?" The advocate wants to say: "Of course not!" but the Socratic method is not without its critics. Many of the critics of the Socratic method are unfamiliar with its use, or have seen it used poorly. At its extremes, the Socratic method has been used cruelly, to embarrass and humiliate students in front of their peers as the instructor engages in a lively game of "hide the ball."[12] The 1970s CBS television program *The Paper Chase* shows the downside quite clearly in the quote with which the mythical law professor, Professor Kingsfield opened each episode: "The study of law is something new and unfamiliar to most of you—unlike any other schooling you've ever known before. You teach yourselves the law, but I train your minds. You come in here with a skull full of mush, and, if you survive, you leave thinking like a lawyer."

Gordon[13] has gone so far as to ask the question: "Is the Socratic method illegal?" In the day and age in which interest in the students' emotional needs seems to trump rigorous instruction, how can we use the Socratic method? Doesn't the very nature of this technique and its dependence on the creation of *aporia* in the student strike at the heart of students' need for self-esteem? Other authors also have related the problems that may accompany the Socratic method, including the ideas that women and minorities are unfairly treated by the process.[1,7,14]

The answer to these objections is relatively simple to state, albeit more difficult to accomplish. Rigor is simply not to be confused with cruelty. Education is not initiation, a hazing process through which students must go. Regrettably, there are still large parts of clinical education in which the instructors feel students must first be "torn down" before they can be correctly educated. Gordon, who asked if the Socratic method was illegal, relates his own experience in this regard as a novice learner.[13] Some clinical instructors are of the opinion that, because they were made to suffer at the hands of their teachers, new students must now experience that same level of suffering. This attitude not only flies in the face of current clinical practice, with its emphasis on the just culture and culture of safety, but it also would comprise a chapter all its own were it to be discussed thoroughly. Let's just agree for the moment that intimidation is inefficient and lacks validity. Your goal is to teach the student how to safely administer an anesthetic. Intimidation teaches the student how not to be yelled at. Making cultural changes in the clinical environment to decrease these behaviors will not be easy. Because our time in instruction is necessarily limited and the amount to be learned so great, is it not in all of our best interests to be efficient in our instruction? Students may need remediation, remonstration, and, unfortunately in some cases, removal from the program. Intentional cruelty masquerading as instruction weakens the ability of nurse anesthesia educational programs to engage in any of these functions, and it ought not to be confused with rigorous but fair Socratic instruction.

In the first part of the chapter, the concept of establishing a tone for education was discussed. Overcoming objections to the Socratic method rests extensively on classroom and clinical culture. Students need to understand the following:

1. They are students as well as professional registered nurses. If they already knew everything, there would be no need to come to class.
2. They will make mistakes during their classroom and clinical recitations that are based on the Socratic method. The mistakes they make are designed to be used to further their education and do not mark them as stupid. (The evaluation of students is discussed extensively in chapter 17 of this text: Socratic method is about instruction, not evaluation.)
3. They ought not to be embarrassed to speak in front of their peers, and denigration of the students by their peers in the classroom will not be tolerated by the Socratic method instructor.
4. Their only goal as students in the classroom is the acquisition of knowledge and judgment that will make them excellent clinicians who are better able to care for their patients.
5. Their only goal in clinical instruction is the use of knowledge and judgment and the honing of skills that results in excellent care of the anesthetized patient.

The program faculty members need to emphasize repeatedly and, more importantly, to model and follow through on these precepts. It is critical that these preceptors continually engage the students during instruction, didactic or clinical.

The final perceived downside is that the Socratic method is a lot of work for the teacher. In this, there can be no argument. It is far less onerous to be the "sage on the stage," pouring data into the heads of our students. The problem is we really cannot be sure what they heard and responded to. Engagement with students using the Socratic method provides the teacher with almost instantaneous feedback regarding the level of knowledge that students have.

Summary

The Socratic method is an extraordinary way of teaching your students how to think for themselves, respond to questions regarding their practice, and explain their rationale behind the clinical decisions they make. It is equally demanding for instructors and students, yet filled with rewards for both. Students are engaged with teachers, self-directed, and growing in confidence with each passing day. Socratic instructors get to make a palpable difference in the lives of their students while continuously monitoring their progression through a demanding program of study. Very few ideas have been subjected to 2,400 years of modification, trial, feedback, and use. The Socratic method is efficient, effective, and fun for teachers and learners. So get out there and ask some questions!

References

1. Pedersen AM. In defense of the oft-maligned Socratic method. *Natl Law J.* New York, NY: Incisive Legal Intelligence; 2006:2.

2. Walker JT, Martin TM, Haynie L, Norwood A, White J, Grant L. Preferences for teaching methods in a baccalaureate nursing program: how second-degree and traditional students differ. *Nurs Educ Perspect.* 2007;28(5):246-250.

3. Buchanan S, ed. *The Portable Plato.* New York, NY: Penguin Books; 1948.

4. Kreeft P. *Philosophy 101 by Socrates: An Introduction to Philosophy Via Plato's Apology.* San Francisco, CA: Ignatius Press; 2002.

5. Paraskevas A, Wickens E. Andragogy and the Socratic method: the adult learner perspective. *J Hospitality Leisure Sports Tourism Educ.* 2003;2(2):10.

6. Green A, Rose W. The professor's dream: getting students to talk and read intelligently. *PS: Political Sci Polit.* 1996;29(4):4.

7. Tucker AA. Leadership by the Socratic method. *Air Space Power J.* 2007;21(20):7.

8. Dreyfus HL, Dreyfus SE. *Mind Over Machine.* New York, NY: The Free Press; 1986.

9. Drucker PF. Brainy quote website. http://www.brainyquote.com/quotes/authors/p/peter_f_drucker.html. Accessed April 19, 2008.

10. Satinover J. *The Quantum Brain: The Search for Freedom and the Next Generation of Man.* New York, NY: John Wiley and Sons; 2002.

11. Samples K. Stand to Reason website. http://www.str.org. Accessed April 18, 2008.

12. Areeda PE. The Socratic method. *Harvard Law Rev.* 1996;109:12.

13. Gordon LA. Is the Socratic method illegal? *Am Surg.* 2003;69(2):181-182.

14. Garlikov R. Using the Socratic method. Rick Garlikov website. http://www.garlikov.com/teaching/smmore.htm. Accessed March 27, 2008.

Chapter 2

A Conceptual Model for Nurse Anesthesia Education

Maura S. McAuliffe, CRNA, PhD, FAAN

Key Points

- This chapter presents a conceptual model for nurse anesthesia education. The model explains the required declarative, procedural, and conditional knowledge components in advanced knowledge acquisition.

- The model demonstrates that acquisition and integration of these knowledge bases are best accomplished using metacognitive strategies during case-based instruction.

- Patient-centered strategic thinking evolves in learners as a result of real-world practice applying theory and principles with a large number and variety of cases.

- Learning to be cognitively flexible, to adaptively reconstruct knowledge to tasks involving new situations, also requires guidance from expert mentors. Mentors can best assist a student to achieve these goals and to progress through the stages of learning by aiming instruction within the student's zone of proximal development.

- Many teaching strategies, such as scaffolded instruction and reflection in action, can be employed in the clinical area; however, in assisting a student to become an independent problem solver, dialogue between student and teacher is essential.

- The conceptual model can be used by students and faculty as an organizing framework to facilitate the outcome of maximizing student learning during clinical experiences. It can also serve as a conceptual framework for educational research and curricula development.

Introduction

Excellence in nurse anesthesia education has been firmly established over the past century. Today's nurse anesthesia educational programs are often viewed by nursing educators as premier graduate-level nursing programs. With the multitude of operating rooms and clinical sites used by nurse anesthesia educational programs in the United States today, practicing nurse anesthetists find they are often involved in clinical teaching at some point in their careers. This chapter presents an educational conceptual framework to provide a vocabulary and principles of clinical instruction to assist nursing educators to do what they do even more effectively.

It is often said that theory guides practice and that practice informs theory. In this chapter, theoretical principles to guide case-based nurse anesthesia education are presented within the framework of a conceptual model. The model demonstrates how student nurse anesthetists, with the aid of expert mentors and using metacognitive strategies, gradually integrate the 3 essential knowledge bases (declarative, procedural, and conditional knowledge) as they become competent and proficient nurse anesthetists. Full integration requires case-based instruction in the clinical area through which learners are aided to view the conceptual terrain from multiple perspectives as they learn to think strategically in providing the best solutions to patient anesthetic challenges. The model can be used by learners, but as importantly, the model demonstrates how faculty can assist learners as they gradually progress through the stages of learning. The model may also serve as a diagnostic tool for identifying problems when student progress is not as anticipated. The model has been tested and used as a conceptual framework in research and curricula development.[1]

Background

The conceptual model of nurse anesthesia education (Figure 2.1) is guided by a constructivist ideology. Constructivism is a collection of theories and ideas about different issues in pedagogy informed by a range of philosophical and epistemological outlooks, each adding a different dimension, but all complementing each other. Learning theories within the constructivist paradigm view all learning as inherently situated, that is, embedded in social and physical environments that reflect real-world complexity. Learning is also viewed as being based on a learner's prior knowledge, which means learners must integrate all newly acquired knowledge into their existing knowledge and skills. Teachers are not viewed as transmitters of knowledge but as guides who facilitate learning. Constructivist philosophy is often seen within teaching modalities employed by the professions.

Although variations in educational curricula exist among and within professions, professional education usually includes 3 types of educational experiences: (1) courses in the basic arts or the basic sciences, (2) courses addressing the profession's typical problems and activities taught in a classroom setting, and (3) the professional initiation—apprenticeship or internship experience. Instruction in each area is essential if students are to learn to think as professionals.[2]

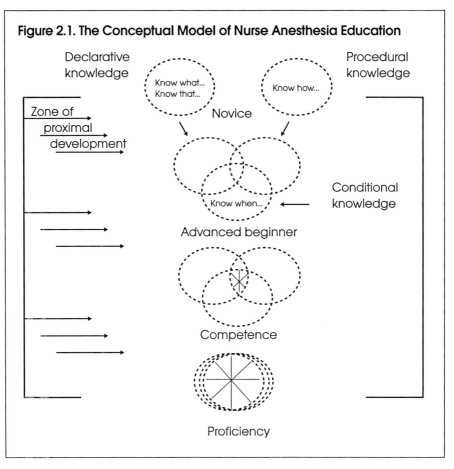

Figure 2.1. The Conceptual Model of Nurse Anesthesia Education

Kuhn[3] described a change in thinking that occurs when a student of physics (novice) learns to think as a physicist (professional). "Looking at a bubble-chamber photograph, the student sees confused and broken lines, the physicist, a record of familiar subnuclear events. Only after a number of transformations of vision does the student become an inhabitant of the scientist's world, seeing what the scientist sees and responding as the scientist does."[3] This transformation of vision that Kuhn refers to results from theory-based instruction coupled with real-life experience. Unfortunately, in many professions, little attention has been given to systematic inquiry of adult educational means and ends.[2] One reason for the lack of empirical studies is that professional education suffers from 2 types of insufficient theory. First, there is no theory of action for the profession to guide educational research.[4] Second, there is little general educational theory of action for instruction. The conceptual model for nurse anesthesia education (Figure 2.1) described in this chapter can serve as an organizing framework for development, refinement, and research in nurse anesthesia educational programs. The 6 stages in the model, which will be discussed later in the chapter, are based on the original framework for skill acquisition developed by Dreyfus and Dreyfus.[5]

Skill Acquisition and Piloting an Aircraft

In the 1970s, when the US Air Force required a theoretical framework to provide an educational structure for training pilots, they turned to Dreyfus and Dreyfus,[5] who developed the theory for skill acquisition. The skill acquisition that occurs in learning to fly aircraft is particularly relevant to nurse anesthesia because they (piloting an aircraft and administering an anesthetic) are often seen as analogous. The takeoff of the aircraft is similar to the induction of anesthesia, the landing to the emergence from anesthesia, and the time during anesthetic maintenance to cruising.

Piloting an aircraft and administering an anesthetic demand continuous processing of information. The pilot's monitoring and scanning of gauges and dials is analogous to the anesthetist's vigilant monitoring of patients while scanning dials and gauges on the anesthesia equipment.[6] The Dreyfus model for skill acquisition developed to assist in pilot training is used to inform the conceptual model of nurse anesthesia education (see Figure 2.1).

Dreyfus and Dreyfus were pioneers in advocating the use of computer-assisted instruction in teaching advanced skill acquisition. This model of instruction had its beginnings in interactive desktop personal computer programs. In the aviation industry, it evolved into the development and use of flight simulators in training pilots. Today, both desktop computer programs and high-fidelity anesthesia simulators are used in many training programs, and simulated instruction in anesthesia and anesthesia crisis management have become widespread.[6,7] Simulated training can provide interactive learning environments where students can apply theoretical principles, coupled with practical skills and critical thinking, in risk-free environments.

The Dreyfus model of skill acquisition has 6 stages: novice, advanced beginner, competent, proficient, expert, and master (Table 2.1). The Dreyfus model illustrates that skill acquisition occurs systematically as students progress through each stage of learning.[8] The *novice* follows rules and is unable to appreciate the unique situational aspects of an experience. The *advanced beginner* has gained some experience, and based on this, begins to recognize situational elements. The *competent* performer uses plans and begins to incorporate his or her point of view into the plans. The *proficient* performer has gained more experience and has a deeper, more involved understanding. The *expert* performer has mastered analytical decision making and has developed intuitive knowledge. In each stage, the learners' sophistication in thinking and monitoring of his or her thinking increases.

Metacognition

An essential element in skill acquisition is the concept of monitoring one's thinking. This concept was further developed by other learning theorists. Flavel[9] coined the term "metacognition" to define the concept in 1977. Metacognition, or monitoring our own thinking, is essential to learning in all education. It enables learners to draw on various thinking strategies and then to accurately assess their current understanding of a situation in light of those strategies. Using metacognitive strategies, learners become aware that they are developing new thinking skills

Table 2.1. Components of Skill Acquisition

Skill level	Components	Perspective	Decision	Commitment
Novice	Context-free	None	Analytical	Detached
Advanced beginner	Context-free and situational	None	Analytical	Detached
Competent	Context-free and situational	Chosen	Analytical	Detached understanding and deciding involved in outcome
Proficient	Context-free and situational	Experienced	Analytical	Involved understanding, detached deciding
Expert	Context-free and situational	Experienced	Intuitive	Involved

(Adapted from Dreyfus and Dreyfus[5] with permission from the Air Force Office of Scientific Research, Arlington, Virginia.)

as problem solvers. The development of these new thinking skills requires real-world and/or realistic-world (simulated) experiences.

The conceptual model of nurse anesthesia education was first grounded in the work of Dreyfus and Dreyfus, then informed by the work of other constructivists and learning theorists whose contributions are described. Effective learning requires the cognitive and control strategies of skill, will, and control (Figure 2.2). Skill subsumes declarative knowledge (knowing what to do) and procedural knowledge (knowing how to do it). Although both knowledge bases are important, they are not sufficient for effective learning. Even knowing when to do it (conditional or strategic knowledge) is not sufficient. Learners must also have the will to learn, that is, they must possess the desire and motivation to learn.[10]

The components of skill, will, and control are interdependent variables, and the extent to which each contributes to successful learning may vary from student to student. Prior success with effective learning strategies assists learners with subsequent learning; however, student motivation is also essential, and students who possess less sophisticated learning strategies can overcome this obstacle and become successful learners. Conversely, highly skilled learners who lack the motivation to learn may be unsuccessful despite that advantage.

Declarative, Procedural, and Conditional Knowledge

In the conceptual model for nurse anesthesia education (see Figure 2.1), the overlapping circles represent the interdependence of declarative, procedural,

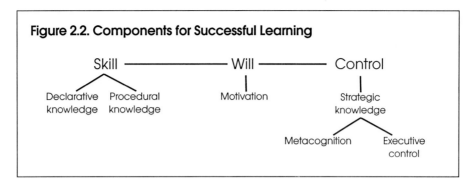

Figure 2.2. Components for Successful Learning

and conditional knowledge that is essential to learning.[11] Declarative knowledge (domain knowledge) is also referred to as systems knowledge.[12] It includes information about task structure and goals, as well as beliefs about our own-ability in relation to those goals.[11] In nurse anesthesia, declarative knowledge includes knowledge of basic sciences such as pharmacology and physiology and knowledge of applied sciences such as principles of nurse anesthesia practice. Much, but not all, of declarative knowledge is taught in the classroom and termed *didactic education*.

Procedural knowledge includes information about the execution of various actions. It is a repertoire of behaviors available to learners who select specific behaviors to attain specific goals. It includes knowledge of how to perform a pro-cedure; for example, intubating the trachea or administering a spinal anesthetic, as well as algorithmic-type knowledge such as knowledge of the American Society of Anesthesiologists' difficult airway algorithm. Procedural knowledge is acquired from direct instruction in conjunction with repeated experience.[11]

Declarative knowledge and procedural knowledge differ from conditional knowledge, in which one must select or execute an action. Conditional knowl-edge describes circumstances of application of procedures. It refers to knowing when and why to take various actions. Conditional knowledge is required to adjust behavior to changing task demands.[11] Conditional knowledge provides rationale for taking various actions and is required for choosing, planning, and evaluating a selected course of action. Conditional knowledge (also referred to as strategic knowledge) includes metacognitive knowledge.[12]

Metacognitive Aspects of Learning

Being aware of being conscious is the defining feature of metacognitive knowl-edge. Its name means a "cognition about cognition." Monitoring our own thinking is essential for successful learning—especially in areas that require complex problem solving.[9] "One is apt to engage in a lot of cognition when there is an explicit demand for it, for example, a vocation that requires one think up and evaluate alternative courses of action, and solve complex problems. More generally there is apt to be more ideation, and more monitoring of that ideation (metacognition), when one is faced with risky decisions, especially if one believes that risk might be reduced by engaging in careful and sustained thought."[9]

Metacognitive knowledge evolves in learners as a result of planned, real-world practice with strategic thinking and technical skills. By enhancing both the frequency and quality of experiences, student insights about learning (metacognitive experiences) evolve.

Complex forms of metacognition place heavy demands on attention and occupy considerable space in working memory.[13] Consequently, student nurse anesthetists are more likely to have these types of experiences when their attention and memory permit; that is, when they have sufficient time to think about their thinking and when they are not in a highly emotional state. A student who is involved in a complex case that involves a critically ill patient may be in a highly emotional state. It is common in this type of situation for the student to be unable to answer simple questions posed by the instructor or to remember the instructor's explanations for decision making. In these instances, the instructor might best assist the student by asking a specific question after the situation has ended. Moreover, postcase conferences can provide opportunities to improve learning, especially when instructors assist students as they reflect on the prior learning situation.

Many learning theorists assert that learners have a central processor, or executive controller, that allows them to perform intelligent evaluations of their own thinking.[14] Student nurse anesthetists should not only be instructed in the use of cognitive strategies but also be instructed in how to use executive control, for example, how to employ, monitor, check, and evaluate their thinking strategies.[15] A common example of instructors teaching a cognitive strategy is teaching students in the use of differential diagnosis. Students are typically taught, for example, how to think about and respond to intraoperative hypotension by using differential diagnoses for hypotension (the etiology may be hypovolemia) as well as use of executive control (provide the patient with a fluid bolus and then reevaluate the situation). Over time, the eventual inculcation of these thinking processes will improve students' abilities to marshal the required knowledge and then construct solutions tailored to the needs of problem-solving situations in the future.

How can anesthesia instructors best assist students to develop and use self-regulatory executive control in their thinking? It has been demonstrated in many real-life situations that interactive learning experiences result in the passing of executive control from teacher to student or master craftsman to apprentice.[16] In this process, teachers are initially viewed as the supportive other, acting first as models and then interrogators. This leads students toward strategic thinking. Eventually, during these interactive processes, the self-regulatory control becomes internalized by the student and the teacher relinquishes control.

Ill-Structured Domains and Learning

Anesthesia knowledge is considered an ill-structured domain. Domains of knowledge are considered to be ill structured when required thinking and problem solving do not have predetermined algorithms. In ill-structured domains, expert mentorship and experience with a wide variety of cases are required for students to develop cognitively flexible processing skills. Also required is a learning environment that will permit knowledge to be learned in various ways and for various purposes.[17-22]

Although students progress incrementally through the 6 stages of learning in the conceptual model for nurse anesthesia education, the teaching and learning that occurs within each stage is not always linear and orderly. This is true of learning that occurs in all ill-structured domains. In ill-structured domains, practitioners must construct actions that are most appropriate and efficient for the task at hand.[17-22] Learning in these disciplines is best accomplished through case-based instruction with the goal of fostering cognitive flexibility.

Cognitive Flexibility

Cognitive flexibility is required for successful performance in ill-structured domains such as anesthesia. This is because the goals of learning must shift from the attainment of superficial understanding of facts to mastery of important aspects of conceptual complexity, and from knowledge reproduction to knowledge use, which is the ability to apply what was taught in new and varying contexts.[17-22]

In introductory learning (most undergraduate learning), the goal is often exposure to subject content or general orientation to a field of study, and learning assessment usually involves simple recognition or recall. In advanced knowledge acquisition, students must attain a deeper understanding of content material, reason with it, and apply it flexibly in diverse situations.[17-22]

The best ways to learn and instruct others to achieve cognitive flexibility for future application are nonlinear and through case-based instruction.[17-22] Although student nurse anesthetists can initially learn the basic concepts in a linear context, eventually emphasis must be shifted from retrieval of intact knowledge structures (eg, recitation of a mnemonic) to construction of new understandings. The goal is case-specific knowledge assembly drawn from multiple sources to address the problem-solving needs of the current situation. To adapt knowledge to tasks involving new situations requires metacognitive executive control strategies (predicting, planning, checking, evaluating, and revising) and flexible knowledge structures.[17-22] A main goal of instruction in nurse anesthesia is to assist the student in developing cognitive flexibility.

To foster development of cognitive flexibility in students, cases must be studied as they occur in their natural, complex situations. By focusing a student's learning at the level of individual cases and then providing experiences with a large number of cases, successful student performance will be enhanced.[17-22]

Seven themes comprise the different facets of cognitive flexibility. In the conceptual model of nurse anesthesia education (see Figure 2.1), these themes are represented by the crisscrossed lines in the middle of the overlapping circles (knowledge domains).

Theme 1: Avoidance of Oversimplification and Overregularization

In advanced knowledge acquisition, educators must emphasize ways that knowledge is not as simple and orderly as it might first seem.[22] In other words, instruction must include measures to demonstrate complexities and to show how the superficially similar can be dissimilar. The problem is that oversimplification can lead to reductive bias. For example, when conceptual elements that are highly interrelated are treated in isolation, learners may miss important parts of their interaction.[17-22]

Teachers are often inclined to oversimplify in an attempt to increase the novice's initial understanding of a concept. The problem with this is that it can instill "habits of the mind" that are later hard to break. It is actually better to introduce complexity early, but in a manageable manner. For example, in teaching students the lower acceptable limits of mean arterial blood pressure for deliberate hypotension, one instructor may simply teach that the safe lower limit is 50 to 55 mm Hg (the lower limit of cerebral autoregulation). Another instructor might initiate a discussion with the student about variables that influence decision making, such as patient positioning, blood pressure measurement relative to the brain, and the patient's underlying diseases (such as sickle cell anemia). Avoiding initial oversimplifications allows students to gain appreciation of complexities in cases and increases the likelihood that learners will take into account more factors when confronted with similar situations in the future.

Another example of the principle of avoiding oversimplification is found in the clinical assignment of anesthesia cases. It is common to see beginning students assigned to the "bread and butter" cases; however, by occasionally assigning them more complicated cases, the instructor will expose them to complexity early, and they will understand that cases may not be as simple as they initially appear. This will not be a wasted experience for students. Although students may not understand all the components, the learning that occurs will be within the context of the complexity of the case. In these instances, instructors are responsible for case management while keeping students engaged by giving them tasks they are able to accomplish.

Theme 2: Multiple Representations

In ill-structured domains such as nurse anesthesia, if cases are treated narrowly in the educational process, the ability to process future cases will be limited. There will be an assumption by students that cases are simpler than they are, and subsequent analysis of new cases will conclude prematurely.[17-22] Also, the learner's reasoning based on precedent cases will result in truncated decision making after only partial analysis of the problem. For example, the etiology of tachycardia can be an inadequate level of anesthesia, and beginning students often observe this during the induction of anesthesia. A student who does not have experience with many cases might reflexively (truncated decision making) increase the concentration of the volatile agent when a patient's heart rate suddenly increases. In this case, the student is not considering the many other things that could be the cause of the tachycardia.

Theme 3: Centrality of Cases

The more ill structured the domain, the poorer the guidance for knowledge application from top-down structures will be. Application of knowledge in ill-structured domains cannot be prescribed in advance by general principles because cases vary greatly with respect to which conceptual elements will be relevant and in what combinations. Overreliance on precompiled knowledge structures such as fixed protocols is a teaching and learning error.[17-22] Certain combinations of drugs work well for typical cases, and beginning students feel more comfortable when given "recipes" for case management; however, experienced nurse anesthetists know that they must always make adjustments to their anesthetic plan and titrate to effect. Students' future decision making and practice skills benefit more when instructors teach them to titrate drugs and tailor anesthetics based on patients' needs instead of giving them prescribed recipes for anesthetic management.

Theme 4: Conceptual Knowledge Is Knowledge in Use

In ill-structured domains, the meanings of concepts are connected to their patterns of use. When use of a concept has a complex and irregular distribution, prepackaged prescriptions for proper activation of the concept cannot be provided.[17-22] A concept has many different uses in cases, and each concept must be tailored to the context of its application. A student may know a fact but may not be able to apply it to a particular case. For example, a student may understand the concept of the carbon dioxide response curve and accurately draw the curve indicating the effect volatile agents and opioids have on it; however, at the end of a case when the student gives a patient a small amount of opioid for postoperative pain control and the patient's respiratory rate declines, the student may not be able to understand the activation of that concept without assistance.

Theme 5: Schema Assembly (From Rigidity to Flexibility)

In ill-structured domains, the goal is to teach students to assemble knowledge from different theoretical and precedent case sources to adaptively fit the situation at hand. Knowledge in nurse anesthesia is used in far too many ways for them all to be anticipated in advance. There must be a shift in learning from retrieval of intact knowledge structures to situation-specific problem solving.[17-22] We sometimes hear students say "We weren't taught that," meaning "We weren't taught exactly that." One learning goal is to foster students' ability to think for themselves and use their knowledge in new ways. It is important for them, as well as for their instructors, to understand and work toward this goal.

Theme 6: Noncompartmentalization of Concepts (Multiple Interconnectedness)

Because of the irregular way various features weave through cases in ill-structured domains, knowledge cannot be neatly compartmentalized. A student strategy frequently encountered in didactic education is relegation of knowledge into separate compartments. For example, students learn anatomy in 1 course and pharmacology in another, often making lists or using mnemonics as study aids to pass examinations. The problem is that students often miss the interconnectedness of concepts and their applications along multiple conceptual and clinical dimensions.[17-23] An example of clinical instructors assisting students with interconnectedness is a case-based discussion about principles of basic science that informed a particular practice decision.

Case-based instruction can highlight important, instructional relationships between aspects of 1 case and aspects of another. Understanding what to do in a given case usually requires reference to more than 1 prototype—the case will be "kind of like this earlier one, kind of like that one." Postcase conferences are a way instructors can assist students in understanding relational aspects of cases. Identifying common denominators among a series of cases is a common teaching strategy. It is also important to highlight aspects of the cases that are different; for example, the patients' differing underlying disease processes, pain tolerance, or body habitus, and how these differing aspects may have influenced case management.

Theme 7: Active Participation

Knowledge cannot be simply handed to student nurse anesthetists. There must be active learner involvement in knowledge acquisition, accompanied by guidance and commentary from expert mentors to help them derive maximum benefit from their experiences. When instructors aim toward the goal of cognitive flexibility, they can build integrated knowledge structures that permit greater flexibility in the ways knowledge can potentially be assembled and used or transferred to different situations. On the other hand, overreliance on automation processes can lead to performance errors. One such error is the continuation of a course of action or strategy when it would be rational to change to an alternative course because conditions have changed (cognitive blockade). Another error might be seen in a person who, lacking cognitive flexibility, adheres to a decision when it has been demonstrated to be a mistake or who persists in a false diagnosis when new information suggests otherwise. A lack of cognitive flexibility can lead a student to consider only part of a problem because he or she is putting information into precompiled knowledge structures that do not fit the situation at hand. To help avoid these types of errors, it is important to teach students to be cognitively flexible so they can adapt their behaviors appropriately to changing situations.

Thinking Out Loud and Gradually Ceding Control

In teaching student nurse anesthetists, it is important to provide opportunities to develop flexible, declarative, procedural, and conditional knowledge structures with cases containing complexity. Clinical instruction must be provided in ways that allow students to gain the most from their experiences.

It takes time to learn to think strategically as a professional because the learner's process of internalization occurs gradually. Initially, teachers control and guide students' activities. Later, they share control over problem-solving functions; the students take initiatives and teachers correct and guide when students make mistakes. Finally, teachers cede control to students and function primarily as a supportive and sympathetic audience. This type of instruction is not unique to nurse anesthesia. Teachers, tutors, and master craftspersons in traditional apprenticeship situations all function as promoters of self-regulation (executive control) by nurturing the emergence of self-control while gradually ceding external control. For example, an instructor confronted with a problem during an anesthetic could model the thought processes used in decision making by thinking out loud. After allowing the student to observe several examples of this strategic thinking, the instructor could then allow the student an opportunity to demonstrate problem-solving strategies. Gradually, after many successful demonstrations, the instructor could cede control of the problem solving to the student. For example, an instructor could think out loud while managing the patient undergoing an abdominal aortic aneurysm resection, during which fluid management can be extremely difficult. The decisions about fluid management, blood volume, and vasodilator therapy are complex and there are no formulas to guide therapy. The aorta is typically cross-clamped to facilitate surgical repair. To prevent hypotension during aortic cross-clamp removal, the vascular space is typically dilated and filled with intravenous fluid so that maximum cardiac output can be achieved. The vasodilator is stopped before declamping and while rapid volume administration is often initiated. By first modeling the decision-making strategies by thinking out loud for the student's first 2 abdominal aortic aneurysm resection cases and allowing the student to be the decision maker in the third case, the instructor gradually cedes external control over problem solving to the student, while correcting and guiding when mistakes are made.

Scaffolded Instruction

Scaffolded instruction is a concept developed to describe the assistance a teacher can offer a learner. The instructor provides initial support, or scaffolding, until the student is ready to be more independent, and then the instructor removes the scaffold when the student is ready. In successful scaffolding, the instructor initially ascertains the students' prior knowledge so that it can be connected to the new knowledge and made relevant to the learner. There are many ways that an instructor can use scaffolding in student learning. Instructors using scaffolding can break the tasks into smaller, more manageable parts; think out loud to verbalize their thinking process when completing tasks; and use questioning, coaching, and modeling to reinforce the learning of concepts. Other methods include the activation of background knowledge by providing tips, strategies, and cues.

Nurse anesthesia instructors frequently use the think-out-loud strategy, which models forms of executive control over thinking and problem-solving activities. The goal is to assist students in becoming successful independent thinkers and problem solvers. Another common strategy is for an instructor to initially use an explicit directive and then be less directive the next time the student needs assistance. Regardless of the specific technique used, scaffolding should be removed, fading gradually, and then completely when the student demonstrates mastery of the task.[23,24] The teacher must keep the learner in pursuit of the task while minimizing the learner's stress. Skills or tasks too far out of reach or tasks that are too simple can lead to student frustration.[24,25]

The Zone of Proximal Development

Central to using scaffolded instruction to assist students to become independent problem solvers is the role of dialogue between teachers and students. The purpose of dialogue is to provide students with just enough support and guidance to achieve goals that are beyond their unassisted efforts. In accomplishing this, teachers must understand the zone of proximal development. This zone is depicted by the arrows to the side in the conceptual model for nurse anesthesia education (see Figure 2.1). Vygotsky, who developed the concept, defines this as the distance between the learners' actual developmental level (determined by independent problem solving) and the level of potential development (as determined through problem solving with the guidance of mentors).[26-28] Once the student has increased knowledge, the level of development expands and the zone of proximal development shifts. Thus, the zone is always changing as the student gains knowledge, and instructors using scaffolded instruction must constantly individualize their interactions with each student in response to the changing zone of proximal development.

It is important that the instructor appropriately assesses the zone of proximal development. Misjudging the zone could lead to underinstruction and boredom or frustration because of instruction beyond the student's abilities. Scaffolded instruction includes the following components[29]:

- Recruitment: The instructor must recruit the student's interest.
- Reduction in degrees of freedom: The instructor must reduce the size of the task to the level that the student can fit with task requirements.
- Direction maintenance: The instructor must keep the student in pursuit of the task.
- Marking critical features: The instructor must accentuate features of the task.
- Frustration control: The instructor must help reduce stress to make the situation less stressful than if the tutor had not been present.
- Demonstration: The instructor must demonstrate an idealization of the task by completing the task or explicating a solution that is beyond the learner's current ability.

Planning and use of instructional strategies such as scaffolded instruction when engaging in clinical teaching will result in a more productive student learning experience and a smoother progression through the stages of learning.

Because all learning begins with the experience of the learner (what the student already knows), it is important to ascertain the student's current knowledge level.

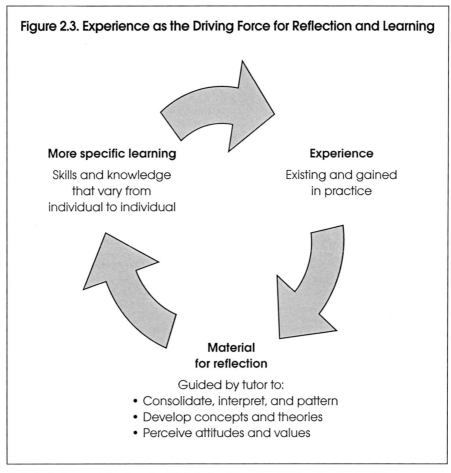

Figure 2.3. Experience as the Driving Force for Reflection and Learning

More specific learning
Skills and knowledge
that vary from
individual to individual

Experience
Existing and gained
in practice

**Material
for reflection**
Guided by tutor to:
• Consolidate, interpret, and pattern
• Develop concepts and theories
• Perceive attitudes and values

(Adapted with permission from the British Further Education Unit, London, England.[30])

In anesthesia, students are experienced critical care nurses who have a wealth of knowledge and experience; however, the first step may be the need to clarify learned misconceptions.

In all cases, students will gain maximally from scaffolded instruction when they have experiences that are then accompanied by reflective activities guided by instructors (Figure 2.3).[30] Nurse anesthesia instructors can best assist students' learning by providing them with experiences (real-world and simulated cases) that require deliberation and action. A method to assist them in analyzing situations is the use of reflection.[31] Schön describes this process as reflection in action.[32,33]

Reflection in Action

Practitioners first make sense of new situations by imposing a structure that often comes through analogy to other previously encountered situations. They then build, through these experiences, a repertoire of examples, images, understandings, and actions. When they encounter a new situation similar to something already present in their repertoire, they bring past experience to bear on the case, which enables them to see an unfamiliar situation as a familiar one. Schön also describes a scaffolding method of assisting students by reflecting their thinking back to them so they better understand their own deliberations.[31,32] The notion of zones of development are recast by Schön as zones of mastery.[32,33] By having the learners engage in reflection, instructors teach them how to be metacognitively aware of their own thinking processes. This has been termed *cognitive apprenticeship* or *collaborative learning* and can lead to important insights for instructors as well as students. Master teachers value learners' expertise and encourage them to take responsibility for their own educational needs. This eventually leads to a sense of empowerment that is important for lifelong learning.[33] Finally, both learners and instructors must be aware that instructors also advance through the stages of a parallel educational model as they progress from novice to master teacher.

The instructor must have a reflective and flexible educational style that is tailored to the individual learner. Learners can enrich an educator's experience in ways that may inform the instructor's own practice. Those who reflect on their teaching styles can become more capable of adjusting their approaches to allow for students' needs and learning styles.[34]

Summary

Nurse anesthesia is a complex domain that requires mastery of a broad range of components that, when combined, reflect the real-world complexity of the field. Prepackaged prescriptions for action do not exist in nurse anesthesia because the diversity of all possible scenarios is impossible to anticipate. The goal of education is for students to acquire a mastery of experiences with a broad range of cases that reflect the complexity of anesthesia practice. To accomplish this, learners must assimilate knowledge from a variety of sources to construct solutions that suit the problem-solving needs of the situation at hand. To achieve a level of successful performance as entry-level providers, student nurse anesthetists need experience applying theory and principles to a large number and variety of cases.

Understanding the stages through which skillful performance develops is important in designing educational programs and materials. This information will facilitate the acquisition of advanced knowledge and cognitive flexibility. To assist learners as they progress through the stages of learning in case-based instruction, it is essential to identify at each stage which capacities the learners have acquired and which ones they may be in a position to attain. The role of the teacher is that of an expert mentor who guides students' learning through reflective deliberations and facilitates their acquisition of higher-order skills. Through this process, expert mentors using appropriate applications of anesthesia and educational theory can assist learners in developing the sophisticated, integrated knowledge structures that are required for adaptation of behavior to rapidly changing situations.

On completion of an educational program, graduate nurse anesthetists will have successfully progressed through the first 4 stages of the model. On completion of the proficiency stage, graduates can safely and independently administer anesthesia as entry-level nurse anesthetists after passing the national certification examination. Some graduates will be content to practice proficiently and will not attempt to progress further. A few will even regress to the stage of competence, still able to safely administer an anesthetic but requiring much direction. Those content to practice at the competent stage will not keep themselves informed of advances in the field. Those graduates who wish to continue to learn about the art and science of nurse anesthesia can develop into expert nurse anesthetists. Expert nurse anesthetists are confident and secure in their practice because they have excellent clinical and critical-thinking skills. Through continued study, expert nurse anesthetists maintain up-to-date declarative, procedural, and conditional knowledge bases.

Some nurse anesthetists will continue their professional growth and achieve the sixth stage, *master*. Those functioning at this level will formally or informally deepen their understanding of nurse anesthesia, usually through intensive study in a specific area. These anesthetists are often the ones who advance the science of the profession through teaching, writing, managing, or conducting research.

References

1. McAuliffe MS. *Case-Based Instruction: An Analysis of Clinical Instruction in Nurse Anesthesiology* [dissertation]. Ann Arbor, MI: University of Michigan Dissertation Services; 1993:1-156.

2. Dinham SM, Stritter FT. Research on professional education. In: Wittrock M(ed). *Handbook of Research on Teaching*. 3rd ed. New York, NY: Macmillan; 1986:952-969.

3. Kuhn TS. *The Structure of Scientific Revolutions*. Chicago, IL: University of Chicago Press; 1970:111.

4. Argyris C, Schön DA. *Theory in Practice: Increasing Professional Effectiveness*. San Francisco, CA: Jossey-Bass; 1974:173-196.

5. Dreyfus SE, Dreyfus HL. A five-stage model of mental activities involved in directed skill acquisition. Unpublished report. University of California at Berkeley: US Air Force Office of Scientific Research; 1980.

6. Friedrich MJ. Practice makes perfect: risk-free medical training with patient simulators. *JAMA*. 2002;288(22):2808-2812.

7. Peile EB, Easton GP, Johnson N. The year in a training practice: what has lasting value? grounded theoretical categories and dimensions from a pilot study. *Med Teach*. 2000;23(2):205-211.

8. Dreyfus SE, Dreyfus HL. *Mind Over Machine*. New York, NY: The Free Press; 1986:122-157.

9. Flavel JH. Speculations about the nature and development of metacognition. In: Weinert F, Kluwe R, eds. *Metacognition, Motivation, and Understanding*. Hillsdale, NJ: Lawrence Erlbaum Associates; 1987:21-29.

10. Weinstein CE, Husman J, Feltovich PJ, et al. Self-regulation interventions with a focus on learning strategies. In: Boekaerts M, Pintrich PR, Ziedner M, eds. *Handbook of Self-Regulation*. San Diego, CA: Academic Press; 2000:727-747.

11. Paris SG, Lipson MY, Wixson KK. Becoming a strategic reader. *Contemp Educ Psychol*. 1983;8(3):293-316.

12. Gott SP. Apprenticeship instruction for real world tasks: the coordination of procedures, mental models, and strategies. In: Rothkopf EZ, ed. *Review of Research in Education*. Washington, DC: American Educational Research Association; 1988:97-169.

13. Flavel JH. Cognitive monitoring. In: Dickson WP, ed. *Children's Oral Communication Skills*. New York, NY: Academic Press Inc; 1981:35-60.

14. Brown AL, Bransford JD, Ferrara RA, et al. Learning, remembering and understanding. In: Mussen PH. *Carmichael's Manual of Child Psychology*. Vol 1. Hoboken, NJ: John Wiley & Sons; 1983:77-166.

15. Brown AL, Campione JC, Day JD. Learning to learn: on training students to learn from texts. *Educ Res*. 1981;10:14-21.

16. Baker L, Brown AL. Metacognitive skills and reading. In: Kamil M, Mosenthal P, Pearson D, Barr R, eds. *Handbook of Reading Research*. New York, NY: Longman; 1984:353-394.

17. Spiro RJ, Jehng JC. Cognitive flexibility and hypertext. In: Spiro R, Nix D, eds. *Cognition, Education and Multimedia*. Hillsdale, NJ: Lawrence Erlbaum Associates; 1990:163-205.

18. Spiro RJ, Feltovich PJ, Jacobson MJ, et al. Cognitive flexibility, constructivism and hypertext: random access instruction for advanced knowledge acquisition in ill-structured domains. In: Duffy T, Jonassen D, eds. *Constructivism and the Technology of Instruction*. Hillsdale, NJ: Lawrence Erlbaum; 1992:57-166.

19. Spiro RJ, Vispoel WL, Schmitz JG, et al. Knowledge acquisition for application: cognitive flexibility and transfer in complex content domains. In: Britton BK, Glynn SM, eds. *Executive Control Processes*. Hillsdale, NJ: Lawrence Erlbaum; 1987.

20. Spiro RJ, Coulson RL, Feltovich PJ, et al. Cognitive flexibility theory: advanced knowledge acquisition in ill-structured domains. In: Ruddel RB, ed. *Proceedings of the 10th Annual Conference of the Cognitive Science Society*. Hillsdale, NJ: Lawrence Erlbaum; 2004:602-616.

21. Jonassen D, Ambruso D, Olesen J. Designing hypertext on transfusion medicine using cognitive flexibility theory. *J Educ Multimedia Hypermedia*. 1992:1(3):309-322.

22. Spiro RJ, Feltovich PJ, Jacobson MI, Coulson RI. Random access instruction for advanced knowledge acquisition in ill-structured domains. In: Duffy T, Jonassen D, eds. *Constructivism and the Technology of Instruction*. Hillsdale, NJ: Lawrence Erlbaum; 1992:57-75.

23. Lipscomb L, Swanson J, West A. Emerging perspectives on learning, teaching, and technology: scaffolding. University of Georgia website. http://projects.coe.uga.edu/epltt/index.php?title=Scaffolding. Accessed April 13, 2009.

24. Zydney JM. Deepening our understanding through multiple perspectives: the effectiveness of scaffolding in a learning environment. Educational Resources Information website. http://www.eric.ed.gov/ERICDocs/data/ericdocs2sql/content_storage_01/0000019b/80/1b/be/65.pdf. Accessed April 13, 2009.

25. Coulson RW, Feltovich PJ, Spiro RJ. *Foundations of a Misunderstanding of the Ultra Structural Basis for Myocardial Failure: A Reciprocating Network of Over-Simplifications (Tech. Rep. No.1).* Springfield, IL: Southern Illinois University School of Medicine, Conceptual Knowledge Research Project; 1986.

26. Vygotsky LS, Cole M, John-Steiner V, Scribner S, Souberman E. *Mind in Society: Development of Higher Psychological Processes.* Cambridge, MA: Harvard University Press; 1978:76.

27. Vygotsky LS, Kozulin A. *Thought and Language.* Cambridge, MA: The MIT Press; 1986:210-256.

28. Dahms M, Geonnotti K, Passalacqua D, Schilk JN, Wetzel A, Zulkowsky M. The educational theory of Lev Vygotsky: an analysis. New Foundations website. http://www.newfoundations.com/GALLERY/Vygotsky.html. Accessed April 13, 2009.

29. Paris SG, Winograd P. How metacognition can promote academic learning and instruction. In: Jones BF, Idol L, eds. *Dimensions of Thinking and Cognitive Instruction.* Hillsdale, NJ: Lawrence Erlbaum Associates; 1990:15-51.

30. British Further Education Unit. *Experience, Reflection, Learning.* London, England: Further Education Unit, Curriculum and Development Unit; 1981.

31. Spencer J. Learning and teaching in the clinical environment. *BMJ.* 2003;326(7389):591-594.

32. Schön DA. *Educating the Reflective Practitioner.* San Francisco, CA: Jossey-Bass; 1990.

33. Schön DA. *The Reflective Practitioner: How Professionals Think in Action.* New York, NY: Basic Books; 1984:128-168.

34. Newman P, Peile E. Valuing learners' experience and supporting further growth: educational models to help experienced adult learners in medicine. *BMJ.* 2000;325(7357):200-202.

Chapter 3

Stressors of Teaching and Learning

Sandra K. Tunajek, CRNA, DNP

Key Points

- Stress is a pressure, force, or substantial strain placed on an individual by certain events or circumstances in life. Individuals respond differently to different types of stressors. Stress may be positive and high energy, or it may be negative.

- The educational preparation of healthcare professionals may be a highly stressful experience for both faculty and students. Psychological burnout may inhibit the ability of faculty to effectively manage periods of change. For student nurse anesthetists, academic information overload and fear of clinical error are the highest stressors.

- Research shows that stress is a major influence affecting performance and interpersonal relationships among faculty and students. Stress may compromise health and well-being in pronounced ways.

- The concept of wellness is gaining nationwide attention as a major factor affecting healthcare professionals and workforce productivity. The increasing focus on patient safety initiatives has highlighted cognitive and physical competence, professional fitness for duty, and impairment issues as emerging interests to public and regulatory agencies.

- Academic and clinical faculty must understand the stress and anxiety that students experience in order to devise the best techniques to help students cope with daily stressors. The characteristics of stress and burnout may impede effective teaching and learning, and they are likely to intensify unless faculty members devise and implement specific interventions.

- In peer support programs, students learn from the perceptions, experiences, and challenges of their fellow students. The creation and success of these programs require a great deal of faculty support.

Introduction

This chapter focuses on the sources of stress for faculty and students, responses to and effects of stress, and coping strategies. Stress is a necessary and unavoidable parallel of daily living and can be beneficial by motivating us to perform necessary tasks. Other types of stress, however, can be harmful. It is not uncommon for graduate students to experience stressful situations, coping issues, and problems during their academic careers. Certainly, working in stressful environments is inherent to a career in the nurse anesthesia profession.

Stressful healthcare work environments and individual well-being are emerging as factors in patient safety. Healthcare institutions are initiating processes for evaluating professional competence and individual fitness for duty. Furthermore, largely in response to productivity and regulatory concerns, facilities including teaching institutions are beginning to introduce stress management and wellness programs. There is ample evidence that students in health professional educational programs experience varying levels of stress; for many students, stress is substantial and is associated with poor academic performance.[1-6]

Research in the medical, dental, and nursing literature indicates that considerable stress is also a factor for graduate level faculty.[2,7,8] Studies in medical specialties have found that stress during residency training affects efficiency, productivity, error rates, and physician burnout.[2,3] The few studies that have investigated nurse anesthesia faculty indicate that a high level of stress is directly related to job dissatisfaction, a heavy workload, and perceptions of lack of authority and control.[8,9]

The studies related to the anesthesia student experience[5,10,11] suggest the major stressors are similar to those in other types of graduate educational programs. However, student nurse anesthetists have an added concern about making clinical errors that may harm patients. Additionally, for most students, the ability to cope is related to the sequencing of clinical time and the year in school.[11,12]

Student nurse anesthetists must adapt to unpredictable workloads; use of new, advanced technology; long working hours; altered sleep and eating patterns; and juggling academic and clinical hours. Adding to the occupational stressors, students must deal with an identity shift from competent registered nurses to novice student anesthetists, often experiencing a perceived loss of control and professional recognition. For many, there is a need for immediate modification in financial status, relocation and long-distance family relationships, and loss of personal time. Furthermore, the student nurse anesthetist is expected to master large amounts of complex material in a short amount of time; perform complex assessments of patient health problems; develop independent, critical reading, listening, and thinking abilities; and clearly articulate problem-solving solutions in a professional, confident manner.[13]

Student nurse anesthetists are highly motivated, achievement-oriented individuals with high expectations. After graduation, they will enter one of the most stressful occupations in healthcare. An attitude of self-reliance, a driven personality, and tendencies to overachieve contribute to a cycle that leads to burnout and further exacerbates stressful circumstances.[14] Finally, students may not be aware of the major impact these pressures can exert on physical and mental health, and resources may not be readily available to assist students in coping with these new stressful experiences.[5,10]

In nurse anesthesia–related studies, a common theme for both students and faculty is the lack of resources,[5,8,15] suggesting an influence on the ability of individuals to cope. Furthermore, the teaching environment may not recognize or encourage the need for resources. More importantly, students may be reluctant to access resources or seek assistance for fear of appearing weak and less capable of achievement, or out of fear of retaliation.[5,6]

Faculty and Student Stress

Stress is a response to change. It is often difficult to define because individuals react to stress very differently. Situations that are stressful for one person may not be for another. Individuals vary widely in their ability to cope effectively with stress.

Faculty Stressors

Of the 3 functions performed by faculty in higher education—teaching, research, and administrative activities—teaching was designated as the most stressful.[2,16] Most of the stressors appear to relate directly to time management and access to resources. The areas causing the most stress for faculty appeared to be excessively high self-expectations, securing financial support for educational programs, having insufficient time and being continually overloaded with work, receiving low pay for work done, lack of time for individual research, interference of work with personal activities, and interruptions and meetings.[7,8,17]

Educators also reported experiencing role ambiguity, intellectual fatigue, physical exhaustion, and loss of morale. Demands to generate revenues, the accelerating competition for grant funding, and the explosion of new technology and emerging biomedical knowledge also contribute to the challenges.[16] Furthermore, the supply of excellent role models and mentors is dwindling as current nurse anesthesia faculty members approach retirement.[15] This compares with similar concerns for faculty in other disciplines of graduate education. At least 20% of faculty reported major depressive symptoms.[18]

Student Stressors

Models that are useful in understanding stress among students are based on the concept that the individual perceives stressful events as "challenging" or "threatening."[19] When students consider their education as a challenge, stress can bring them a sense of competence and an increased capacity to learn. Competence is the internal drive to be effective and master the environment and is associated with academic performance. When education is seen as a threat, however, stress can elicit feelings of helplessness, self-doubt, and a foreboding sense of failure.[19,20]

Adult students entering graduate education can experience a reaction similar to shock as they attempt to adjust to the multiplicity of new responsibilities while organizing their time and dealing with changes in their relationships at home.[20,21]

In the general population, research on graduate students' stress is a fairly recent phenomenon. Evidence from several studies suggests that academic performance is the most critical concern of students, especially first-year students, and that the problems perceived to be the most intense sources of stress are examinations and grades, financial concerns, and fear of failure on specific assignments.

Among student nurse anesthetists, academic information overload and fear of clinical error are the highest stressors.[11] A comparison study between graduate nurse anesthetists and general nursing graduates found that student nurse anesthetists have significantly higher scores on excitement seeking and addictive tendencies ($P = .002$).[22] Excitement seeking, by definition, describes an individual's preference for quantity and intensity of interpersonal relationships and is a facet of extraverted personalities. Because the neurochemistry is not well understood, ongoing research in drug and alcohol abuse is investigating the association of personality, excitement seeking, and addiction tendency.[23]

Another process in nurse anesthesia schools that also can cause stress is the subtle, but pervasive, process of being socialized into a profession. Students take the new skills they are learning, absorb these skills and undergo a transformation in their sense of identity. The transformation of a nurse into a Certified Registered Nurse Anesthetist (CRNA) is an adjustment to a new role, which, if successful, creates the new status of belonging to a unique social group.[24] Peer expectations and adherence to these high standards of professional conduct during the educational process is an additional stressor.

Neumann et al[25] found that emotional exhaustion greatly influences student performance and affects personal commitment. The degree to which students experience emotional fatigue depends on individual flexibility, engagement in learning, student-faculty contact, and the perception of stress. Regarding the latter, one study indicated a considerable mismatch between faculty and students in their perceptions of students' stressors and reactions to stressors.[12] The faculty members perceived the students to experience a higher level of stress and to display reactions to stressors more frequently than the students actually perceived they were experiencing stress. However, both groups identified work overload and variability in faculty expectations as the major perceived stressors.

Burnout

Burnout is a distinctive kind of job-related stress that inhibits the person's capacity to function effectively.[6] Research indicates that individuals engaged in the helping professions or human services are especially susceptible to burnout. Although burnout, with its accompanying emotional exhaustion and dissatisfaction, has prompted much study as it relates to management and business, it is not well documented in the anesthesia literature. The educational processes for healthcare professionals, which appear to accept fatigue as a condition of teaching and learning, have not recognized that burnout exists for both students and faculty. Some academic health centers are beginning to address the issue, but there are severe gaps in supportive mechanisms that facilitate effective coping.

Burnout is not just a temporary condition, but an unhealthy situation that can turn productive, enthusiastic workers into detriments to their profession, their colleagues, and themselves. Burnout usually affects the most able individuals, those who are the most competent and committed, feel the most strongly about the value of what they do, and set high expectations for themselves.

Some stress is to be expected in education and has been found to be motivational. Yet, how much, and what may be counterproductive, has not been well researched in the anesthesia literature. However, it is clear that burnout and stress among students affects academic performance.

Burnout among faculty inhibits the ability to effectively lead programs, particularly during periods of change. Teaching can generate a high level of stress and fatigue and can lead to burnout. Academic demands, financial difficulties, family problems, and the relationships between students and faculty advisers were cited as the biggest contributors to stress and burnout.[7] Factors contributing to overall stress are noted in Table 3.1.

One of the greatest challenges in education is effectively managing teaching loads and schedules. This includes time for family, friends, personal endeavors, nourishing the soul, reflection, renewal, and reinvigoration. Demands are increasing with more work, more students, and less free time. The increased demands and workloads result in teachers having less time for preparation, teaching, and interaction with students. Unfortunately, student interaction may be one of the first things that overworked instructors decrease, affecting the attitudes, self-esteem, and motivation of both faculty and students. If unable to fulfill all expected activities, faculty may feel increased pressure, experiencing greater stress. Regrettably, the prevalence of stress and burnout syndromes reported among practitioners, residents, and students in nursing and medicine studies shows that stress is associated with depression, alcohol and drug use, relationship difficulties, anxiety, and even suicide.[3,23]

Table 3.1. Sources of Perceived Faculty Stressors

Having a heavy workload (combined clinical and classroom teaching).

Retaining failing students or dealing with difficult students.

Meeting research requirements.

Providing individual clinical supervision.

Teaching those who have learning disabilities and attention-deficit disorders.

Using new technologies.

Increasing diversification of expertise.

Dealing with campus politics and meeting the economic necessities of the institution.

Dealing with changes in administrative demands or administrative leadership.

Lacking financial and personnel support.

Having time pressures and deadlines.

Dealing with inequities and inequalities.

Personality Type and Stress

Stress is connected with major changes in personal or work-related environments. In general, adverse physical and emotional consequences usually result from the way an individual perceives particular events or conditions. Too many changes at one time, either positive or negative, can overload an individual's capacity to adapt successfully and may result in a variety of illnesses. Stress depends on the individual's perception of the situation. Thus, what may be stressful to one person may be excitingly challenging and stressful in a positive way to another. Even to the same person, the same event can be stressful at one time and stimulating at another time. How someone responds to stress depends on the environment, the magnitude of the stressor, the person's self-perceived ability to handle the stressor, the person's physical condition, and more often, the habitual response.[26]

Stress can be self-imposed by setting too high standards or having unrealistic expectations regarding one's abilities. Situational stressors include time constraints, lack of resources, threats to emotional or physical well-being, challenges beyond an individual's ability to respond, or conflicts between personal values and the values of others. Additionally, individuals with type A personalities, who exhibit a high degree of self-control, impatience, competitiveness, inability to relax, orientation to achievement, and denial of failure, appear to be more prone to stressful reactions.[2,26,27]

There are many personality frameworks that offer insights into differences among people. One of the most researched theories is the Myers-Briggs Type Indicator, which refines personality into 16 types. This theory holds that people take in information and make decisions differently, which are 2 key processes in education. These variations in behavior are quite orderly and consistent. More and more career counselors, educators, and academic centers are using personality testing to determine specialty choice for medical professions.[28]

Determining a person's natural personality type is frequently complicated by lifelong learning experiences. After the onset of puberty, adult learning begins to overlay the core personality, which is influenced by genetics and environment. For some people, this learning serves to strengthen the natural core of what is already there, but with others, it produces multiple facets to personality. The broad categories reflect tendencies toward extraversion or introversion. Overlaying these basic traits are decision-making and communication styles. Extraverted personalities tend to be characterized by sociability, assertiveness, talkativeness, and activity. Extraverted people tend to prefer large groups to small gatherings. Facets of the extraverted personality include warmth, gregariousness, assertiveness, activity, excitement seeking, and positive emotions. Introverted personalities tend to be independent, reserved, and even-paced. They typically value solitude and display their emotions with less exuberance.

Impact of Stress on Learning

The influences of behavioral, individual, cognitive, and environmental factors determine how people interact and learn from each other.[29] The effects of stress on learning and memory, both facilitating and impairing influences, are well described in the literature,[26] and authors note that good stress can be invigorating and empowering. With good stress, energy peaks, memory sharpens, chemicals producing pleasure increase in the brain, and senses are heightened. Sustained stress can damage the hippocampus, the area of the brain critical to learning and memory. The body makes no distinction between immediate, pleasurable, or acutely threatening stress and chronic physical and psychological stress. Additionally, an individual's personality or frame of mind when encountering stress may influence the health effects of stress.

The brain interprets what is potentially threatening and therefore stressful and determines the individual's behavioral and physiological responses. Behavioral responses may include the fight or flight response, overeating, smoking, drinking to excess, and losing sleep at night. Thus, lifestyle and behavior are key contributors to being stressed out.

The literature documents that both increased and decreased stress responses can profoundly affect cognition and behavior.[30] The amygdala and hippocampus portions of the brain interpret what is stressful, then regulate appropriate responses by controlling the release of glucocorticoids and activating the sympathetic nervous system. Uncontrollable stress impedes hippocampal memory, and stress-induced alterations contribute to memory impairments.[30,31] Increased glucocorticoid levels also impair memory function, disrupt problem solving, and weaken spatial recognition memory. The response to stress involves the active release of hormones and other mediators that produce adaptation to acute stress. Subsequent pathophysiology results when the same mediators are dysregulated over long periods.

In the hippocampus and prefrontal cortex (the center of emotion) repeated stress causes dendrites to shrink and spine synapses to decrease in number. In the basolateral amygdala, stress causes increased dendritic branching and synapse density, essentially leading to a constant state of fear. As remodeling of neural circuitry occurs, mediators are under repeated stress, leading to impaired memory, increased anxiety, aggression, and impaired attention. The body further reacts by compromising the immune system and the cardiovascular system, resulting in long-term health effects.[26]

Stress affects cognition in a number of ways, acting rapidly via catecholamines and more slowly via glucocorticoids. The activation or arousal of the stress systems leads to a cluster of behavioral and physiological changes that are consistent and predictable, including increased alertness, vigilance, improved cognition, and focused attention.[32]

The relationship between changes in arousal and motivation is often expressed as an inverted-U function (also known as the Yerkes-Dodson law). The basic concept is that, as arousal level increases, performance improves, but only to a point, beyond which the increases in arousal lead to deterioration in performance.[30,32]

Anxiety involves cognitive and somatic components. Cognitive anxiety (worry) is characterized by negative expectations, lack of concentration, and images of failure, whereas somatic anxiety refers to physical symptoms such as nervousness and tension.

People monitor their environments and, through the appraisal process, interpret situations as harmful or threatening.[19] Stress occurs when people feel inadequate to meet the challenge. Coping consists of adaptive resources to meet the demands and cognitive and behavioral efforts to manage the demands. This theory has been enhanced by the role that control plays in the appraisal, in which perception of control tends to reduce the negative emotional responses. This concept involves cognitive, physiological, and overt behavioral components and is the basis for recognizing, preventing, and coping interventions.

Signs of Stress-Related Problems

Historically, the physical changes in response to stress were an essential adaptation for meeting natural threats. Likewise, in today's world the stress response can be an asset for raising levels of performance during critical events such as graduate school, job interviews, or important meetings, or in situations of actual danger or crisis. However, if stress becomes persistent, all parts of the body's functional ability (eg, brain, heart, lungs, blood vessels, and muscles) become chronically overworked or underworked. This may produce physical or psychological damage over time. Short-term acute stress can also be harmful if it leads to inappropriate behaviors.

Stress is not itself an illness but is a condition that can give rise to real illness. Various psychological and behavioral changes affecting work performance and interpersonal relationships may be noticed by colleagues, including inability to concentrate, overworking, irritability or aggression, becoming withdrawn or unsociable, or reluctance to accept constructive criticism and advice. The long-term consequences of stress include cynicism, apathy, depression, emotional exhaustion, hostility, alcohol and substance abuse, obsessive-compulsive disorders, and other dissociative behavioral patterns.

It is estimated that 10% to 15% of all healthcare professionals will misuse drugs or alcohol at some time during their careers in an attempt to deal with stress. Specialties such as anesthesia, emergency medicine, and psychiatry appear to have higher rates of substance abuse, most likely related to baseline provider personalities and functioning in a highly stressful, risk-prone environment with easy access to drugs.[23,33] The concepts of substance misuse and addiction are not new to the medical and nursing communities. It is considered the most common occupational hazard for anesthesia practice.[34] The nurse anesthesia profession has addressed the problem since the early 1980s, offering educational resources, peer support, and more recently, the American Association of Nurse Anesthetists Wellness Program to assist CRNAs and students.[34,35] Substance abuse and chemical dependency among nurse anesthetists have been reported in the literature at the rate of 10%[36] and perhaps as high as 18%.[23]

Colleagues are often the first to recognize an impaired practitioner and the last to address the concern. Often, they will make excuses, overlook obvious symptoms, and cover up for mistakes. This attitude and enabling behavior by coworkers is prevalent throughout the profession and contributes to the ongoing concerns for professional well-being. The substance abuse problem among nurse anesthesia professionals, along with prevention recommendations and treatment modalities, is extensively documented by Quinlan[34] in *A Professional Study and Resource Guide for the CRNA.*

Despite focused educational efforts, prevention, and awareness initiatives, consistent mechanisms to address intervention, treatment, and reentry into the workforce are lacking.[33] Established policies and procedures must be developed, understood, and adhered to if students and nurse anesthetists are to recognize the problem and take necessary action in assisting themselves and their colleagues. An analysis of the addictive disease process, behaviors, consequences of abuse, and recommendations for implementing educational programs, interventional policies, and tools to deal with the impaired professional can be found in the highly recommended text, *Substance Abuse Policies for Anesthesia,* by Higgins Roche.[32]

Advanced practice nurses have a high incidence of disciplinary action by regulatory boards, and impaired nurse anesthetists are at risk for loss of license and ability to practice. Although many states have alternative disciplinary programs that address the impaired professional,[23,35] there is great variability in these models. Moreover, institutional, state, and federal guidelines to address impaired professionals often include conflicting ethical and legal components.

Healthcare professionals face the stigma and prejudices associated with addiction, as well as loss of license, careers, and, all too often, their lives. It is therefore imperative that faculty, students, and professional colleagues understand the stressors, risks, and coping mechanisms related to working in this profession.

Faculty and staff are often the first to recognize students who are in trouble. Awareness of the damaging effects of stress and learning is critical to dealing with the potential unmanageable and ineffective coping mechanisms that may contribute to inappropriate behaviors as well as the resulting bad consequences. It is prudent to look for a cluster of signs or signals that appear within a similar time frame. Recognizable indicators that students may be experiencing more stress than they can cope with are listed in Table 3.2.

Table 3.2. Recognition of Student Problems

Student-stated need for assistance

Changes in academic or clinical performance

Physical symptoms of exhaustion, loss of or increased appetite, headaches, crying, and sleeplessness or oversleeping

Withdrawal, sudden crying, unexplained anger, or unusual irritability

Misuse of alcohol, drugs, or other compulsive behavior

Reference to suicide

Concerns related to racial or ethnic identity or sexual orientation

Marked change in personal lives, such as death of a family member or close friend, the end of an important relationship, divorce, and changes in family responsibilities

---

When a student's mood, behavior, and appearance have changed or are inconsistent with previous observations, it may indicate that the student is having problems. Often, students will use alcohol or drugs to cope with excessive stress and discover that the substance use becomes a problem in itself. Excessive drinking, drug use or dependence, and self-destructive behaviors are almost always indicative of underlying problems. Nurses are 4 times more likely to commit suicide compared with people working outside medicine, and doctors are twice as likely to kill themselves compared with people working in other professions.[23] Regardless of the circumstances, students should be referred to appropriate professionals, and any reference to suicide should be taken seriously.

Distance Education Factors

As advances in technology change the face of education, a growing number of faculty are moving into a teaching environment that is geographically independent of both students and colleagues. The separation by distance of student and teacher removes a vital link of communication between these 2 parties. Isolated students experience anticipatory stress related to a perceived lack of support and technical assistance.[37] The isolation may have an impact on behavioral issues and academic achievement. Students need access to faculty for feedback on academic courses as well as contact with instructors to serve as a support system if stress becomes a problem.[25]

Distance learning takes away much of the social interaction that would be present in traditional learning environments. Geographical isolation has been identified as one of the major problems for distance students.[37,38] This may lead to feelings of inadequacy and insecurity and a lack of confidence in their own abilities.[37,38] Of particular importance is the lack of staff training in course development, technology, and redesign of existing materials for distance students.[15] Perhaps the biggest problem for distance programs is the change in teaching styles from face-to-face instruction to that of a mentor, tutor, and facilitator.

It is critical that the support needs of these faculty and students be identified and addressed. Unfortunately, the literature offers little evidence of research into the experiences of the distance educator. Although there is general recognition that managing students is a demanding and often stressful aspect of conducting a distance course, faculty support is most often limited to technical and instructional design support.[16,39] There is little or no attention given to the totality of the experience of teaching at a distance and what the impact is on a social or personal level from the faculty perspective. McLean[16] also found a secondary factor that can directly influence the stress levels and job satisfaction of clinical faculty operating exclusively at a distance: uncertainty about the scope of teaching in this environment.

Increasingly, nurse anesthesia education is heavily involved in distance education, and clinical rotations have created an organizational structure that unbundles both the student and instructor from their traditional roles. Both student and instructor stress is connected to workload and to self-imposed expectations about performance and achievement. Distance education is an around-the-clock endeavor. It is important for program administrators to recognize this stress and to realize that, if faculty members are unable to temper it themselves, burnout is likely. The challenges faced by faculty teaching exclusively at a distance are not entirely different from those of their on-campus counterparts, but the form those challenges take and the avenues by which they are managed are necessarily changed in distance learning.[16]

If students try strategies for coping and still experience the negative aspects of stress, then faculty should encourage students to seek professional counseling or therapy. In times of major crisis, debriefing strategies and encouraging students to express feelings are paramount. These suggestions will more likely be received and acted on if a good relationship between teacher and student already exists and if teachers understand what stress is and the ramifications of their dealing poorly with a student's inability to cope. Students should be encouraged to contact the facility employment assistance program if one exists.

Coping Strategies

Active coping refers to a style characterized by solving problems, obtaining information, seeking social support or professional help, changing environments, planning activities, and reframing the meaning of problems. Research indicates that students and nurse anesthetists develop multiple mechanisms to deal with daily stress.[5,10,11]

Student nurse anesthetists are adult learners who must acquire extensive critical knowledge, experiences, and personal growth to become competent professionals. Much of that knowledge is gained through anxiety-producing situations in which the consequences can have a substantial impact on patients. Therefore, the clinical instructor needs to be aware of the traits and anxiety tendencies of students in order to devise the best techniques to help students cope with the day-to-day stressors.

Positive and Negative Coping

Coping strategies can be separated into 2 categories: positive and negative. Positive or functional coping strategies consist of family support, social support, religion, exercise, spirituality, mentoring, and talking to friends. The specific coping skills may include establishing good study habits, managing time wisely, learning positive self-talk, learning how to relax, forming or joining a student support group, getting plenty of sleep, and eating right.[5] Negative or dysfunctional coping strategies help to perpetuate problem situations. The inappropriate behavior may reduce stress immediately but can have profound lifelong implications and also become addictive. These habits are difficult to change. Negative coping methods include isolation, use of drugs or alcohol, workaholic tendencies, violent behavior, angry intimidation of others, binge eating, and other types of self-destructive behavior (eg, attempting suicide).

The type of strategies that students use to cope with their problems will affect their well-being as well as influence their academic performance. Recently, mechanisms for stress reduction through the use of meditation, particularly for control of pain, have been introduced to patients with positive results. These techniques are being adopted by healthcare institutions, introducing processes to support coping strategies among employees. Furthermore, these innovations are now emerging in medical schools and nursing education communities as support for students and residents.[3,40]

A critical issue concerning stress among students is its effect on learning. Individuals under low and high levels of stress learn the least, and those under moderate stress learn the most. Solutions suggested for reducing stress in students include instruction in recognizing learning styles[41] and informing students in advance of the difficulties they might face as well as encouraging them to develop their own strategies to achieve personal goals. Sapolsky[26] recommends prevention by learning to recognize the signs of stress and what situations trigger it.

The Council on Accreditation of Nurse Anesthesia Educational Programs' standards require accountability of the schools in regard to the students, including fair and equitable processes, nondiscrimination, and limits on hours worked.[42] Policies must include a mechanism to address complaints, grievances, and student concerns. Students should be informed of the program's policies and processes.

Stress is necessary to challenge students to learn. Approaches are needed that reduce the negative aspects of stress that lessen students' learning and performance. The key to reducing stress is providing students with a feeling of control over their education, information about what to expect, and feedback to improve their performance. Students who do not feel helpless will adopt their own coping strategies.[21]

For faculty, the challenge is in recognizing stress and meeting the learning needs of students. For students, it is dealing with the changes and stressors of nurse anesthesia education. Studies show that, for students, a sense of humor and a support system are probably the best stress reducers there are for dealing with new situations.[43,44] Students also should remember that faculty members have their own set of stressors to deal with on a daily basis and may at times feel overwhelmed.

Humor

Studies have shown the health benefit of humor.[43] A good hearty laugh can help to reduce stress, lower blood pressure, elevate mood, boost the immune system, improve brain function, protect the heart, make people feel closer to others, and foster instant relaxation. Humor is cathartic, can reduce fear and anxiety, offer alternative perspectives, and simply make people feel good. Research has shown that laughter decreases stress hormones and increases infection-fighting antibodies. Humor has been recognized by nurse researchers as a therapeutic intervention known to have positive psychological and physiological outcomes for patients.[44] Although sometimes overlooked, humor may be useful to the graduate student for mediating stress. It can facilitate moving into new roles, promote insight, help bring new situations into perspective, and promote more effective coping.

Despite the fact that humor and laughter have tremendous clinical potential, little attention has been given to the subject of using humor in graduate and postgraduate education. Wanzer and colleagues[45] noted that the inclusion of humor does not ensure that learning will occur. However, the appropriate and timely use of humor can augment teaching by increasing students' interest and attention and by reducing anxiety about subjects such as statistics and research methods. Humor reduces stress; increases motivation; improves morale, enjoyment, comprehension, interest, and rapport; and facilitates the transfer of knowledge and socialization into the profession.

The role of humor in education continues to be debated, and empirical studies have mixed results. Sapolsky[26] asserts that humor is vital to encourage critical thinking in students. Furthermore, humor has the potential to be a powerful method of motivating students and increasing cognitive ability. Studies of brain activity show that people who engage in humor exhibit similar brain activity as people who are engaged in divergent thinking.[43] Laughter has also been theorized as serving as a social function to help people identify with a group. Humor is an acceptable way of releasing tension and nervous energy.

Active and Reactive Coping

Coping strategies can be either active or reactive. Active coping (dealing with the actual stressful situations or events) can be strengthened by providing students with clear expectations, early success, and positive support.[19] Authoritarian behavior of the instructor has an important influence on student motivation and autonomy and must be balanced with support and caring. Both are interrelated with student satisfaction.

Reactive coping (dealing with one's own thoughts and feelings) can be facilitated by offering accessible professional and peer counseling, student support groups, and adequate faculty advising. Faculty should attempt to challenge students, but not so much that they lose their motivation, spontaneity, and initiative.

The following suggestions can help minimize sources of student stress: communicate explicit expectations and responsibilities for students; develop a positive interactive relationship with students; allow students to have at least a modicum sense of control over their student roles; treat students as individuals rather than as a generalized whole; and assist students to learn stress-coping strategies.

Although institutions of higher education have recognized the varied needs for support that must be provided to undergraduates, there is a lack of support for graduate students who face issues that are different but no less complex or challenging. Similarly, there are few graduate educator support systems available to address faculty stress.[2] Methods of coping commonly used by faculty may be classified into 2 major categories: primarily preventive strategies and primarily combative strategies, as shown in Table 3.3.

Preventive and combative strategies are active coping mechanisms. There are many healthy ways to manage and cope with stress. Many strategies focus on changing the situation or changing the individual's reaction. Preventive strategies concentrate on maintaining realistic self-expectations, recognizing unproductive stress-inducing ways of behaving, and learning to monitor stress-related symptoms

Table 3.3. Methods of Faculty Coping

Preventive

Avoid stressors by developing more nurturing relationships, finding a more suitable job, and attempting to create a more rewarding work environment.

Manage the expectations and demands made on oneself.

Change stress-inducing ways and recognize unproductive behaviors.

Augment personal coping resources.

Combative

Monitor stress by being aware of stress-related symptoms.

Marshall personal resources.

Take action to reduce the stressor by being assertive and refusing inappropriate requests for additional responsibilities.

Develop tolerance for unavoidable stress by cognitively restructuring the situation.

Lower stress-arousal or block it out.

and triggering events. Combative strategies are active measures that promote assertive approaches to reducing stress. Positive actions to assist in managing stress include cognitive restructuring techniques; developing personal resources, positive attitudes, and resilience; and actively finding alternative ways of responding to stressful situations.

Peer Support

Among protective resources that build positive coping strategies are social support relationships. Social support has been associated with beneficial outcomes for both mental and physical health. Support comes from a number of places, but peer support is the single most effective mechanism for both faculty and students. Students seek out the support of their significant others, families, advisors, and mentors, but the largest number of students—more than 80%—turn to their peers. The students' satisfaction levels for graduate student groups and peer support groups (where available) show them to be among the highest valued resources.[5]

A peer support program can take several forms. It might consist of a formal group of volunteer graduate students who meet regularly with students and work with department faculty. An informal "big buddy" mentorship program that partners every first-year graduate student with an experienced upperclassman also exists at some institutions. One-on-one mentorship programs can be found as well. As a first contact, the peer is often able to direct the student to a more knowledgeable faculty member or other individual resource, and provide the student with the encouragement needed to seek help. All of these programs rely on the fact that students feel much more comfortable discussing their concerns with a peer they trust than they do with faculty, administrators, or mental health providers. Even more valuable, however, is that these programs allow students to get support without having to explicitly ask for it.[46,47]

Peer credibility tends to be based on firsthand knowledge and expertise. The strength of peer support groups lies in enhancing the effectiveness of existing

Table 3.4. Student Coping Strategies

Ask faculty members to help you set academic priorities.

Break the work into pieces by setting small goals.

Study in groups to prevent burnout and feeling isolated.

Use relaxation techniques, such as meditation and deep-breathing exercises.

Manage time wisely.

Join a student support group.

Learn positive self-talk.

Take care of yourself by getting enough sleep and exercise.

Ask for help.

counseling systems and providing a supporting link for successful self-care and improved health and wellness.[34]

Peer support programs, by definition, involve student-student interactions; however, the creation and success of these programs will require a great deal of faculty support, including seeking out interested clinical instructors and recent graduate students. Students must know that their advisors and their department both support participation and involvement in peer support programs. In a national study on the lifestyles of graduate students, most students placed a high value on good relationships that enable students to learn from the perceptions, experiences, and challenges of their comrades.[6] These relationships also provided an emotional release from academic intensity.

Program directors should keep in mind that the goal is not to eliminate all stress but to help students develop a variety of skills to cope with the negative aspects of stress. Table 3.4 lists some specific student coping strategies.

If students try strategies for coping and still experience the negative aspects of stress, faculty should encourage students to seek professional counseling or therapy. This suggestion will more likely be received and acted on if a good relationship between the teacher and student already exists.

A preventive approach involves giving people realistic warnings, recommendations, and reassurances. There is little research in the field of higher education that describes how best to inform students about the challenges. More research is needed to identify why and how teacher–student relationships deteriorate and how to help faculty construct more successful relationships. Conversely, students should make efforts to behave respectfully toward faculty, staff, and peers and should willingly take responsibility for their behavior.

Critical Incident Stress Debriefing Programs

Although occupational stress exists in all work situations, the intensity and emotional demands of the healthcare environment place exceptionally high performance expectations and stress on healthcare providers, including students. Stress associated with dramatic, emotionally overwhelming situations, known as critical incidents, can

Table 3.5. Reactions to Crisis	
Type of reaction	**Common reactions**
Emotional	Fear, anger, guilt, grief, or anxiety
Mental	Difficulty concentrating, confusion, or nightmares
Physical	Headaches, dizziness, fatigue, or stomach problems
Behavioral	Sleep problems, loss of or increased appetite, isolation, or restlessness

overcome professionals' normal coping mechanisms. A critical incident is any event that causes an unusually intense stress reaction. The distress people experience after such an event limits their ability to cope, impairs their ability to adjust, and negatively affects the work or learning environment. Examples of traumatic events that produce such reactions include death (including suicide) of a patient, a coworker, or student; a serious illness; or a violent or threatening incident in the work setting.

Critical incident stress debriefing (CISD) is a process that prevents or limits the development of posttraumatic stress in people exposed to these major incidents.[48] Professionally conducted debriefings help people cope with and recover from the aftereffects of a critical incident. Not only does CISD enable participants to understand that they are not alone in their reactions to a stressful event, it also provides them with an opportunity to discuss their thoughts and feelings in a controlled, safe environment. Optimally, CISD should occur within 24 to 72 hours of a critical incident.

Crisis intervention has several purposes. It aims to reduce the intensity of an individual's emotional, mental, physical, and behavioral reactions to a crisis (Table 3.5). It also helps individuals return to their level of functioning before the crisis, develop new coping skills, and eliminate ineffective and inappropriate ways of coping, such as social withdrawal, isolation, and substance abuse.

European anesthesiologists have published guidelines for dealing with the aftermath of anesthetic catastrophes and advise against underestimating the psychological impact on staff following the death or serious injury of an operative patient.[49] Now being introduced into hospital settings, CISD offers a coping option for anesthesia departments and other clinical settings for assisting students and faculty when faced with a major stressful situation.

Summary

The nurse anesthesia profession needs a proactive, supportive, structured process designed to assist student nurse anesthetists in dealing with the multiple stressors inherent to their education.

Nurse anesthesia educational leaders should keep in mind that the goal is not to eliminate all stress but to help students develop a variety of skills to cope with the negative aspects of stress related to education. The guiding principle of stress reduction is a preventive approach so that the negative aspects of stress can be avoided. Raising awareness and giving students realistic warnings, recommendations, and reassurances supported by constructive feedback improves faculty-student relationships. Although the faculty cannot be responsible for the overall well-being of students, faculty members do have a responsibility to recognize signs of stress and to help students deal with a stressful issue in a constructive manner.

Faculty should provide active intervention, establish student support groups, and employ mechanisms to reduce stress. For example, faculty can avoid continual reference to the National Certification Examination, provide positive and frequent feedback in a constructive and honest manner, specify expectations, and assist students to understand that learning clinical skills and new technologies are progressive steps on the path to success.

As the role of graduate education in our society continues to evolve, the needs of graduate students are changing, too. Support for student nurse anesthetists can no longer be restricted to academic and financial issues. The program must also consider how it might help students deal with the pressures and stresses of graduate school.

The profession's recent move toward mandatory doctoral education for entry into practice has the potential to further increase the workload and challenges for programs, students, and faculty. Faculty who are stressed will be less effective in what they do. Stress can obstruct teaching and empathetic listening. Tension and ill health can undermine job performance. Most of all, faculty should not only have a thorough understanding of stress but also demonstrate the ability to implement appropriate practices in their own lives, thus modeling positive stress management for their students. Healthy stress management is one of the most important lifelong learning skills that any individual may acquire.

Students should be proactive and advocate for their educational program to address self-care issues because the management of stress is associated with less professional burnout, greater job satisfaction, enhanced academic performance, and better mental and physical health. It is also important for graduate students to take active steps to remain healthy and fit for duty.

As healthcare practitioners, the more we know and understand about stress, the more proactive we all can become in achieving balance and perspective in our professional careers. Stress prevention and coping strategies are important to understand if we are to have meaningful discussions regarding health and well-being with all those who participate in education, be they students, teachers, administrators, or policy makers.

References

1. Beck DL, Hackett MB, Srivastava R, McKim E, Rockwell B. Perceived level and sources of stress in university professional schools. *J Nurs Educ.* 1997;36(4):180-186.

2. Benjamin L, Walz GR. *Counseling Students and Faculty for Stress Management.* Ann Arbor, MI: University of Michigan, Education Resources Information Center (ERIC), Clearinghouse on Counseling and Personnel Services; 1987:ED 279 917.

3. Finkelstein C, Brownstein A, Scott C, Lan YL. Anxiety and stress reduction in medical education: an intervention. *Med Educ.* 2007;41(3):258-264.

4. Jones MC, Johnston DW. Reducing distress in first level and student nurses: a review of the applied stress management literature. *J Adv Nurs.* 2000;32(1):66-74.

5. Perez EC, Carroll-Perez I. A national study: stress perception by nurse anesthesia students. *AANA J.* 1999;67(1):79-86.

6. Repak N. Emotional fatigue: coping with academic pressure. Grad Resources website. http://www.gradresources.org/articles/emotional_fatigue.shtml. Accessed March 27, 2009.

7. Shirey MR. Stress and burnout in nursing faculty. *Nurse Educ.* 2006;31(3):95-97.

8. Martin-Sheridan D. Factors that influenced six nurse anesthesia programs to close. *AANA J.* 1998;66(4):377-384.

9. McCall WG, Alves SL, Brooks DY, Fallacaro MD, Gray GC, Ritter D. An analysis of factors influencing nurse anesthesia educational program director turnover: 1976-77. *AANA J.* 1997;65(6):537-542.

10. Kless JR. Use of a student support group to reduce student stress in a nurse anesthesia program. *AANA J.* 1989;57(1):75-77.

11. Wildgust B. Stress in the anesthesia student. *AANA J.* 1996;64(3):272-278.

12. Misra R, McKean M, West S, Russo T. Academic stress of college students: comparison of student and faculty perceptions. *Coll Student J.* 2000;34: 236-245.

13. Tunajek S. Student stress: a question of balance. *AANA NewsBull.* 2006;60(5):20-21.

14. Kendrick P. Comparing the effects of stress and relationship style on student and practicing nurse anesthetists. *AANA J.* 2000;68(2):115-122.

15. Horton BJ. The importance of mentoring in recruiting and retaining junior faculty. *AANA J.* 2003;71(3):189-195.

16. McLean J. Forgotten faculty: stress and job satisfaction among distance educators. University of West Georgia Distance Education Center website. 2006. http://www.westga.edu/~distance/ojdla/summer92/mclean92.htm. Accessed April 1, 2009.

17. Davies MA, Spence Laschinger HK, Andrusysyn MA. Clinical educators' empowerment, job tension, and job satisfaction: a test of Kanter's Theory. *J Nurses Staff Dev.* 2006;22(2):78-86.

18. Owens BH, Herrick CA, Kelly JA. A prearranged mentorship program: can it work long distance? *J Prof Nurs.* 1998;14(5):78-84.

19. Lazarus R. *Psychological Stress and the Coping Process.* New York, NY: McGraw-Hill; 1966.

20. McKinzie C, Altamura V, Burgoon E, Bishop C. Exploring the effect of stress on mood, self-esteem, and daily habits with psychology graduate students. *Psychol Rep.* 2006;99(2):439-448.

21. Hodgson C, Simoni J. Graduate student academic and psychological functioning. *J Coll Student Dev.* 1995;36(3):244-253.

22. McDonough JP. Personality, addiction and anesthesia. *AANA J.* 1990;58(3):193-200.

23. Baldisseri MR. Impaired healthcare professional. *Crit Care Med.* 2007;35(2 suppl):S106-S116.

24. Waugman WR. Professional roles of the Certified Registered Nurse Anesthetist. In: Foster SD, Jordan LM, eds. *Professional Aspects of Nurse Anesthesia Practice.* Philadelphia, PA: FA Davis Co; 1994:11-19.

25. Neumann Y, Finley-Neumann EF, Reichel A. Determinants and consequences of students' burnout in universities. *J Higher Educ.* 1990; 61(2):565-580.

26. Sapolsky RM. *Why Zebras Don't Get Ulcers: The Acclaimed Guide to Stress, Stress-Related Disease and Coping.* 3rd ed. New York, NY: WH Freeman; 2004.

27. Bandura A. *Social Foundations of Thought and Action: A Social Cognitive Theory.* Englewood Cliffs, NJ: Prentice-Hall; 1986.

28. Burges N. Personality and medical specialty choice: a literature review and interpretation. *J Career Assess.* 2002;10(3):362-380.

29. Sandi C, Pinelo-Nava MT. Stress and memory: behavioral effects and neurobiological mechanisms. *Neural Plast.* 2007;16(6):1-20.

30. Lupien SJ, Fiocco FA, Wan AN, et al. Stress hormones and human memory function across the lifespan. *Psychoneuroendocrinology.* 2005;30(3):225-242.

31. McEwen BS, Sapolsky RM. Stress and cognitive function. *Curr Opin Neurobiol.* 1995;5(2):205-216.

32. Higgins Roche BT. *Substance Abuse Policies for Anesthesia.* Winston-Salem, NC: All Anesthesia; 2007.

33. Tunajek S. Peer support: validity and benefit. *AANA NewsBull.* 2007;61(5):29-31.

34. Quinlan D. Peer assistance: part I and part II. In: Foster S, Faut-Callahan M, eds. *A Professional Study and Resource Guide for the CRNA.* Park Ridge, IL: American Association of Nurse Anesthetists; 2001:425-484.

35. Bell DM, McDonough JP, Ellison JS, Fitzhugh EC. Controlled drug misuse by Certified Registered Nurse Anesthetists. *AANA J.* 1999;67(2):133-140.

36. Molinari DL, Dupler A, Lungstrom N. Stress of nursing students studying online. In: Rodgers P, Berg G, Boettecher J, Howard C, Justice L, Schenk K, eds. *The Encyclopedia of Distance Learning, Teaching, Technologies, and Applications.* Vol 3. Hershey, PA: Idea Group; 2005:1666-1673.

37. Gates GS. Teaching-related stress: the emotional management of faculty. *Rev Higher Educ.* 2000;23(4):469-490.

38. Cragg C, Andrusysyn MA, Humbert J. Experiences with technology and preferences for distance learning delivery methods in a nurse practitioner program. *J Distance Learning.* 1999;14(1):31-39.

39. Bower BL. Distance education: facing the faculty challenge. University of West Georgia Distance Learning Center website. 2001. http://www.westga.edu/~distance/ojdla/summer42/bower42.html. Accessed May 4, 2009.

40. Kabot-Zinn J. Mindfulness-based interventions in context: past, present, and future. *Clin Psychol Sci Pract.* 2003;10(2):144-156.

41. Garcia-Otero M, Teddlie C. The effect of knowledge of learning styles on anxiety and clinical performance of nurse anesthesiology students. *AANA J.* 1992;60(3):257-260.

42. Standards for Accreditation of Nurse Anesthesia Educational Programs. Park Ridge, IL: Council on Accreditation of Nurse Anesthesia Educational Programs; 2006:10.

43. Fry WF. Humor and the brain: a selective review. *Int J Humor Res.* 2002;15(3):305-333.

44. Robinson V. *Humor and the Health Profession: The Therapeutic Use of Humor in Health Care.* 2nd ed. Thorofare, NJ: Slack; 2004.

45. Wanzer MB, Frymier A, Wojtaszczyk A, Smith T. Appropriate and inappropriate uses of humor by teachers. *Commun Educ.* 2006;55(2):178-196.

46. Singh B. Peer support: taking advice from a friend. *MIT Faculty Newslett.* 2006;18(4):184-189.

47. Whittemore R, Rankin SH, Callahan CD, Leder MC, Carroll DL. Peer advisor experience providing social support. *Qual Health Res.* 2000;10(2):260-276.

48. Dyregrov A. The process in psychological debriefings. *J Trauma Stress.* 1997;10(4):589-605.

49. Gazoni FM. Life after death: a resident's perspective. *Anesth Patient Safety Found Newslett.* 2006;21(1):7-8.

Chapter 4

Legal Issues for Educators

Mary Jeanette Mannino, CRNA, JD

Key Points

- Applicable laws come from many different types of governance and should be well researched and updated often to ensure the best understanding and most accurate compliance.

- In-depth screening and frequent evaluation are important parts of maintaining a student program.

- A clear understanding of the student's capabilities, duties, and roles is important to a successful and safe learning environment.

- Students should be supervised by appropriate parties at all times to avoid legal issues.

- It is important to know who is the "captain of the ship" and in what situations this applies. Legal liability can be perceived in many ways, so documentation and knowledge are key.

- Certified Registered Nurse Anesthetists should be taught how the law applies to them and their businesses. They should be aware of their responsibilities and roles. They should have an accurate understanding of contract law, common business practice, and negotiation technique.

Introduction

There are many components to understanding the legal aspects of nurse anesthesia education, including the rights and responsibilities of the university, the faculty, the students, clinical rotations, and the profession. As in many other areas of nursing, there are myths and misunderstandings regarding the law and its application to practice.

Because nurse anesthesia education and practice are based on the scientific method, it is frequently difficult for educators, practitioners, and students to understand the "shades of gray" that encompass legal study and conclusions. While science is generally very current and frequently tested, the law is often years behind clinical practice and is ever evolving. Legal precedents may be shattered, laws may be enacted with a political and economic genesis, and appeals may be lengthy and expensive.

Although not comprehensive in its scope, this chapter will emphasize the important areas of concern regarding the law and anesthesia education. It is not intended to replace legal counsel from individual institutions or to be considered legal advice. Rather, a look at some of the applicable laws and analysis of relevant legal cases will provide educators and students with a frame of reference and resources to answer some of the major legal questions.

Sources of Law

There are 4 sources of American law: constitutional law, administrative law, statutory law, and common law. In addition, each state has a separate constitution and procedures for enacting and enforcing its own laws.

In nurse anesthesia education, there may be some overlap in federal and state constitutional law. For example, civil rights and discrimination may be covered by both entities. Except for federal jurisdiction areas such as the military, the Native American system, and the District of Columbia, the US government generally does not get involved in licensure and other administrative legal areas that are relegated to state jurisdiction.

However, the federal government does have considerable legal influence over educational funding, grants, and healthcare reimbursement. In recent years we have seen major changes in Medicare reimbursement for anesthesia services. In the late 1980s, a federal law was passed allowing Certified Registered Nurse Anesthetists (CRNAs) to receive direct reimbursement from Medicare for anesthesia services. Subsequently, rule changes regarding reimbursement for supervision of nurse anesthesia students were enacted. The issue of reimbursement for nurse anesthetists by a medically directing physician anesthesiologist is addressed in the Tax Equity and Fiscal Responsibility Act of 1982[1] (TEFRA). This issue has generated considerable confusion and concern about reimbursement issues influencing standard-of-care determination. While reimbursement is beyond the scope of this chapter and is in itself a complicated issue, it is important for educators to be familiar with current law and to ensure that there is no fraudulent billing in the name of the students or the program.

Each state has the duty to protect its citizens and has set up licensure boards to develop criteria for licensees, including setting educational standards and enforcing rules and regulations. Most state nurse practice acts identify nurse anesthesia as legal and may identify the educational and certification requirements. A common misconception is that the boards of nursing exist to protect and promote nursing. In reality, the boards' duty is to the public and to assure them that an individual licensed by the state has met requirements.

Most anesthesia programs (except US military and Veterans Health Administration programs) require students to maintain a basic nursing license and be in good standing with the state. After graduation and certification, state nursing boards may require a practitioner to have a separate designation as a nurse anesthetist. The American Association of Nurse Anesthetists (AANA) State Government Affairs Division[2] is an excellent resource for information on the requirements of each individual state.

Common Law

Historically, common law is a holdover from British rule. It has been called "judge-made law" and is based on the law of precedent. There are also instances when the facts of a case are distinct from all previous cases and the court will form an opinion as a "matter of first impression." Many of the cases reviewed and analyzed in this chapter are based on common law.

Case Law

State and federal courts publish many decisions based on issues relative to interpretation of statutes, rules, and regulations. Many of the antitrust cases argued by nurse anesthetists have been a result of the need to determine whether there was a violation of federal antitrust laws in denying privileges to CRNAs.

Postsecondary Education Law

Academic law has evolved also, as colleges and universities have moved from totally private institutions to those that are federally funded. Recent examples include faculties that have elected to be part of collective bargaining units and athletic regulations that have been expanded to include women.

Whether or not postsecondary law has been codified, institutions have set up their own governances, due process procedures, and rules. As universities become more research oriented with federal and private funding support, additional legal and ethical standards apply.

Nurse anesthesia educational programs additionally must comply with the standards established by the Council on Accreditation of Nurse Anesthesia Educational Programs (COA). This places an additional burden for educators to ensure that there is no conflict between the university and the COA.

Hospital/Facility Law

Nurse anesthesia education includes a major clinical component requiring facilities where the students learn the technical skills necessary in the practice of anesthesia.

It is in the clinical area where many students and educators realize that technical skills are as important as academic foundation. Depending on the structure of the program, students may complete a "front-loaded" program in which the academic study precedes the clinical study, or a combined program in which classes and the clinical portion are held simultaneously.

It is incumbent upon the program administrators and clinical coordinators to have a strong understanding of the hospital and anesthesia department standards, rules, and regulations. These include operating room policies, infection control, and use of equipment and supplies. Each facility will have its own method of documentation of the course of an anesthetic, and the students must be aware of this information and the importance of compliance. It is best that the faculty attempt to protect the students from anesthesia department politics and reimbursement issues.

Education Law Regarding Student Status

The university and appropriate department will have admission standards for application to nurse anesthesia programs. Although these standards are required by the COA, many programs establish higher standards and admission requirements. These standards must be in writing and the applicants must have a thorough understanding of the content.

Institutional admission standards require assurance that legal criteria are met. These include: (1) the selection process must not be arbitrary or capricious; (2) the institution is bound under a contract legal theory to adhere to its published admission policies; and (3) according to Standard 5, the institution may not discriminate on the basis of race, color, religion, age, gender, national origin, marital status, disability, sexual orientation, or any factor protected by law.[2]

While there is a paucity of case law specifically regarding nurse anesthesia education, the following is a case regarding student status and dismissal from an anesthesia program.[4]

The plaintiff, "JJ" (Plaintiff) brought action against "SCU and BH" nurse anesthesia program (Program) alleging violations of Title II of the Americans with Disabilities Act as well as a state common law claim for negligent misrepresentation, breach of contract and promissory estoppel. (Promissory estoppel is a legal doctrine in contract law, whereby there may be reliance made on the terms of the contract.)

The facts show that the plaintiff was admitted to the program in 1999. The program was of two years duration with the graduates being awarded a master's degree from the university and a certificate of Nurse Anesthesia from the hospital.

After completing the academic program, the plaintiff began the clinical portion and was scheduled to graduate in May 2001. At some point in March 2001, the plaintiff's performance level in the clinical area began to decline due to extreme anxiety. On March 8, 2001, the plaintiff met with the medical and program directors to discuss his clinical performance. After that meeting, a memorandum was prepared stating that the student appeared to be suffering the effects of an acute stress response or some form of chronic anxiety disorder and professional counseling and/or psychological evaluation were recommended. In the memorandum, it was questioned whether or not he was capable of successfully attaining his educational goals.

About three weeks later, the plaintiff once again met with the directors and was informed that his clinical work had been suspended. At that time they provided him with three options: (1) continue his academic course of study in order to complete the requirements for a Masters of Science from the university and take a leave of absence from the clinical phase until September 1, 2001, when he would be able to restart the nine month clinical phase; (2) continue the academic course of study and completely resign from the Program; or (3) completely resign from both further academic study and the program. The plaintiff chose the first option, took a leave of absence and returned to the program, September 2001. On December 11, 2001, however, the plaintiff was dismissed from the Program.

Alleging that at no time was he offered any type of professional counseling or a psychological evaluation, he filed a legal action for emotional distress and requested compensatory and punitive damages.

To argue his case, the plaintiff entered into evidence the student handbook that states that the faculty and administration of the program "will assist a student whenever possible…." The plaintiff contended that despite this clause in the handbook and despite the defendant's knowledge of his physical disability, the Program failed to accommodate him during the three-month period between his return from his leave of absence until the time he was dismissed from the Program.

The court of appeals dismissed all of the plaintiff's allegations, but there are legal lessons that are important to anesthesia educators.

Legal Lessons: The student handbook and clinical evaluations will be used as evidence in legal proceedings regarding student actions, such as probation and dismissal. If at all possible, students who have difficulty with the clinical portion of the program should be identified early and remedial action should be taken.

Supervision of Students

Supervision of students in the clinical area is a legal concern for the supervising CRNAs, anesthesiologists, and institution. It is frequently easier to administer the anesthetic oneself than to supervise a student. Also, supervising anesthesia providers are concerned that a worthwhile learning experience for the students may not always be in the best interests of the patient.

This is another area in which common sense should outweigh any legal concerns. No harm should be allowed to happen to a patient, under any circumstances. However, there are many situations in which there may be different ways to administer an anesthetic to a patient for a certain procedure. It is reasonable to expect that the student has researched these various options, has a clear understanding of the pros and cons, and is prepared, both academically and technically, to perform the procedure. If a student is not prepared to justify use of the technique and to plan appropriately for it, it may be prudent for him or her to be relieved of direct administration of the anesthetic.

There have been some legal cases that directly address the issue of supervision of nurse anesthesia students. Clinical faculty and program administrators should be aware of the outcomes of these cases and apply the lessons learned when dealing with similar situations.

From a legal perspective, there are various components of the supervision issue that may create problems and, from a risk management perspective, be dealt with in advance. These include assignment of students appropriate to educational level and patient physical status, level of supervision needed, student preparation for cases, identification of high-risk patients and procedures, medical record documentation, ability of the student to troubleshoot a problem, and evaluation of the student after the procedure.

No chapter on the legality of supervision of nurse anesthesia students would be complete without a discussion of the *Central Anesthesia Associates v Worthy* case.[5] Although it is an old decision, several key elements of the legal supervision of student nurse anesthetists are addressed. It involves an institution in Georgia where anesthesiologist assistants practice along with CRNAs and MD anesthesiologists, and where student nurse anesthetists receive clinical experience. Georgia law addressed the legality of nurse anesthesia practice in a statute that stated:

> ...anesthesia may lawfully be administered by a Certified Registered Nurse Anesthetist, provided such anesthesia is administered under the direction and responsibility of a duly licensed physician with training and experience in anesthesia."
>
> The facts show that a woman gave birth without anesthesia and without complications. The next day she underwent a tubal ligation which was performed by her obstetrician/gynecologist assisted by an intern employed by the hospital. A professional corporation consisting of anesthesiologists administered the anesthesia through a registered nurse enrolled as a student nurse anesthetist in a school operated at the hospital by the anesthesiologists' corporation. At the time of induction, the student nurse anesthetist was under the supervision of a physician's assistant employed by the corporation. During the tubal ligation procedure, Mrs. Worthy suffered a cardiac arrest resulting in brain damage.
>
> In the subsequent malpractice suit, the issue of whether or not an anesthesia assistant could legally supervise a CRNA student arose. The court ruled that the statute did not permit anesthesia assistant supervision of student nurse anesthetists.

Legal Lesson: From an educator's perspective, careful adherence to state law regarding supervision is critical.

Vicarious Liability

Students, faculty, surgeons, and administrators frequently discuss who is liable and who pays in a medical malpractice suit. This topic is based on myths and history, rather than current legal doctrine. There are several ways to look at this topic, including legal precedent, history, custom, and procedural strategy.

Historically, this issue is related to the "captain-of-the-ship" doctrine and has been expanded in recent years to include economic concerns and politics. The case that defined the captain of the ship was a 1949 case,[6] in which a hospital could not be sued for the acts of its employees because of charitable immunity. The court ruled that a private practice physician could be sued because immunity did not apply to him and that he was considered the captain of the ship.

In the current medical malpractice arena, hospitals no longer have charitable immunity and can be sued for the acts of their employees under the laws of agency. Yet the issue of the surgeon's assumed liability for hospital employees and independent contractors continues to be discussed in the anesthesia community. Unfortunately, the misused term "supervision" has made this topic even more controversial.

Because this topic has many facets, this chapter will address only a few of them and will not attempt to include reimbursement and political issues; however, there is a difference, depending on whether the party named in a lawsuit is an anesthesia student or a CRNA. Furthermore, the assumed liability of others for the acts of a CRNA is related to the employment status and contractual language.

Agency Law

Under the laws of agency, generally the employer is responsible for the acts of the employee that are performed within the scope of the employment. Because of the unusual nature of anesthesia practice, a CRNA has many employment options, including being employed by a facility (hospital or ambulatory surgery center), a medical group, or a CRNA group, or being self-employed. Because of the need for nurse anesthetists, many CRNAs practice in several different arrangements at the same time. This becomes an issue because of the need to ensure there is malpractice insurance coverage. Because many of the employment opportunities for CRNAs are different than for nursing, students need to be educated about the job market and on the pros and cons of the various relationships.

Whether one is a student or CRNA, knowledge of the current law on vicarious liability and the ability to successfully argue its application to practice is critical to the individual and the profession. This topic will provoke emotional arguments that make no legal or financial sense. However, a surgeon's ego may interfere with his or her understanding of the law when it comes to the captain-of-the-ship analogy.

There have been a number of legal rulings on the issue, most stating that the surgeon is not automatically the captain of the ship. For example, in *Lauro v Knowles,*[7] the plaintiff (Lauro) sought to impose captain-of-the-ship liability for an eye injury she received in the operating room.

> Dr. Knowles operated on the plaintiff to alleviate carpal tunnel syndrome in her
> right wrist. He performed the surgery at St. Joseph Hospital (hospital). There was

an anesthesiologist and a student registered nurse anesthetist involved in providing anesthesia. When the plaintiff awoke from anesthesia, she suffered from a corneal abrasion of her right eye. The injury was allegedly sustained in connection with the administration of anesthesia.

Dr. Knowles testified at his deposition that he assumed plaintiff was prepped and had already been given anesthesia when he walked into the operating room. He said that he had nothing to do with the administration of anesthesia or with the anesthesiology team stationed at the head of the operating table. Rather, he claimed, these functions were the responsibility of the anesthesiologist and the other members of that team who were present. The Rhode Island court agreed with other jurisdictions that it must be a finding of fact that the surgeon exercised control over the anesthesia process and in this case there was no evidence of that control.

Other cases have affirmed the importance of the surgeon exerting control over anesthesia in order to be legally considered captain of the ship. *Parker v Vanderbilt University*[8] and *Franklin v Gupta*[9] briefly state this case to clarify. In *Franklin v Gupta*, the Maryland court noted that the operating room environment is changing to a point where the surgeon can no longer have actual control over technical equipment and the people who operate it.

From a practical standpoint, it is wise for all parties to understand that the surgeon will not be liable for the acts of the nurse anesthetist unless he or she has participated in the anesthetic. This statement assumes the nurse anesthetist understands that he or she is responsible and liable for his or her own acts and must have sufficient insurance coverage.

Contract Law

Contracts are part of daily commerce and may be found in all aspects of one's professional career. Knowledge of contract law is essential to program directors, faculty, and students. It is usually prudent for contracts to be written or reviewed by an attorney who is familiar with state law and the area of interest specific to the subject. It is also prudent for everyone to know how to read a contract, have an understanding of the terms, and be aware of the legal remedies if there is a breach.

A contract is a legally enforceable agreement between 2 or more parties that creates an obligation to do or not to do certain things. For a contract to be legal, the parties must be legally competent to enter into a contract and there must be mutual agreement of the terms. Although there are situations in which verbal contracts are legal, for the purposes of this chapter we will assume that the terms of the agreement have been put into writing.

Because a written contract can appear to be complicated, many people do not take the time to carefully read and understand their legal obligations. Most contracts contain certain standard clauses that are modified to suit the special needs of the circumstances. The clauses that may be seen in a contract that are of interest to the nurse anesthesia profession include name and purpose of contract, parties, recitals (statements of background, often containing "whereas" clauses), starting date, length of contract, terms of relationship, duties of each party, termination clause, covenants, applicable law, remedies for breech or nonperformance, and signatures and dates signed.

Special Types of Contracts

Although the standard clauses appear in most contracts, there will be certain articles that are specific to each type of contract. Each institution and individual has different contractual needs. Tables 4.1 through 4.3 contain examples that may be relevant to educators and students. The following case is illustrative of a student requesting not to fulfill the terms of a posteducation agreement.[10]

> A Hospital entered into a contract with its then-employee registered nurse (AC), by which the hospital agreed to provide tuition assistance for anesthesia school. The terms of the contract included tuition assistance in the form of a monthly stipend and health and dental insurance, while AC was in anesthesia school.
>
> The contract provided that if AC works for the Hospital for a period of five years after completion of her studies, her loan would be forgiven. The agreement also stated that if she failed to rejoin the hospital as an active employee after graduation, she would be responsible for paying the hospital for the advances, plus accrued interest.
>
> When she graduated from her anesthesia program, she sought employment elsewhere because it appeared that there were no nurse anesthetist positions available at the Hospital. The Hospital brought a breach of contract action against the nurse anesthetist, seeking repayment for the money given. The nurse anesthetist responded, stating that the Hospital breached the contract by failing to offer her a position as a nurse anesthetist.

Table 4.1. University and Clinical Site Contracts

Duties of university

Prepare students for clinical sites.

Appoint clinical coordinators.

Provide salary of clinical coordinators.

Provide malpractice insurance for students.

Duties of clinical site

Supervise students.

Participate in clinical conferences.

Participate in clinical evaluation of students.

Provide stipend (if any).

Stipulate department policies and procedures.

Ensure student participation in clinical site activities.

Table 4.2. Student Contract for Stipend Assistance

Obligations of student

Graduate from accredited anesthesia program.

Pass certification examination.

Work for facility or group for a specified period of time.

Fulfill all obligations.

Obligations of facility/group

Provide stipend at agreed amount at specified time.

Guarantee employment upon student graduation and certification.

Specify or negotiate employment salary and benefits specified or negotiated at employment.

Specify buyout terms if student is unable to fulfill obligation.

Table 4.3. Employment and Contract Between CRNA and Hospital

Obligations of CRNA

Maintain license and certification.

Maintain hospital privileges in good standing.

Provide anesthesia services to surgical and obstetrical patients at the hospital.

Provide perianesthesia services, including preanesthesia and postanesthesia assessment.

Provide postoperative pain management.

Maintain anesthesia equipment.

Order anesthesia supplies.

Provide hospital billing office with appropriate information to allow for billing.

Be available for anesthesia services Monday through Friday and every other weekend.

Obligations of hospital

Provide state-of-the-art anesthesia equipment and monitors.

Provide anesthesia supplies and medications.

Provide operating room and postanesthesia care unit personnel to assist in anesthesia procedures.

Provide salary and benefits.

- Annual salary of $_____
- Benefits to include _____paid days off and _____days and $_____for professional activities and such as continuing education
- Full investment in pension program
- Health insurance for family
- Malpractice insurance
- Clinical privileges through medical staff with due process right

A trial court ruled in favor of the hospital awarding them $29,879.84 plus interest for a total of $43,396.49. The nurse anesthetist appealed this ruling.

The Court of Appeals, in affirming the trial court's decision in favor of the hospital, discussed the fact that in order for a contract to be valid, both parties must agree to its terms. Part of the higher court's analysis was the fact that according to the writing of the contract, the nurse agreed to remain an employee of the hospital, but not necessarily as a nurse anesthetist. Since there was not an anesthesia position available at the time, the appellant had the option of working as a nurse under the terms of financial agreement.

Legal Lessons: This case points out how the terms and the *intent* of the contract must be understood. The nurse anesthetist relied on a *verbal* assurance that the hospital would provide her with a nurse anesthetist position; however, the final decision for hiring would be made by the physician anesthesiologist director of the department. Students should be counseled to understand the importance of any financial agreement for tuition assistance and the payback terms. This case is a good example of an unexpected outcome for the student who fully expected to be employed as a nurse anesthetist and not as a nurse to fulfill the payback terms of her agreement.

A student must understand the professional and ethical considerations of breaching a contract or failing to fulfill the terms or essence of the agreement. As professionals, nurse anesthetists are held to high standards in business and clinical practice. Although an act may not be illegal or worthy of a lawsuit, poor judgment on the part of the anesthetist can have long-lasting effects on the individual's professional career.

Noncompete Clauses

Clearly the most misunderstood areas of contracts are noncompete clauses. Although these covenants may be upheld by the law, they may depend on the jurisdictions and facts surrounding their inclusion. As more CRNAs become business owners, having such a clause may be a good business decision in preventing employee or subcontractor anesthetists from underbidding or otherwise attempting to get the contract.

Noncompete clauses generally have 2 components: time and distance. A typical clause may read, "after conclusion of this contract, for whatever reason, the anesthetist will not provide anesthesia services in a 50-mile radius of the hospital for 2 years." These clauses restrict competition with the original group or hospital.

Whether to sign or modify a noncompete clause depends on the individual's circumstances, the anesthesia market, and the negotiating skills of all parties. Gene Blumenreich,[11] AANA general counsel, has presented a very balanced approach to this subject and his paper is a good topic of classroom discussion. In his article, he discusses several approaches to negotiating these particular clauses. Blumenreich recommends that nurse anesthetists understand the legal implications of these covenants and makes suggestions how they may be used as a bargaining tool in employment contract negotiations.

Negotiations

It is imperative that anesthetists develop negotiation skills to assist with the various business and practice options and opportunities. These skills are useful when the anesthetist is obtaining a contract for employment or private practice or membership in an HMO, PPO, or other managed care entity. This section will describe the negotiation process and assist the reader in developing the necessary skills to negotiate a business contract effectively. Negotiation is a process through which parties determine whether an acceptable agreement can be reached. Information is exchanged and evaluated and used as the basis for final decisions.

Effective negotiation involves the gathering and exchange of information to assess the parties and the potential for agreement. This information includes the positions, needs, interests, and goals of the parties. Most negotiations in an anesthesia business will probably be performed by the anesthetist or spokesperson for a group; however, there may be circumstances when an attorney or consultant may be retained for that purpose. Learning how to be an effective negotiator may make the difference in a successful business venture and is one of the most critical elements as practice situations change.

Characteristics of an Effective Negotiator

In a survey of business leaders, characteristics of an effective negotiator were identified in their order of importance (Table 4.4).

Table 4.4. Characteristics of an Effective Negotiator

Preparation and planning skills

Knowledge of subject matter being negotiated

Ability to think clearly and rapidly under pressure and uncertainty

Ability to express thoughts verbally

Listening skills

Judgment and general intelligence

Integrity

Ability to persuade others

Patience

Decisiveness

Ability to earn respect and confidence of opponent

General problem-solving and analytic skills

Self-control, especially of emotions and their visibility

Insight into other's feelings

Persistence and determination

Ability to perceive and exploit available power to achieve objective

Insight into hidden needs and reaction of own and opponent's objective

Ability to lead and control members of own team or group

Experts often cite planning as one of the most critical aspects in successful negotiations. In the planning process, careful attention must be given to the purpose of the contract, goals of the parties, national and local market trends, financial considerations, and underlying agendas. A strategy should be developed and parameters established. An effective system for planning successful negotiations using a 14-step process is suggested (Table 4.5).

Table 4.5. Effective Steps in Planning Successful Negotiations

1. Gather information before the negotiation.
2. Determine your goals.
3. Identify issues.
4. Analyze the market and customary terms.
5. Assess strengths and weaknesses.
6. Estimate the other party's bottom line and opening position.
7. Consider win/win outcomes.
8. Set the opening position.
9. Set the bottom line.
10. Choose strategies and tactics.
11. Consider concessions and tradeoffs.
12. Determine an agenda.
13. Analyze timing.
14. Choose the mode of communication.

Teaching Law to Student Nurse Anesthetists

Legal classes are often taught as part of the curriculum in nurse anesthesia programs. Law may be taught as a separate course or integrated in other classes such as professional aspects. For the best understanding, the class should be taught to senior students. Students who have not been in the clinical area have little basis for understanding standards of anesthesia practice. Because most schools do not teach much about the business of anesthesia, this is a good opportunity to include it in the curriculum. Since nurse anesthetist practice is unique in many respects, this course should not be taught in a class that includes other advanced practice nurses. The purpose of this course is not to teach law to the anesthesia students but to teach how the law is applied to the profession and practice. It is especially important for the students to understand the legal basis for CRNA practice and how the law is constantly evolving.

It is also important to teach this class based on CRNA practice instead of student practice where rules of supervision are different. Students must be made aware that there are state laws and institutional policies and procedures that may be different from those at their educational clinical sites. The AANA is the best resource for information and legal rulings relating to CRNA practice. Students and graduates should be very familiar with the Legal Briefs column that appears in the *AANA Journal* and information on the public side of the AANA website at www.aana.com.

Included in this chapter as Appendix 4.1 is the syllabus from the Law and Medicine class required for the anesthesia students at Gonzaga University in Spokane, Washington. The content is updated every year, so current cases and rulings will be applicable. Because nurse anesthesia programs are at a master's degree level, this class is taught with student participation and an emphasis on analysis of facts and practical application (Appendix 4.1).

Summary

Teaching law to nurse anesthesia students is a challenge because of the changing political, legal, and economic environment. There are also many individuals and institutions who will use legal excuses or threats to influence CRNA practice. If the students, graduates, and faculty understand the basic tenets of law and know where to find resources, the entire profession will benefit.

References

1. Tax Equity and Fiscal Responsibility Act of 1982, HR 4961, 97th Congress, 1982.

2. AANA State Government Affairs website. http://www.aana.com/Advocacy.aspx ?ucNavMenu_TSMenuTargetID=49&ucNavMenu_TSMenuTargetType=4&uc NavMenu_TSMenuID=6&id=131. Accessed January 23, 2009.

3. Kaplan WA, Lee BA. *The Law of Higher Education.* 3rd ed. New York, NY: John Wiley and Sons; 1995:337.

4. *Johnson v Southern Connecticut State University,* 29 NDLR 64 (104 LRP) (Connecticut, 2004).

5. *Central Anesthesia Associates v Worthy,* 333 SE2d 829 (1985).

6. *McConnell v Williams,* 361 Pa 355 (1949).

7. *Lauro v Knowles,* 739 A2d 1183 (RI, 1999).

8. *Parker v Vanderbilt University,* 767 SW 2d 412, (TN, 1988).

9. *Franklin v Gupta,* 81 MD App. 345, 567 A 2d 524, (MD, 1990).

10. *Sweetwater Hospital Association v Carpenter,* No. E2004-00207-COA-R3-CV (TN, Ct App, 2005).

11. Blumenreich G. Nurse anesthetists in the middle: covenants not to compete. *AANA J.* 1998;66(6):541-544.

Appendix 4.1. Class Outline, Gonzaga University, Spokane, Washington Law and Medicine

Credits: 2
Instructor: Mannino, CRNA, JD
Resource material: Provided by instructor
                        (please bring to class)

Teaching methods:

- Lectures
- Analysis of video deposition
- Anesthesia legal case review
- Moot court
- Preparation and negotiation of anesthesia services

Objectives:

- Compare civil and criminal law from the anesthesia perspective.
- Trace an anesthesia lawsuit through the legal system.
- Discuss the importance of the nurse practice act in anesthesia practice.
- List the three components of informed consent.
- Describe how a consent is a defense against battery.
- List the factors of negligence and relate each one to anesthesia practice.
- Discuss the ways standard of care is determined.
- Describe the legal parameters of products liability.
- List the reasons why a contract is important to the anesthetist.
- Prepare a sample contract for anesthesia services.
- Describe four economic principles and relate them to anesthesia practice.
- Compare practice options available to nurse anesthetists.

Outline:

American legal system

> How laws are made
> Court system
> Common law
> Constitutions
> Adversary system

Anatomy of a lawsuit

> Preliminary stage
> Trial
> Appeals
> Disposition (settlement)
> Arbitration

Statutory and regulatory law

> Nurse Practice Acts
> Other statutes
> Administrative law related to licensure
> Legal basis for nurse anesthesia practice

Criminal law and anesthesia

> Practicing medicine without a license
> Criminal battery

Consent law

Consent as a defense to battery
Informed consent
Consent for research

Negligence

Elements of negligence
Anesthesia practice and negligence
Litigation of anesthesia cases
Res ipsa loquitur
Prevention of anesthesia lawsuits
Defense of anesthesia lawsuits

Vicarious liability

Captain-of-the-ship doctrine
Supervision and implied liability
Practical aspects of vicarious liability

Employment law

Practice options for nurse anesthetists
Employment rights

Other areas of law

Product liability
Antitrust law
Intentional torts

Contract law

Purpose of contracts
Types of contracts
Elements of an employment contract
Contract for anesthesia services
Negotiations
Review of other anesthesia-related contracts

Anesthesia economics

Economic principles
Reimbursement for anesthesia services
Third-party payment

Case presentations and final examination projects

Suggested Resources

1. Blumenreich GA. Legal Briefs column. *AANA Journal.*
   These columns, written primarily by the AANA general counsel, are some of the best resources for current legal cases regarding nurse anesthetists and should be mandatory reading for both students and CRNAs.

2. Kaplan WA, Lee BA. *The Law of Higher Education.* 3rd ed. San Francisco, CA: Jossey-Bass; 1995.
   This is a comprehensive resource and reference for all legal aspects of higher education. There is no specific area for anesthesia or related clinical education; however, it can be useful for general university legal issues.

3. University libraries

University libraries are some of the best resources for legal research and assistance to students and faculty. A law library connected with the university (or a local library), this is also an excellent source of information.

4. The AANA website. www.aana.com.

This website has invaluable information regarding legal, education, practice, and reimbursement issues.

Resources for Effective Negotiations

Cohen H. *You Can Negotiate Anything.* Secaucus NJ: Lyle Stuart/Citadel Press; 1980. This book is frequently quoted in other books on negotiations. It is considered to be one of the best books on negotiation techniques.

Ilich J, Jones BS. *Successful Negotiating Skills for Women.* Reading, MA: Addison-Wesley; 1981.

Jandt FE, Gillette P. *Win-Win Negotiating.* New York, NY: John Wiley & Sons; 1985.

Leeds D. *Smart Questions: A New Strategy for Successful Managers.* New York, NY: McGraw Hill; 1987. This book uses the power of questions in the negotiating process. It is very readable and contains valuable information for the nonprofessional negotiator.

Levin E. *Negotiating Tactics.* New York, NY: Fawcett; 1980.

Mannino MJ. *The Business of Anesthesia: Practice Options for Nurse Anesthetists.* Park Ridge, IL: AANA Publishing; 1994.

Schoenfield M, Schoenfield R. *Legal Negotiations: Getting Maximum Results.* Colorado Springs, CO: Shepards/McGraw-Hill; 1988. This book is primarily written for lawyers who do all types of negotiations on behalf of their clients. It is useful reference in that it is well organized and presents a systematic approach to negotiating.

Chapter 5

Educational Requirements for Nurse Anesthesia Programs

Francis Gerbasi, CRNA, PhD

Key Points

- The Council on Accreditation of Nurse Anesthesia Educational Programs establishes the standards and requirements that all accredited nurse anesthesia programs must meet.

- The standards and requirements are developed with input from the community of interest (eg, Certified Registered Nurse Anesthetist educators and practitioners, student nurse anesthetists, healthcare administrators, and the American Association of Nurse Anesthetists Board of Directors).

- Quality assessment by programs' continuous self-study and review is an essential requirement.

- Monitoring student achievement includes benchmarks that a program must meet for Certification Examination pass rates, attrition, and employment rates.

- Accreditation requirements include but are not limited to program administrators' qualifications and responsibilities, student admission requirements, and the curriculum (eg, didactic and clinical).

Introduction

When the National Association of Nurse Anesthetists was established in 1933, a primary goal of its Bylaws was to develop nurse anesthesia educational objectives.[1] Over the years, the commitment of leaders in the nurse anesthesia profession has taken nurse anesthesia education from apprenticeships to the award of graduate degrees at accredited universities. In 1998, all nurse anesthesia educational programs were awarding master's degrees. In 2008, programs had started to move toward awarding professional doctorate degrees. This chapter will provide the reader with a better understanding of the 2004 standards used to accredit nurse anesthesia programs and how programs demonstrate compliance with the requirements.

Educational Standards

Educational requirements for all accredited nurse anesthesia educational programs are governed by the Council on Accreditation of Nurse Anesthesia Educational Programs' (COA) Standards for Accreditation of Nurse Anesthesia Educational Programs.[2] The COA is the only accrediting agency recognized by the US Department of Education (USDE) and the Council for Higher Education Accreditation (CHEA) to accredit nurse anesthesia educational programs at the master's, post-master's certificate, and doctorate degree levels.

The standards and criteria are measures used by the COA to assess the quality of nurse anesthesia education. The COA's standards address 5 areas: (1) governance, (2) resources, (3) program of study, (4) program effectiveness, and (5) accountability. These 5 areas address the operation of the program; the curriculum; the quality of student, alumni, and faculty achievement; and the program's accountability and integrity to its communities of interest.

To be considered for COA accreditation, a nurse anesthesia program must demonstrate that it develops and implements the necessary mechanisms to comply with the standards and criteria. An example of how programs demonstrate compliance with effectiveness standards is the development and implementation of a systematic evaluation process that includes assessment of didactic and clinical instruction, the learning environment, the competence of graduates, and the program's resources. The standards are developed with input from the stakeholders that are affected by them, including Certified Registered Nurse Anesthetist (CRNA) practitioners and educators; student nurse anesthetists, administrators and faculty; hospital administrators; state boards of nursing; members of the councils on certification, recertification, and public interest in anesthesia; and the American Association of Nurse Anesthetists Board of Directors. A major revision of the standards normally takes 4 to 5 years.

In addition to establishing standards for nurse anesthesia programs, the COA is responsible for developing the policies and procedures used to implement the standards. Policies and procedures are used to foster educational quality and to facilitate implementation of the Standards for Accreditation of Nurse Anesthesia Educational Programs.[2] Policies and procedures are also established to meet the requirements of external agencies and to safeguard the rights, responsibilities, and interests of students, faculty, administrators, the profession, the public, and other members of the community of interest. Substantive revisions that could have a major effect on programs are subject to review, hearing, and comment by the COA's community of interest. Nurse anesthesia programs are expected to follow the Accreditation Policies and Procedures in carrying out their educational activities and submitting accreditation-related requests to the COA.[3]

It is essential that program administrators and faculty have a good understanding of current accreditation standards, policies, and procedures. The Standards for Accreditation of Nurse Anesthesia Educational Programs and the Accreditation Policies and Procedures are posted on the members-only side of the AANA website (https://www.aana.com).

In addition, the COA publishes a Program Directors' Update 3 times each year. The Program Directors' Update provides program administrators and faculty with information regarding changes in accreditation and education requirements. Each nurse anesthesia program is assigned an accreditation and education specialist. The specialists provide support for the programs in processing programs' accreditation-related activities such as continued accreditation reviews and requests for new clinical sites. Program administrators are encouraged to contact their program's assigned COA accreditation and education specialist with any questions regarding the accreditation standards, policies, and procedures.

General Requirements for Nurse Anesthesia Programs

Accreditation of nurse anesthesia programs provides quality assurance concerning the educational preparation of nurse anesthetists through continuous self-study and review. Accredited programs are required to perform ongoing evaluation and assessment to determine their integrity and educational effectiveness. Each program must continuously monitor and evaluate its didactic and clinical curriculum, including curriculum content, admissions policies, faculty, and clinical sites used for student educational experiences. The common methods that programs use to meet this requirement include student evaluations of the didactic and clinical instruction, exit student evaluations of the program, alumni evaluations, and employer evaluations of the graduates. These aspects of programs are evaluated periodically by the COA to determine their compliance with accreditation standards[1] and their relevance to anesthesia practice.

The COA's process for the accreditation of a nurse anesthesia program is focused on ensuring the program's compliance with the accreditation standards. The process as identified in the COA's Accreditation Policies and Procedures is consistent with the USDE and CHEA recognition requirements. The first step in the process for a new nurse anesthesia program is for the sponsoring institution to file a letter of intent with the COA. The letter of intent must be from the chief executive officer (CEO) of the sponsoring institution and reflect the institution's legal authority to grant the degree and its commitment to provide the necessary resources to establish a program that meets accreditation requirements. Established nurse anesthesia programs must have the CEO submit a letter indicating that the sponsoring institution has the legal authority to grant the degree.

Following the COA's acceptance of the letter of intent, both new and established programs start an accreditation review process. The process includes the submission of evidence of eligibility, a self-study, and on-site review. The on-site review is conducted by experienced nurse anesthesia educators and practitioners approved by the COA to serve as on-site reviewers. Only after all of these activities have been completed will the program be reviewed by the COA. The COA reviews all of the documentation and makes an accreditation decision based on the program's ability to demonstrate compliance with the standards. The length of accreditation awarded can be from 2 years to 10 years. The COA's decisions regarding the length of accreditation awarded are based on guidelines and criteria that include a program's compliance with the standards.

It is important to note that the accreditation decision process does not consider workforce issues (eg, assessment of supply and demand for CRNAs in the state). This would be inconsistent with USDE and CHEA recognition requirements that the accreditation process and decision be focused on a program's ability to demonstrate compliance with accreditation standards. In addition, considering the supply and demand for CRNAs in the state would have antitrust implications for the COA.

Ongoing monitoring of accredited programs is accomplished through submission of annual reports and progress reports to the COA for review. Annual reports provide data regarding the conducting institutions and programs, including the names of university and program officials, degrees offered, and the academic units in which nurse anesthesia programs are housed. In addition, programs report student attrition and graduate employment rates. The COA can request that a program provide a progress report for a variety of reasons, such as concerns identified by students and faculty on program or clinical site evaluations and partial compliance or noncompliance with the standards and criteria.

Monitoring Student Achievement

The COA requires that programs document student achievement in multiple ways. Indicators of student achievement include identifying the number of students who complete the program, the number of graduates who pass the National Certification Examination for Nurse Anesthetists (NCE) in accordance with the COA's Certification Examination Policy, and the number of graduates who secure employment within 6 months after graduation. In addition, each program must conduct graduate (alumni) and employer evaluations to assess the program's ability to prepare nurse anesthetists who are competent and capable of functioning in a variety of anesthesia settings.

In 2003, the COA implemented the monitoring of a program's pass rates on the NCE. Programs must demonstrate that graduates take the NCE and pass it in accordance with the COA pass rate requirement.[4] The mandatory pass rate is 80% of a composite of the previous 5 years' national Council on Certification of Nurse Anesthetists pass rate for first-time takers. Programs must meet or exceed the

COA mandatory pass rate. Programs that fall below the mandatory pass rate are placed on monitoring. If improvement is not demonstrated within a specified time by increasing a program's pass rates above the mandatory rate, the program's accreditation is subject to revocation.

In 2007, the COA implemented the monitoring of a program's attrition and employment rates.[5] Programs are required to report student attrition and employment rates on the COA annual report. Attrition rates higher than 20% and employment rates less than 80% based on a 5-year average require programs to provide status reports to the COA. If improvement is not shown within a specified time, a program's accreditation is subject to revocation.

Programs must demonstrate that they meet national benchmarks for each of these 3 outcome measures (ie, Certification Examination pass rate, attrition, and employment rates). This stringent evaluation process helps to ensure the effectiveness of nurse anesthesia education and the COA's compliance with USDE recognition requirements for accrediting agencies.

Program Administrator Requirements

Standard I Criteria A4 and A5 of the Standards for Accreditation of Nurse Anesthesia Educational Programs require that nurse anesthesia programs employ CRNAs who have graduate degrees in the roles of program administrator and assistant program administrator.[2] The program administrator must have the responsibility and authority for the administration of the program. Administration of a nurse anesthesia program includes the management of faculty and students, fiscal program management, maintenance of COA accreditation and other higher education accreditation requirements of the university, faculty continuing education, and program evaluation, at a minimum. The program administrators must have earned a graduate degree from an institution of higher education accredited by a nationally recognized accrediting agency. A doctorate degree is preferred for CRNA program administrators; however, it is not required at this time. All CRNA clinical coordinators must have a master's degree by 2014. Program administrators must provide the COA with an official transcript demonstrating compliance with this requirement.

Admission Requirements

The standards identify the minimum admission requirements applicants must meet for acceptance in a nurse anesthesia program. Standard III Criterion C13 requires applicants admitted to a nurse anesthesia program be graduates of an accredited school of nursing, possess a bachelor's degree, hold current licensure as a registered nurse, and have at least 1 year of professional experience in an acute care setting. Most applicants have acquired clinical experience that exceeds the 1-year minimum.

Requirements for the Didactic Curriculum

The didactic curriculum of nurse anesthesia programs is governed by the standards and provides students the scientific, clinical, and professional foundation upon which to build sound and safe clinical practice. Based on the COA's 2007 Annual Report data, most nurse anesthesia programs range from 60 to 75 graduate semester credits in courses pertinent to the practice of anesthesia.[6] The standards identify the basic nurse anesthesia curriculum and prerequisite course requirements such as anatomy, physiology, pathophysiology, pharmacology, chemistry, biochemistry, physics, professional aspects, equipment, technology, pain management, research, and clinical conferences (Table 5.1).[2] Courses in anesthesia practice provide content such as induction, maintenance, and emergence from anesthesia; airway management; anesthesia pharmacology; teaching of regional anesthesia techniques; and anesthesia for special populations such as obstetric, geriatric, and pediatric patients. Students are instructed in the use of anesthesia machines and other related biomedical monitoring equipment and are evaluated didactically using such traditional evaluation methods as examinations, presentations, care plans, and papers.

Table 5.1. Standards for Accreditation of Nurse Anesthesia Educational Programs: 2004 Minimum Curriculum Course Requirements

Courses	Minimum no. of contact hours
Pharmacology of anesthetic agents and adjuvant, drugs including concepts in chemistry and biochemistry	105
Anatomy, physiology, and pathophysiology	135
Professional aspects of nurse anesthesia practice	45
Basic and advanced principles of anesthesia practice, including physics, equipment, technology, and pain management	105
Research	30
Clinical correlation conferences	45

Nurse anesthesia programs must be able to show that they provide an extensive, educationally sound curriculum combining both academic theory and clinical practice. Evidence includes student, faculty, alumni, and employer evaluations. The curriculum should be provided in a logical manner. Classroom and clinical experiences should be sequential, starting from basic and moving toward more advanced knowledge and skills as the student progresses in the program. The policies and procedures of each program should use outcome criteria to promote student learning while enhancing the program's quality and integrity.

The methods used to provide nurse anesthesia education are changing as new technologies such as distance education and simulation are being applied in higher education. Based on the COA's 2008 Annual Report, more than 44% of nurse anesthesia programs use some form of distance education in providing didactic instruction.[6] The distance education offerings vary from several core nursing courses to programs in which the majority of the didactic curriculum is provided using distance education. Standard III Criterion C11 requires distance education programs and courses to achieve the same outcomes as traditional educational offerings. Programs must be approved by the COA prior to offering distance education. Program administrators should follow the established accreditation policies and procedures for submission of distance education requests.

The majority of programs use some form of simulation.[6] Simulation offerings vary from use of manikins to demonstrate regional anesthesia techniques to full body simulators. At present, simple models and simulated experiences may be used to satisfy the minimum case requirements for placement of central venous pressure catheters and fiberoptic airway management techniques.[2]

Requirements for the Clinical Curriculum

The standards establish a program's minimum requirements for the clinical curricula and help ensure that graduates are prepared to administer all types of anesthesia, including general, regional, selected local, and conscious sedation to patients of all ages for all types of surgeries. The clinical curriculum should ensure students are taught to use all currently available anesthesia drugs, to manage fluid and blood replacement therapy, and to interpret data from sophisticated monitoring devices. In addition, students should obtain experience in the insertion of invasive catheters, the recognition and correction of complications that occur during the course of an anesthetic, the provision of airway and ventilatory support during resuscitation, and pain management.

Supervised clinical experience provides student nurse anesthetists with the opportunity to incorporate didactic anesthesia education into the clinical setting. During their clinical anesthesia experience, students must be supervised by CRNAs or anesthesiologists who are immediately available. The clinical supervision ratio of students to instructors must be coordinated to ensure patient safety and should not exceed 2 graduate students to 1 CRNA or anesthesiologist. To meet the standards and be eligible to take the NCE, a student must have performed a minimum of 550 anesthetics, which must include specialties such as pediatric, obstetric, cardiothoracic, and neurosurgical anesthesia.[2]

Programs should establish processes to accurately track and evaluate students' clinical experiences and performance. Clinical evaluations should include both formative and summative assessments. Clinical faculty should remember that programs rely on accurate and complete assessment of the students' clinical performance.

Requirements for Doctorate Degrees

In June 2007, the AANA Board of Directors unanimously adopted the position of supporting doctoral education for entry into nurse anesthesia practice by 2025. This decision was based on more than 2 years of investigation to thoroughly explore the interests and concerns surrounding doctoral preparation of nurse anesthetists. The COA has established additional criteria for practice and research-oriented doctorate degrees. Nurse anesthesia programs must obtain COA approval for courses that prepare CRNAs to obtain degrees (ie, CRNA completion programs) when the certificate or degree title references anesthesia or a significant component of the curriculum includes anesthesia-related material. In addition, programs moving from a master's degree for entry into practice to a doctorate degree are required to obtain COA approval.

As of July 1, 2008, there are 4 nurse anesthesia programs that offer post-masters doctorate degrees for nurse anesthetists: the Rush University College of Nursing Nurse Anesthesia Program, the Virginia Commonwealth University Department of Nurse Anesthesia, the University of Pittsburgh School of Nursing Nurse Anesthesia Program, and the Texas Wesleyan University Graduate Programs of Nurse Anesthesia. At its May 2008 meeting, the COA approved the first entry into practice professional doctorate degree program at the Charleston Medical Center School of Nurse Anesthesia in Charleston, West Virginia.

Summary

Nurse anesthesia education has flourished for more than a century by continuing to meet increasingly stringent educational standards. Advancements in nurse anesthesia education have helped form the foundation of the nurse anesthesia profession. As programs move from master's to doctorate degrees for entry into nurse anesthesia practice, it will be important that program administrators and faculty continue to ensure that programs meet accreditation requirements and that graduates have the knowledge and skills to provide safe, high-quality anesthesia care to patients.

References

1. National Association of Nurse Anesthetists. *Constitution and Bylaws.* Park Ridge, IL: American Association of Nurse Anesthetists; 1933.

2. Standards for Accreditation of Nurse Anesthesia Educational Programs. Park Ridge, IL: Council on Accreditation of Nurse Anesthesia Educational Programs; 2004.

3. Accreditation Policies and Procedures. Park Ridge, IL: Council on Accreditation of Nurse Anesthesia Educational Programs; 2007.

4. Gerbasi F. Program Directors' Update, Issue Thirty-Nine. http://www.aana.com/uploadedFiles/Credentialing/Accreditation/COA_Resources/issue39_0503.pdf. Accessed February 2, 2008.

5. Implementation of Policies for the Monitoring of Nurse Anesthesia Programs' Attrition and Graduate Employment Rates. Park Ridge, IL: Council on Accreditation of Nurse Anesthesia Educational Programs; May 2007.

6. Council on Accreditation of Nurse Anesthesia Educational Programs Annual Report. Park Ridge, IL: Council on Accreditation of Nurse Anesthesia Educational Programs; 2008.

Chapter 6

Evidence-Based Practice and the Nurse Anesthetist: Making the Connection

Lisa J. Thiemann, CRNA, MNA
John J. McFadden, CRNA, PhD

Key Points

- Evidence-based practice is critical to improving patient outcomes.

- Implementation of evidence-based practice requires a thorough assessment of the best available evidence.

- Evidence exists in many forms; the strength and applicability of evidence requires practitioner judgment.

- In contrast to research utilization, evidence-based practice incorporates the experience and judgment of the healthcare practitioner and the patient's desires.

- Evidence-based practice requires several key skill sets to be successful.

- Adoption of evidence-based practice may pose challenges; however, the rewards for patients are substantial.

Introduction

This chapter will give a historical background of evidence-based practice (EBP), define EBP, and discuss the reasons for and against use of EBP. It also will outline the steps of the EBP process, describe how to implement an evidence-based approach to clinical practice, and explain how to appraise the strength of evidence-based literature.

Beginnings of Evidence-Based Practice

Certified Registered Nurse Anesthetists (CRNAs) have a long-standing history of delivering high-quality anesthesia services. Evidence-based practice facilitates a clinician's ability to provide high-quality care while integrating multiple aspects of the patient's and the patient's family preferences.

The widely cited Institute of Medicine (IOM) report titled, *To Err Is Human: Building a Safer Healthcare System,* which attributed some 98,000 US deaths to medical errors, served to awaken the American public to the risks associated with healthcare.[1] As a result, healthcare consumers and purchasers began to question the quality of care rendered and, therefore, the continued competence of its practitioners. In a follow-up IOM report titled, *Health Professions Education: A Bridge to Quality,* the following recommendation was issued:

> Department of Health and Human Services (DHHS) and leading foundations should support an interdisciplinary effort focused on developing a common language, with the ultimate aim of achieving consensus across the health professions on a core set of competencies that includes patient-centered care, interdisciplinary teams, evidence-based practice, quality improvement, and informatics.[2]

With the issuance of the Health Professions Education report, multiple communities of interest have embraced the IOM's call for EBP competence. This support may be viewed through the proliferation of clinical practice guidelines, which are based on the analysis and summary of quantitative reports, or the implementation of hospital and clinician-level performance measures based on available evidence.

Evidence of the rapid proliferation of the evidence-based concept in the literature is demonstrated by Alper et al,[3] whose MEDLINE search in 2003 using the keywords *evidence based* returned almost 54,000 citations. More than 42,000 of these were published since 1993. This rapid expansion of knowledge available to the clinician is daunting. In an evidence-based approach to care, in which a clinician is expected to continually apply the best evidence to the care of patients, the activity of continually assessing the best available evidence becomes challenging. For example, Alper et al[3] estimated the time it would take for a physician trained in medical epidemiology to evaluate all primary care–related literature to exceed 620 hours each month.[3] This is equivalent to more than 15 full-time jobs based on a 40-hour workweek.

Choudry and colleagues[4] assessed the proposition that physicians with more clinical practice experience may be less likely to render high-quality patient care. Their results revealed that, as experience increased, clinical performance decreased, bringing into question the accuracy of the belief that a more experienced practitioner will provide the highest quality care. Heater et al[5] reported a 28% improvement in patient outcomes when care is rendered based on best and latest evidence.

The half-life for the nursing profession is estimated to be between 2 and 5 years.[6] Professional half-life is defined as the point at which half of a practitioner's beginning knowledge becomes dated as a result of changes in the field or is simply forgotten. Due to the rapidly changing healthcare arena, practitioners entering into practice today may be competent; however, that competence may not be long lasting.[7] Rapidly changing medical and technological advances can have a major impact on a healthcare practitioner's explicit knowledge base in a short time. In this world of healthcare quality measurement, it is critical that CRNAs become well versed in the application of an EBP approach to care.

Understanding the Evidence-Based Practice Movement

Nurse anesthetists, like other healthcare providers, make decisions as part of their daily practice. Each patient encounter generates a host of clinical questions that require thoughtful answers. The uniqueness of every patient undergoing an anesthetic requires decision making to be an ongoing, continuous process. How do nurse anesthetists gather and interpret data, draw conclusions, reference the most up-to-date scientific data, and ensure that the right action plan is constructed for each patient? How does a practitioner meet the need for information to make the correct decisions? Although it may appear to the untrained eye that the clinical nurse anesthetist is on autopilot after induction and before emergence, a commitment to vigilance requires nonstop observation, decision making, and reaction during the provision of care.

Making a decision is a cognitive and emotional activity that involves selecting one pathway over others in an attempt to solve a problem and achieve a desired outcome. The many factors that influence a decision include bias and preconceptions, previous experiences, logic and reasoning, values and ethics, available resources, emotions, and knowledge. Some authors theorize that personality or even genes may also influence how an individual makes decisions. Clearly, decision making is a dynamic, complex phenomenon that involves many attributes. In healthcare, the practitioner balances input from many of these variables. In addition, clinical decision makers may rely on input from other colleagues, published research articles and textbooks, product literature, or even gut instinct. The weight placed on any one of these variables will vary depending on the decision at hand and its urgency.

When did the process for decision making in healthcare become an area of interest? Some trace the origins of the decision-making process to the start of the scientific revolution in the mid-1500s when Copernicus published *On the Revolution of the Heavenly Bodies* and Vesalius published *On the Structure of the Human Body*. This era marked a transition in the way science was conducted and how complex questions about life were answered. Simply relying on the views of authority figures (the received view) or tradition was no longer acceptable. Other experts, however, prefer to consider the focus on using data for decision making as a more sophisticated, recent trend. Specifically, in the medical profession, Archie Cochrane,[8] an epidemiologist who has roots in Scotland and England, has been credited with beginning the evidence-based movement with the publication of his book, *Effectiveness and Efficiency: Reflections on Health Services*. His ideas and support eventually led to the development of the Cochrane Centres for evidence-based medical research; The Cochrane Collaboration, an international not-for-profit and independent organization that produces and disseminates systematic reviews of healthcare interventions; and The Cochrane Library, which consists of a collection of evidence-based medicine databases.

Several terms have been used to label the process of using data to support making decisions in healthcare. The expression *evidence-based medicine,* which began appearing in the medical taxonomy in the early 1990s, has been attributed to the McMaster Medical School in Hamilton, Ontario. McMaster's methodologies were put into practice through the development of the Evidence-Based Medicine Working Group, led by David L. Sackett, MD, and Gordon Guyatt, MD. The group is now called the Evidence-Based Clinical Practice Working Group.[9] Sackett became the founder of the Centre for Evidence-Based Medicine in Oxford, England. Throughout the 1990s, interdisciplinary teams were being established by the US Agency for Health Care Policy and Research in an attempt to develop evidence-based clinical guidelines. This agency was later renamed the US Agency for Healthcare Research and Quality. It continues to serve as a clearinghouse for clinical guidelines (http://www.guideline.gov). This development in medicine has influenced other professions, including nursing, to adopt the evidence-based model. Other terms currently associated with the process include *evidence-based practice, evidence-based nursing, evidence-based healthcare,* and *evidence-based nurse anesthesia practice.* The basis for all of these terms is the same: using data from research to support making clinical decisions, rather than basing clinical care on tradition and authoritative dictates.

A Common Definition for Evidence-Based Practice

One universal definition of EBP does not exist, and EBP does not equal research utilization. Research utilization involves the application of a single research study to clinical practice, whereas EBP involves a thorough assessment of the relevant landscape to optimize patient outcomes. Many authors have completed important work to refine the concept of evidence-based medicine or practice over the years. Many scholars offer their own definitions of EBP, each emphasizing different attributes.

Sackett and coauthors[10] see evidence-based medicine as "the integration of best research evidence with clinical expertise and patient values." Sackett et al offer additional definitions. *Patient values* are the "unique preferences, concerns and expectations each patient brings to a clinical encounter and which must be integrated into clinical decisions if they are to serve the patient."[10] *Best research evidence* is "clinically relevant research, often from the basic sciences of medicine, but especially from patient-centered clinical research into the accuracy and precision of diagnostic tests (including the clinical examination), the power of prognostic markers, and the efficacy and safety of therapeutic, rehabilitative, and preventive regimens."[10] *Clinical expertise* is defined as "the ability to use our clinical skills and past experience to rapidly identify each patient's unique health state and diagnosis, their individual risks and benefits of potential interventions, and their personal values and expectations."[10]

Sigma Theta Tau International proposes that *evidence-based nursing practice* is "an integration of the best evidence available, nursing expertise, and the values and preferences of the individuals, families, and communities who are served."[11] Pravikoff et al[12] offer this definition: "Evidence-based practice is a systematic approach to problem solving for health care providers, including RNs, characterized by the use of the best evidence currently available for clinical decision making, in order to provide the most consistent and best possible care to patients." As the definition of EBP evolves, the main constituents of the definition remain stable: a decision-making process for clinicians that considers research data, clinician expertise, and patient input.

The Changing View of Science

Like other scientists, nurses have a history of searching for cause-and-effect relationships to guide the decision-making process in providing care. Florence Nightingale exemplified this process by combining her understanding of mathematics, the classics, and her knowledge about hospital care to conduct studies about urban and hospital sanitary conditions. Statistical analysis was the basis for her correlations between mortality and lack of ventilation, lack of natural light, and overcrowded conditions, as described in her work *Notes on Hospitals*.[13] These cause-and-effect studies led her to be considered the first biostatistician.[14]

Nightingale based her ideas about nursing on the scientific theories of her time and paralleled the ideas of the medical community. Positivism was the dominant philosophy of science of the time. The ontology of positivism is that the world is real and knowable and exists independent of the observer. Positivists believe the world is governed by natural laws resulting in cause-and-effect relationships, and the world is predictable. The goal of this worldview is to uncover truths and facts as quantitatively derived relationships between variables. Like her contemporaries, Nightingale was convinced of the power of this approach to science coupled with the use of statistics.

As the profession evolved, nursing scholars questioned the congruence of the profession's holistic foundation with the positivist approach to science. How can the human health experience be reduced to measurable concepts independent of historical, cultural, social, and personal contexts? A reductionist approach can become so dissociated from the object that the approach is attempting to explain that it no longer provides useful information. In addition to predicting and controlling the relationships among variables, there is a recognized need to explain and understand the meaning of the phenomena of human health through a postmodern approach. This can only be done in the context in which these phenomena occur. As a profession that involves intimate relationships between unique individuals with varying life experiences, nursing is well suited to the postmodern worldview. This is the paradigm that helps shape the dualism between the science and art of nursing.

So where does this leave today's nurse anesthetist who is attempting to make rapid decisions about life-and-death situations? There is no doubt that quantitative research using the scientific method and a positivist approach provides knowledge about many biophysical processes in which the profession is involved. This knowledge is invaluable to the nurse anesthetist. The limitation of these approaches is that they can never fully explain what an individual experiences when faced with the transition between health and illness and the various aspects involved in receiving modern healthcare. A context-dependent, postmodern approach may be used when trying to understand the interpersonal relationships involved in providing nurse anesthesia care. These methods add richness to capturing the experiences of people as they receive healthcare. A plurality of approaches will enrich the profession so that knowledge development is supported with a solid understanding of the lived human experience. And so the phrase embraced by the modern scholar applies: "the question drives the method."

As a result of the multiple approaches to generating knowledge and research data, it is a challenge for most healthcare providers to identify and apply the appropriate data or set of evidence needed to make a decision. Searching a knowledge base, weeding through the available science, reflecting on one's own clinical expertise, and contemplating the uniqueness and singularity of the patient and situation at hand require a formidable skill set.

Several scholars have identified barriers that exist for nurses to accomplish this task. These barriers include lack of time, limited resources, undeveloped skills in data searching and the research process, inexperience in applying the evidence, and patient noncompliance.[15-18] These challenges are not necessarily unique to nurses, but applicable to a wide range of healthcare providers, including nurse anesthetists.

Identifying the appropriate data and applying it to the situation at hand is one of the more demanding tasks involved in clinical decision making. Some decisions made by nurse anesthetists allow for creativity; no one approach emerges as best. Providing reassurance in the preoperative holding area or discussing a medical error that has occurred are examples of situations that demand judgment, concern about the individual patient's needs, and other considerations that are context-dependent. Other decisions, however, leave less room for the imaginative spirit. Choosing a dose of an intravenous agent or managing a rare coexisting disease during administration of a general inhalation anesthetic may allow for some ingenuity, but generally these situations require data that have been tried and tested. It is a challenge finding the right blend of evidence types to make decisions in nurse anesthesia practice. Thus, nurse anesthetists and most healthcare providers consider a variety of research approaches—quantitative analysis, qualitative analysis, and mixed method approaches—and integrate these findings with their own judgment and the desires of the patient to make decisions about how to provide care.

Wyszewianski and Green[19] described 4 types of physician practitioners with regard to use of available evidence. These descriptions are of interest to the nurse anesthesia profession and may be applicable as well.

1. The seeker actively engages the professional literature and readily accesses electronic as well as print collections. This type of practitioner usually embraces the concept of an evidence-based approach to care, in that the individual easily translates information gleaned from the literature into practice. The seeker actively engages in independent evidence appraisal.

2. The receptive practitioner, in similar fashion, will apply new information to the clinical setting; however, this information must originate from a respected and trusted source rather than from an independent assessment.

3. The traditionalist will place greater weight on experience, skill, and authoritative advocates for change when making clinical decisions or considering an alteration to clinical practice. The final type of practitioner that Wyszewianski and Green[19] described is the pragmatist.

4. The pragmatist shares in the belief that clinical practice is grounded in a scientifically sound foundation; however, pragmatists are less likely to adopt practices if they view them as being disruptive to the flow of care or as having an impact on patient satisfaction.

Practicing nurse anesthetists and registered nurses pursuing graduate studies in the field may derive benefits by comparing these approaches with their own personal approaches to reviewing the available evidence and incorporating it into practice.

Evidence-Based Practice: Why or Why Not?

There are several reasons that support the need to use research results or evidence when making a decision that affects another person's health and well-being. The recent focus on error reduction by the IOM has promoted healthcare practices that are based on sound scientific knowledge. Accrediting and regulatory agencies, including the Magnet Recognition Program by the American Nurses Credentialing Center, also promote the use of evidence-based decisions in practice. This promotes scholarship in clinical practice. In many ways, the EBP movement attempts to minimize the distance between scholarship and practice, between researcher and clinician. That is, knowledge generators and knowledge users must share perspectives more consistently.[20]

The ethical principle of autonomy, or self-determination, requires that a patient provide informed consent before receiving healthcare. Informed consent involves frank, open discussion about risks, benefits, outcomes, and alternatives of care. These discussions between provider and patient cannot occur without some evidence supporting a care decision. Decisions regarding treatments and interventions should include the goal of being cost-justifiable because funding and resources for healthcare are not limitless. Use of healthcare resources needs to be supported by data that defend an intervention's benefit and cost-efficiency. Lastly, patients and payers, as consumers of healthcare, have the right to be aware of the processes that a provider uses and the outcomes achieved. In the broadest sense, these are aspects considered when evaluating quality of care.

Evidence-Based Practice: Implementation Considerations

Not everyone views EBP as a panacea for ending the healthcare industry's woes. Holmes and coworkers[21] cautioned against having a false sense of security in believing that quantitative, positivist research serves as the strongest evidence available for decision making. In fact, Holmes et al[22] highlighted hidden political concerns of EBP. They suggested that the creation of practice guidelines can discipline, govern, and regulate nursing work yet suppress creativity and critical thinking. Finally, unless practitioners possess the skills to read, evaluate, weigh, and apply research, the process is not effective. This skill deficit sets up a disconnect between research and practice. This ultimately may inhibit a practitioner's resourcefulness and his or her ability to synthesize and integrate knowledge.[23]

The adoption of an evidence-based approach to clinical practice often faces numerous barriers. According to Pravikoff et al,[12] there are 2 main types of barriers healthcare practitioners may encounter when attempting to implement an EBP. A practitioner may experience personal barriers that impede the implementation of EBP. These barriers may include such things as a diminished value or knowledge for research into practice, a lack of database search skills (including internal database structure or function understanding), lack of computer skills necessary to conduct searches, access-related issues (eg, computer, library, or database), difficulties understanding the literature, or an inability to evaluate and synthesize the literature.

In addition to personal barriers, there are also institutional barriers that pose a challenge to the implementation of an evidence-based framework supporting clinical practice. The facility may not place importance on adopting an EBP. It may lack the necessary budget or support services to accomplish this approach, or the institution may not hold the philosophical belief in the positive ramifications of adopting an evidence-based approach to care. In a recent study of medical residents, Windish et al[24] discovered that most residents lacked the necessary knowledge to interpret statistics published in the medical literature. Although the sample size was small, the study is telling in a healthcare era with widespread support for an evidence-based approach to patient care.

Just as there are barriers to the implementation of an evidence-based approach to care, there are also facilitators to the adoption of this care approach, both internally and at the organizational level. According to Fineout-Overholt et al,[25] these facilitators may include fostering the relationships between academic and clinical settings, the commitment of facility administration, or the identification of a mentor to foster the development of evidence-based skills in healthcare practitioners.

Given these inhibiting and facilitating factors, how will practitioners transition into an EBP? Diffusion describes the process by which an innovation or information is communicated over time among members of a group. Diffusion occurs in a fashion graphically similar to a sigmoid curve, such that early adopters of the innovation fall to the lower-left portion of the curve and late adopters to the upper right. According to Dearing,[26] the characteristic "S" shape of the curve results from modeling of the innovation in the field over time, as influenced by the group's leaders.

Rogers'[27] diffusion of innovations theory has been used to study research transfer and dissemination of information. Diffusion theory requires several key components, which include an innovation; adopters; a group or system with leaders and perceived pressure to adopt the innovation; personal adoption processes, which include innovation awareness and implementation; and a diffusion system. Balas and Boren[28] report that it takes more than 17 years to translate research findings into widespread clinical practice. Rogers[27] discusses 5 attributes of an innovation that may affect the rapidity with which it is adopted.

1. The perceived advantages (eg, cost) of the innovation
2. The degree of fit the innovation holds with current processes (eg, how well the innovation integrates into the existing system)
3. The degree of observable outcomes
4. The degree of commitment to the innovation that the adopter requires (eg, can the adopter later choose not to implement the innovation or must the adopter be dedicated to the innovation)
5. The innovation's degree of complexity[29]

Many practitioners may not adopt an innovation until hearing of a colleague's success in implementing the innovation.[30] Considering EBP as an innovation within this context may help explain why it has been slow in achieving widespread adoption.

Table 6.1. Evidence-Based Process Steps

1. Form a PICO question.
2. Identify and retrieve best available evidence.
3. Appraise the evidence.
4. Integrate clinical expertise and patient values and needs with research.
5. Evaluate intervention's effectiveness.

PICO indicates patient population, intervention of interest, comparison intervention or status, and outcome.

The Nuts and Bolts of Evidence-Based Practice

Many models exist or are in development to describe the process for EBP. Melnyk and Fineout-Overholt[31] describe 5 critical steps that form the foundation for the process of EBP (Table 6.1).

1. Convert the need for information into an answerable question. The question should address the population of interest, the intervention of interest, the condition of interest, the outcome of interest, and a timeframe. The authors suggest the acronym PICO for focusing the formation of the question. This step and the second step often benefit from the assistance of an experienced librarian or researcher.
2. Identify and collect the best evidence that addresses the question.
3. Critically evaluate or appraise the evidence. Consider the validity, reliability, rigor, relevance, and clinical applicability of what is known about the issue. Determine the gaps vs the consistencies in the evidence available.
4. Integrate the research with clinical expertise and the unique values and needs of the patient.
5. Evaluate the effectiveness and efficiency of the intervention and the process.

To be successful in applying an evidenced-based process to clinical practice, a clinician must follow a fairly structured process, which begins with formation of a clinical question. To uncover all existing evidence that relates to a clinical question, it is imperative that the clinician frame the question appropriately. If the question is too broad, a clinician may have difficulties working through the abundance of literature returned while conducting a database search.

As suggested by Melnyk and Fineout-Overholt,[31] the use of the PICO (patient population, intervention of interest, comparison intervention or status, and outcome) format may be helpful. One PICO-style example is as follows: In the pediatric patient (patient population), how effective is dexamethasone (intervention) vs ondansetron (intervention comparison) in preventing nausea (outcome)? Practitioners may consider the addition of an appropriate timeframe when framing the questions (ie, PICOT).

The next step a practitioner must take is to locate the evidence. This step requires access to electronic databases such as PubMed, EMBASE, or Cumulative Index of Nursing and Allied Health Literature (CINAHL). Clinicians must select the most appropriate database to maximize their success in uncovering the existing evidence. A practitioner must become familiar with types of studies to which each database will afford access. For example, CINAHL contains nursing, allied health, and biomedicine studies. In comparison, PsycINFO contains citations in the field of psychology or the psychological aspects of related disciplines. In addition to selecting an appropriate database, the ability to identify key search terms is important. Practitioners must be savvy at selecting the search keywords that have the greatest potential to uncover the existing literature. Several helpful evidence-based Internet resources are listed in Table 6.2.

Table 6.2. Useful Resources in Evidence-Based Medicine

Resource	Website
Centre for Evidence-Based Medicine (CEBM)	http://www.cebm.net
Joanna Briggs Institute (JBI)	http://www.joannabriggs.edu.au
Agency for Healthcare Research and Quality (AHRQ)	http://www.ahrq.gov/
Cochrane Collaboration	http://www.cochrane.org/
PubMed database	http://www.ncbi.nlm.nih.gov/pubmed/
Ovid Technologies	www.ovid.com

Once the practitioner has successfully conducted a literature search associated with the clinical question at hand, the practitioner must undergo a thorough assessment of that literature. Generally, evidence that is quantitative in nature, systematic reviews or meta-analyses on the associated topic, considered to be the strongest evidence, provided the reviews or metaanalyses are rigorously conducted. Randomized clinical trials are usually considered the next evidence tier, followed by (in order of importance) cohort studies; case-control studies; case series; case reports; and ideas, editorials, or opinions. From a historical perspective, qualitative studies have played less of a role in the EBP movement; however, the healthcare arena has recently begun to embrace the value that qualitative reports can add to an EBP approach.

Ranking the Evidence: Strong vs Weak

When examining the body of research around a given topic, it is necessary to sift through the data and information to separate stronger sources from weaker ones. The investigator must ascribe value to each piece of evidence and determine if it is appropriate for the question at hand. This step is wrought with implications not only for the researcher and the practitioner but also for educators and policy makers. In essence, this step holds the power to continue a current practice or change a clinician's care decisions.

The strength of a research study or other source of data is not based on the conclusion reached but rather on the extent to which appropriate methodology is used to conduct the study or generate the source. To minimize the influence of bias when accomplishing this goal, experts in evidence-based research recommend the use of a ranking system. Many examples of ranking systems are available from various sources such as governmental agencies, academic centers, and health systems. The type of data examined drives the style of the ranking system. Once a body of research has been ranked, the ranking labels then can be used by practitioners to make decisions.

Most existing ranking systems, or taxonomies, are designed according to type of research design (ie, quantitative or qualitative studies). In general, the Agency for Healthcare Research and Quality recommends that assessing the strength of a body of evidence should include 3 domains[32]:

1. *Quality:* The extent to which a study's design, conduct, and analysis has minimized selection, measurement, and confounding biases (internal validity)
2. *Quantity:* The number of studies that have evaluated the question, overall sample size across studies, magnitude of the treatment effect, and strength from causality assessment, such as relative risk or odds ratio
3. *Consistency:* Whether investigations with both similar and different study designs report similar findings (requires numerous studies)

In general, most evidence ranking and grading systems used in today's literature will use 1 of 3 coding systems. These coding systems may be letters, numbers, or a combination of letters and numbers (eg, 1a or IIb). The difficulties posed by these coding systems are that they are often not universally reproducible and must be adapted based on the question at hand and the types of literature that will answer the question at hand. An example of an evidence ranking methodology is provided in the Appendix at the end of this chapter.[33]

Critical appraisal of the quantitative literature requires addressing questions such as the following:

- Are the results of the study valid?
- Are the results reliable?
- Will the results apply to this patient population?

The postmodern paradigm associated with qualitative research has yielded many evaluative techniques and criteria. The evolution of these criteria are exemplified in the seminal writings of Guba and Lincoln,[34] among others.[35-40] Although no single method is "right," a trustworthy qualitative work includes—but is not limited to—assessment of such concepts as credibility (eg, accuracy of researcher actions), transferability (ie, results meaningful to other populations), dependability (eg, under similar circumstances another researcher would reach the same conclusions), and confirmability (eg, conclusions rooted in data).

Tools have been developed to assess documents such as guidelines (eg, the Appraisal of Guidelines Research and Evaluation [AGREE] instrument), randomized controlled trial reports (eg, Consolidated Standards of Reporting Trials [CONSORT], and meta-analyses of randomized controlled trials (eg, Quality of Reporting of Meta-analyses [QUORUM]. These tools were developed to assist the practitioner in evaluating the quality of that particular piece of evidence (eg, guideline).

A Note About Rigor

The rigor of a research study refers to the extent that error or bias has been minimized. Quantitative and qualitative research have different methods of assessing rigor because the 2 approaches have different philosophical underpinnings, methods of data collection, and techniques for analysis. To assess the rigor of all studies (quantitative, qualitative, or mixed methods) using the same ranking system will overlook the variation among these research methods, and it risks the erroneous evaluation of the studies as deficient. To that end, many experts propose multiple frameworks for evaluating research, based on the nature of the research itself.

Relationship Between Evidence-Based Practice and Ethics

Most nurses associate ethics with clinical nursing practice. The ethical dilemmas of modern nursing practice include the use of genetic information, distribution of healthcare resources, application or refusal of advanced technology, and safeguarding confidential information. But ethics extends to research and EBP as well. The principles of autonomy, beneficence, nonmaleficence, justice, veracity, and fidelity frame the duties that nurses have to patients in implementing a decision-making process.

Every decision made in nursing involves risk. Some decisions that aim to be beneficial are instead actually harmful. Certainly, some decisions involve inconsequential risks; others, however, may affect quality of life. A thoughtless conversation, inconsiderate approach, or negative comment may invoke psychological or emotional hurt. A wrong decision that involves pharmacology, timing, or an invasive procedure may lead to suffering, pain, or even death. These all serve as examples that counter the principles of nonmaleficence and beneficence. Patients also have a right to expect that their healthcare providers are competent, that they disclose the facts behind their care choices, and that they are efficient and cost-effective in their care. Not doing so contradicts the principles of fidelity, veracity, and autonomy.

Nurses who engage in decision making without adequate evidence are operating in a state of ignorance, basing interactions, treatments, and practices on no facts or false information. Nurses have a moral imperative, therefore, to use evidence to support their care decisions. If evidence is lacking, nurses have a duty to collect and share evidence. It is simply unethical for a nurse to base clinical decisions on false assumptions or inaccurate knowledge.

Other ethical questions are associated with the use of research and the implementation of an EBP approach. Are there adequate safeguards to protect individual patient information when sharing case reports and small sample studies? How will evidence be used and who will benefit? For example, a policy-making group could be enticed to use weak evidence to support a decision that decreases healthcare costs at the expense of improved patient outcomes for a small patient population. A pharmaceutical company could base a marketing strategy on a weak study that leads providers and patients to make choices based on false assumptions. These examples require consideration of the ethical principle of justice as the rights of an individual or group are balanced against the rights of another individual or group. And lastly, the temptation exists for practitioners to apply the steps of EBP as a formula for resolving ethical dilemmas. Use of recipes or algorithms alone cannot replace the thoughtful, situation-specific debate of ethical principles by bioethics committees and similar groups. To do so would violate the spirit of considering the individual patient's needs and practitioner's expertise that is germane to high-quality healthcare decision making.

Summary

The discourse regarding the risks and benefits of employing an EBP process for decision making in any healthcare specialty, including nurse anesthesia, is bound to continue as long as the process exists. Just as the scientific method has evolved since its inception in the 16th century, the EBP model will evolve and will continually be refined. No professional should embrace the process because it is the popular trend in healthcare. Instead, the conscious decision to subscribe to the process should be made because it is in the best interests of the patients for whom they care. The real challenge for nurse anesthetists who practice evidence-based nurse anesthesia will be in embracing multiple ways of knowing and synthesizing the best evidence with clinical judgment and honoring the singularity of each patient entrusted to their care.

Appendix 6.1. Oxford Centre for Evidence-Based Medicine Levels of Evidence (May 2001)[33]

Level	Therapy/prevention, etiology/harm	Prognosis	Diagnosis	Differential diagnosis/symptom prevalence study	Economic and decision analyses
1a	SR (with homogeneity[a]) of RCTs	SR (with homogeneity[a]) of inception cohort studies; CDR[b] validated in different populations	SR (with homogeneity[a]) of level 1 diagnostic studies; CDR[b] with 1b studies from different clinical centers	SR (with homogeneity[a]) of prospective cohort studies	SR (with homogeneity[a]) of level 1 economic studies
1b	Individual RCT (with narrow confidence interval[c])	Individual inception cohort study with >80% follow-up; CDR[b] validated in a single population	Validating[d] cohort study with good[e] reference standards; or CDR[b] tested within 1 clinical center	Prospective cohort study with good follow-up[f]	Analysis based on clinically sensible costs or alternatives; SRs of the evidence; and including multiway sensitivity analyses
1c	All or none[g]	All or none case series	Absolute SpPins and SnNouts[h]	All or none case series	Absolute better-value or worse-value analyses[i]
2a	SR (with homogeneity[a]) of cohort studies	SR (with homogeneity[a]) of either retrospective cohort studies or untreated control groups in RCTs	SR (with homogeneity[a]) of level >2 diagnostic studies	SR (with homogeneity[a]) of level 2b and better studies	SR (with homogeneity[a]) of level >2 economic studies
2b	Individual cohort study (including low-quality RCT; eg, <80% follow-up)	Retrospective cohort study or follow-up of untreated control patients in an RCT; derivation of CDR[b] or validated on split-sample[j] only	Exploratory[d] cohort study with good[e] reference standards; CDR[b] after derivation, or validated only on split-sample[j] or databases	Retrospective cohort study, or poor follow-up	Analysis based on clinically sensible costs or alternatives; limited review(s) of the evidence, or single studies; and including multiway sensitivity analyses
2c	"Outcomes" research; ecological studies	"Outcomes" research		Ecological studies	Audit or outcomes research
3a	SR (with homogeneity[a]) of case-control studies		SR (with homogeneity[a]) of level 3b and better studies	SR (with homogeneity[a]) of level 3b and better studies	SR (with homogeneity[a]) of level 3b and better studies
3b	Individual case-control study		Nonconsecutive study, or without consistently applied reference standards	Nonconsecutive cohort study, or very limited population	Analysis based on limited alternatives or costs, poor-quality estimates of data, but including sensitivity analyses incorporating clinically sensible variations
4	Case-series (and poor-quality cohort and case-control studies[k])	Case-series (and poor-quality prognostic cohort studies[l])	Case-control study, poor or non-independent reference standard	Case-series or superceded reference standards	Analysis with no sensitivity analysis
5	Expert opinion without explicit critical appraisal, or based on physiology, bench research, or "first principles"	Expert opinion without explicit critical appraisal, or based on physiology, bench research, or "first principles"	Expert opinion without explicit critical appraisal, or based on physiology, bench research, or "first principles"	Expert opinion without explicit critical appraisal, or based on physiology, bench research, or "first principles"	Expert opinion without explicit critical appraisal, or based on economic theory or "first principles"

Grades of Recommendation[m]

A	Consistent level 1 studies
B	Consistent level 2 or 3 studies or extrapolations from level 1 studies
C	Level 4 studies or extrapolations from level 2 or 3 studies
D	Level 5 evidence or troublingly inconsistent or inconclusive studies of any level

(Reprinted with permission from the Centre for Evidence-Based Medicine, Oxford, England.)

SR indicates systematic review; RCT, randomized clinical trial; CDR, clinical decision rule; CI, confidence interval.

[a] By homogeneity, we mean a systematic review that is free of worrisome variations (heterogeneity) in the directions and degrees of results between individual studies. Not all systematic reviews with statistically significant heterogeneity need be worrisome, and not all worrisome heterogeneity need be statistically significant. Studies displaying worrisome heterogeneity should be tagged with a "−" at the end of their designated level.

[b] A CDR is an algorithm or scoring system that leads to a prognostic estimation or a diagnostic category.

[c] See note [b] for advice on how to understand, rate, and use trials or other studies with wide confidence intervals.

[d] Validating studies test the quality of a specific diagnostic test, based on prior evidence. An exploratory study collects information and trawls the data (eg, using a regression analysis) to find which factors are significant.

[e] Good reference standards are independent of the test, and applied blindly or objectively applied to all patients. Poor reference standards are haphazardly applied, but still independent of the test. Use of a nonindependent reference standard (where the test is included in the reference, or where the testing affects the reference) implies a level 4 study.

[f] Good follow-up in a differential diagnosis study is >80%, with adequate time for alternative diagnoses to emerge (eg, 1-6 months for acute, 1-5 years for chronic).

[g] Met when all patients died before the prescription (Rx) became available, but some now survive on it; or when some patients died before the Rx became available, but none now die on it.

[h] An "Absolute SpPin" is a diagnostic finding whose Specificity is so high that a Positive result rules in the diagnosis. An "Absolute SnNout" is a diagnostic finding whose Sensitivity is so high that a Negative result rules out the diagnosis.

[i] Better-value treatments are clearly as good, but cheaper, or better at the same or reduced cost. Worse-value treatments are as good and more expensive, or worse and equally or more expensive.

[j] Split-sample validation is achieved by collecting all the information in a single tranche, then artificially dividing this into "derivation" and "validation" samples.

[k] By poor-quality cohort study, we mean one that failed to clearly define comparison groups and/or failed to measure exposures and outcomes in the same (preferably blinded), objective way in both exposed and nonexposed individuals and/or failed to identify or appropriately control known confounders and/or failed to carry out a sufficiently long and complete follow-up of patients. By poor-quality case-control study, we mean one that failed to clearly define comparison groups and/or failed to measure exposures and outcomes in the same (preferably blinded), objective way in both cases and controls and/or failed to identify or appropriately control known confounders.

[l] By poor-quality prognostic cohort study, we mean one in which sampling was biased in favor of patients who already had the target outcome, or the measurement of outcomes was accomplished in <80% of study patients, or outcomes were determined in an unblinded, nonobjective way, or there was no correction for confounding factors.

[m] Extrapolations are where data are used in a situation that has potentially clinically important differences from the original study situation.

Source: Bob Phillips, Chris Ball, Dave Sackett, Doug Badenoch, Sharon Straus, Brian Haynes, and Martin Dawes, November 1998.

References

1. Kohn LT, Corrigan JM, Donaldson MS. To err is human: building a safer health system [electronic version]. National Academies Press website; 2000. http://www.nap.edu/catalog/9728.html. Accessed June 20, 2005.

2. Greiner AC, Knebel E, eds. Health professions education: a bridge to quality [electronic version]. National Academies Press website; 2003. http://www.nap.edu/books/0309087236/html. Accessed June 20, 2005.

3. Alper BS, Hand JA, Elliott SG, et al. How much effort is needed to keep up with the literature relevant for primary care? *J Med Libr Assoc.* 2004;92(4):429-437.

4. Choudry NK, Fletcher RH, Soumerai SB. Systematic review: the relationship between clinical experience and quality of health care. *Ann Intern Med.* 2005;142(4):260-273.

5. Heater BS, Becker AM, Olson RK. Nursing interventions and patient outcomes: a meta-analysis of studies. *Nurs Res.* 1988;37(5):303-307.

6. Lysaght RM, Altschuld JW. Beyond initial certification: the assessment and maintenance of competency in professions. *Eval Program Plan.* 2000;23:95-104.

7. Lundgren BS, Houseman CA. Continuing competence in selected health care professions. *J Allied Health.* 2002;31(4):232-240.

8. Cochrane A. *Effectiveness and Efficiency: Reflections on Health Services.* London, England. Nuffield Provincial Hospital Trust; 1972.

9. Sackett D, Richardson WS, Rosenberg W, Haynes RB. *Evidence-Based Medicine: How to Practice and Teach EBM.* New York, NY: Churchill Livingstone; 1997.

10. Sackett DL, Straus SE, Richardson WS, Rosenberg W, Haynes RB. *Evidence-based Medicine.* Edinburgh, Scotland: Churchill Livingstone; 2000.

11. Evidence-based nursing position statement. Sigma Theta Tau International Honor Society for Nursing website. Revised July 6, 2005. http://www.nursingsociety.org/aboutus/PositionPapers/Pages/EBN_positionpaper.aspx. Accessed March 31, 2009.

12. Pravikoff DS, Tanner AB, Pierce ST. Readiness of US nurses for evidence-based practice. *Am J Nurs.* 2005;105(9):40-51.

13. Nightingale F. *Notes on Hospitals.* London, England. Parker and Son; 1859.

14. Cohen IB. Florence Nightingale. *Sci Am.* 1984;250:128-133.

15. Gerrish K, Ashworth P, Lacey A, et al. Factors influencing the development of evidence-based practice: a research tool. *J Adv Nurs.* 2006;57(3):328-338.

16. Fink R, Thompson CJ, Bonnes D. Overcoming barriers and promoting the use of research in practice. *J Nurs Adm.* 2005;35(3):121-129.

17. Olade R. Evidence-based practice and research utilization activities among rural nurses. *J Nurs Scholarsh.* 2004;36(3):220-225.

18. McKenna HP, Ashton S, Keeney S. Barriers to evidence-based practice in primary care. *J Adv Nurs.* 2004;45(2):178-189.

19. Wyszewianski L, Green LA. Strategies for changing clinicians' practice patterns: a new perspective. *J Fam Pract.* 2000;49(5):461-464.

20. Reed PG, Lawrence LA. A paradigm for the production of practice-based knowledge. *J Nurs Manage.* 2008;16(4):422-432.

21. Holmes D, Murray SJ, Perron A, McCabe J. Nursing practice guidelines: reflecting on the obscene rise of the void. *J Nurs Manage.* 2008;16(4):394-403.

22. Holmes D, Murray SJ, Perron A, Rail G. Deconstructing the evidence-based discourse in health sciences: truth, power and fascism. *Int J Evidence-based Health Care.* 2006;4:180-186.

23. Hudson K, Duke G, Haas B, Varnell G. Navigating the evidence-based practice maze. *J Nurs Manage.* 2008;16(4):409-416.

24. Windish DM, Huot SJ, Green ML. Medicine residents' understanding of the biostatistics and results in the medical literature. *JAMA.* 2007;298(9):1010-1022.

25. Fineout-Overholt E, Melnyk BM, Schultz A. Transforming health care from the inside out: advancing evidence-based practice in the 21st century. *J Prof Nurs.* 2005;21(6):335-344.

26. Dearing JW. Evolution of diffusion and dissemination theory. *J Public Health Manage Pract.* 2008;14(2):99-108.

27. Rogers EM. *Diffusion of Innovations.* 5th ed. New York, NY: Free Press; 2003.

28. Balas EA, Boren SA. *Managing Clinical Knowledge for Healthcare Improvements: Yearbook of Medical Informatics.* Bethesda, MD: National Library of Medicine; 2000.

29. Rabin BA, Brownson RC, Haire-Joshu D, Kreuter MW, Weaver NL. A glossary for dissemination and implementation research in health. *J Public Health Manage Pract.* 2008;14(2):117-123.

30. Davies BL. Sources and models for moving research evidence into clinical practice. *J Obstet Gynecol Neonatal Nurs.* 2002;31(5):558-562.

31. Melnyk BM, Fineout-Overholt E. *Evidence-Based Practice in Nursing and Healthcare: A Guide to Best Practice.* Philadelphia, PA: Lippincott Williams & Wilkins; 2005.

32. West S, King V, Carey TS, et al. *Systems to Rate the Strength of Scientific Evidence.* Rockville, MD: Agency for Healthcare Research and Quality; 2002. Evidence Report/Technology Assessment 47.

33. Welcome to CEMB. Centre for Evidence-Based Medicine website. May 2001. http://www.cebm.net/?0=1025/?0=1025. Accessed July 2, 2008.

34. Guba EG, Lincoln YS. *Effective Evaluation: Improving the Usefulness of Evaluation Results Through Responsive and Naturalistic Approaches.* San Francisco, CA: Jossey-Boss; 1981.

35. Lincoln YS. Emerging criteria for quality in qualitative and interpretive research. *Qualitative Inquiry.* 1995;1:275-289.

36. Lincoln YS, Guba EG. Paradigmatic controversies, contradictions, and emerging confluences. In: Denzin NK, Lincoln YS, eds. *The Landscape of Qualitative Research.* 2nd ed. Thousand Oaks, MI: Sage; 2003:253-291.

37. Rolfe G. Validity, trustworthiness and rigour: quality and the idea of qualitative research. *J Adv Nurs.* 2006;53(3):304-310.

38. Sandelowski M. The problem of rigor in qualitative research. *Adv Nurs Sci.* 1986;8(3):27-37.

39. Sandelowski M. In response to: deWitt L, Ploeg J. Critical appraisal of rigor in interpretive phenomenological nursing research. *J Adv Nurs.* 2006;55(5):643-645.

40. Schwandt TA. Farewell to criteriology. *Qual Inquiry.* 1996;2:58-72.

Chapter 7

Medicare as a Second Language: Policy and Payment Issues for CRNAs and Educators

Pamela K. Blackwell, JD

Key Points

- Medicare has a direct impact on Certified Registered Nurse Anesthetists' payment and on the environment in which they practice.

- Specific payment and policy terms, rules, and regulations are used by Medicare to regulate anesthesia payment and practice.

- Nurse anesthesia educators and student nurse anesthetists should have the Medicare knowledge necessary to better advocate for themselves, their profession, and their patients at the federal, state, and local levels.

- Medicare pays Certified Registered Nurse Anesthetists for anesthesia services using the anesthesia conversion factor, the anesthesia payment formula, and various payment models, including medically directed and nonmedically directed anesthesia services, the Medicare Rural Pass-Through Program for anesthesia, and other services.

- Nurse anesthesia educators, student nurse anesthetists, and Certified Registered Nurse Anesthetists should be able to differentiate between the Medicare Part A physician supervision requirement and billing for Medicare Part B medically directed and nonmedically directed anesthesia services.

- Nurse anesthesia educators and student nurse anesthetists should know how to bill Medicare for teaching student nurse anesthetists how to provide anesthesia and other services.

Key points continue on page 110.

- Certified Registered Nurse Anesthetists, nurse anesthesia program educators, and student nurse anesthetists must play an active role in developing quality anesthesia measures for pay-for performance programs.

- Learning to "speak Medicare" will provide nurse anesthesia educators with the knowledge necessary to prepare student nurse anesthetists to better address the practice management and business aspects of anesthesia practice related to Medicare.

Disclaimer

The content of this chapter is intended as background information to address questions you may have. It should in no way be construed as legal advice.

Introduction

Learning a new language can be an intimidating, frustrating, confusing, and humbling experience. Travelers quickly learn that not understanding the language can leave them at a substantial disadvantage. Without knowing the local lingo you are unable to communicate who you are, what you need, and where you want to go, or learn how much it will cost to get there. The same can be said of healthcare professionals who find themselves struggling to make their way through the uneven and treacherous terrain of anesthesia reimbursement without fluency in Medicare.

Medicare is the single largest payer of healthcare services, so it is wise for all healthcare professionals, including Certified Registered Nurse Anesthetists (CRNAs), to learn Medicare as a second language. It is to the advantage of CRNAs to learn to speak Medicare early, when they are in nurse anesthesia educational programs, so they will be prepared to handle the practice management and business aspects of anesthesia.

How is Medicare like a second language? All languages have vocabulary words and Medicare's vocabulary comes in the form of acronyms (eg, CMS, SGR, CPT). Medicare has formulas that determine how CRNAs are paid for their services, just as languages have formulas to conjugate verbs. Medicare also includes legal language similar to those words in all languages that have distinct meanings depending on the context in which they are used. Finally, as with all languages, learning Medicare is a process that takes patience and practice and the rewards of mastering it are great. Professionals who "speak Medicare" will have a greater understanding of the healthcare system and greater freedom and ability to advocate for themselves, their profession, their patients, and the students they teach in the clinical setting.

This chapter provides the vocabulary and instruction to start you on your way to speaking Medicare. It is organized according to a series of frequently asked questions posed by your fellow CRNAs, student nurse anesthetists, hospital administrators, faculty, and other healthcare providers.

Frequently Asked Questions

Have You Had Your Medicare Latte Today?
How Big Is the Medicare Program?

In 2006, approximately $2.17 trillion was spent on healthcare in the United States, which is approximately 16% of the US gross domestic product (GDP).[1] Close to half of US health expenditures are funded by taxpayer dollars and are paid by public sources such as Medicare, Medicaid, and various state and local programs. Medicare costs equate to 19% of the US budget, totaling $420 billion per year. This is equivalent to every person in the United States contributing $1,375 per year to Medicare.[2] In everyday terms this is equal to every person in the United States purchasing 508 coffee lattes per year, 1.3 lattes per person every day.[2] If you add in Medicaid expenditures, the per-person contribution increases to $2,458 per year. Compared with 2004, Americans are now spending $733 more per person for Medicare and Medicaid (Figure 7.1).

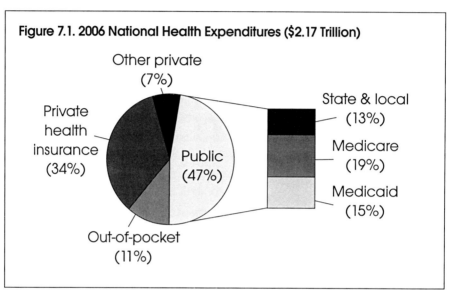

Figure 7.1. 2006 National Health Expenditures ($2.17 Trillion)

(Adapted from Centers for Medicare & Medicaid Services website.)

Why Should Medicare Matter to Me as a CRNA?

Many graduate nurse anesthetists beginning their careers as CRNAs find that the majority of their patients are Medicare beneficiaries. According to a 2007 Government Accountability Office study, CRNAs tend to be the predominant anesthesia providers in healthcare facilities where there are more Medicare beneficiaries.[4] This means that for many CRNAs, a substantial portion of their paycheck is paid by Medicare. Nurse anesthetists are also the predominant anesthesia providers in veterans hospitals and in the US Armed Forces.

The CRNAs of tomorrow will work in a healthcare system burdened by increasing demands for healthcare services but with fewer financial resources to meet those demands. Medicare and Medicaid face major financial challenges that will likely have an impact on the amount of funding available to pay for anesthesia services. The exponential growth in healthcare costs as well as the growth in the number of Medicare beneficiaries as the Baby Boomer generation reaches retirement will render ineffective many efforts to curb costs and will increase pressure to find ways to contain expenditures. These cost increases make CRNAs and all healthcare providers vulnerable to Medicare reimbursement cuts.

What is the Sustainable Growth Rate and How Does it Determine How CRNAs Are Paid for Medicare Services?

For many years, physicians and other clinicians have faced cuts in Medicare reimbursement under the physician fee schedule (PFS) as a result of the sustainable growth rate (SGR) formula. Developed by Congress and implemented by Medicare, the SGR is used to contain annual healthcare spending for provider services. One of the problems with the SGR is that it does not accurately account for the real cost of healthcare services in that changes in annual Medicare spending are tied to the GDP growth rather than healthcare growth and inflation. From 2007 to 2017, GDP growth is estimated at approximately 4.8% per year, but healthcare inflation is estimated to be 6.7%.[3] In recent years, when faced with having to cut provider reimbursement, Congress decided to override the SGR formula and permit spending above the targeted amount. Providers, including CRNAs, have experienced substantial payment cuts, but not as large as those they would have experienced if Congress had not acted to reduce the amount of the annual cuts called for by law. For example, in 2008, had Congress not acted, Medicare Part B providers would have experienced a 10% cut in payments rather than remaining at approximately the 2007 payment level.[5] In the future, all Medicare Part B providers, including CRNAs, face a 20% cut in their payments in 2010 and an additional 5% each year for many years thereafter to make up for overspending that occurred from 2004 to the present.[6] Over time, this could amount to an approximate reduction in anesthesia payments of 35% by 2012.

Many CRNAs and other providers remain concerned that cuts in reimbursement will result in a reduction in patients' access to services. Despite the recent reimbursement cuts, the Medicare Payment Advisory Commission (MedPAC), which advises Congress on Medicare issues, has found that Medicare beneficiaries generally have appropriate access to provider services despite reimbursement cuts in recent years. The commission has also found that the number of providers who become and remain participating Medicare practitioners continues to increase[7]; however, MedPAC has expressed concerns that consecutive annual cuts could, over time, threaten beneficiary access to provider services.[7]

With guidance from the American Association of Nurse Anesthetists (AANA) Federal Government Affairs Office in Washington, DC, CRNAs have played a crucial role in encouraging Congress to override the SGR cuts by building professional relationships with their US senators and representatives over many years.

CRNAs and Direct Medicare Part B Payment

Since 1986, under Medicare Part B, CRNAs can bill Medicare directly for their anesthesia services and can bill and be paid for 100% of the PFS amount for their services just as an anesthesiologist can.[8] Physician supervision of CRNAs, as under Medicare Part A, is not a requirement for CRNAs to bill and be paid directly by Medicare for their services. Nurse anesthetists do not have to work with an anesthesiologist under Medicare Part B medical direction payment rules to bill and be paid directly by Medicare for their services. In all states, CRNAs can bill Medicare directly for providing *nonmedically directed* services.

What Is the Anesthesia Payment Formula?

The anesthesia payment formula includes 3 components: base units, time, and the anesthesia conversion factor. This formula is used by Medicare to determine how much Medicare will pay CRNAs and anesthesiologists for their anesthesia services.

Base units are the value of the service measured in units based on the complexity of the service. A more complex service has higher base units than a less complex service.

Time is the period of time in which the anesthesia provider was providing the patient anesthesia services, including the time the anesthesia provider spent monitoring a patient during surgery. The time component is unique to anesthesia services and is based on the idea that the surgeon and not the anesthesia provider controls the length of the surgical case. When CRNAs or other healthcare professionals provide services other than anesthesia, such as analgesia and pain management, time is not a component of their payment formula. Healthcare professionals including CRNAs who provide nonanesthesia-related services also use a different conversion factor than the anesthesia conversion factor. The nonanesthesia-related payment formula includes only base units and a conversion factor.

The *anesthesia conversion factor* converts the value of the anesthesia provider's services into a dollar amount. The anesthesia conversion factor varies, depending on the SGR for that year as well as on the geographic area in which a provider practices. For instance, in an area where wages are higher, the conversion factor would also be higher to better correlate with the wages and cost of living in that area. Likewise, where the wages are lower, the conversion factor is lower. The formulas are shown in Table 7.1.

Table 7.1. The Anesthesia Conversion Factor

Nonmedically directed service

The CRNA can bill for $202.50—100% of the PFS.

10 units (base units + time) × $20.25 = $202.50

Medically directed service

The CRNA and anesthesiologist can each bill for $101.25—50% of the PFS.

10 units (base units + time) × $10.13 = $101.25

(2008 national average anesthesia conversion factor.)

What Is the Difference Between Medical Direction and Physician Supervision of CRNAs?

Medical Direction Under Medicare Part B

The 7 medical direction steps are listed in the Code of Federal Regulations (Table 7.2).[9] Medically directed anesthesia services specify the activities that a medically

Table 7.2. The 7 Requirements to Bill for Medical Direction

1. Perform a preanesthetic examination and evaluation.

2. Prescribe the anesthesia plan.

3. Personally participate in the most demanding aspects of the anesthesia plan including, if applicable, induction and emergence.

4. Ensure that any procedures in the anesthesia plan that he or she does not perform are performed by a qualified individual as defined in operating instructions.

5. Monitor the course of anesthesia administration at frequent intervals.

6. Remain physically present and available for immediate diagnosis and treatment of emergencies.

7. Provide indicated postanesthesia care.

(Adapted with permission from the Code of Federal Regulations.[9])

directing physician must perform to be paid for anesthesia services. The physician *must* perform all 7 medical direction steps (and document that he or she has performed all 7 medical direction steps) to be eligible to bill for medical direction. A physician can medically direct up to 4 concurrent anesthesia cases. According to Medicare, the medical direction requirements are merely payment requirements for anesthesiologists and are not quality-of-care standards.[10]

For a medically directed service in which a CRNA and anesthesiologist are working together, the CRNA may bill Medicare directly for 50% of the PFS amount for the service and the anesthesiologist can bill Medicare directly for the other 50% of the PFS amount for the service. Figure 7.2 and Figure 7.3 illustrate medical direction ratios. For a medically directed service, the person billing for the anesthesia service uses the QX, QY, or QK modifier on the CMS 1500 claims form to denote to Medicare that the service was medically directed and that 50% of the PFS can be billed for the CRNA and 50% of the PFS can be billed to the anesthesiologist. The Q modifiers are used to denote the type of anesthesia provider who provided the anesthesia service.

For each patient, the physician must follow the 7 medical direction steps. The idea of medical direction was initially introduced in the Tax Equity and Fiscal Responsibility Act of 1982 (TEFRA), which became law. Its provisions for medical direction are found under the Social Security Act.[11] The actual medical direction steps were developed by the Health Care Financing Administration, which is now the Centers for Medicare & Medicaid Services (CMS), with input from the AANA and the American Society of Anesthesiologists. The medical direction steps were created to address the potential for fraudulent billing by anesthesiologists for multiple concurrent cases.[12] The TEFRA indicated a need to ensure that anesthesiologists demonstrate that they provided certain services as a part of a given anesthetic case to qualify for payment.[12]

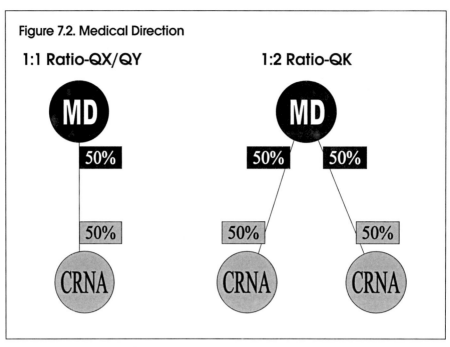

Figure 7.2. Medical Direction

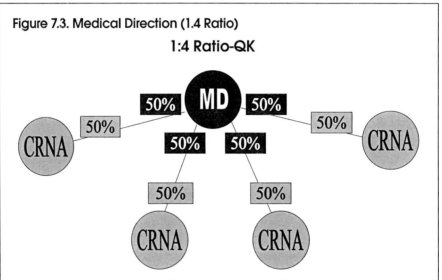

Figure 7.3. Medical Direction (1.4 Ratio)

Nonmedical Direction Under Medicare Part B

Under Medicare Part B, a *nonmedically directed* service is one in which the CRNA provides the anesthesia service. For nonmedically directed cases, the CRNA can bill the case at 100% of the PFS and the anesthesiologist cannot bill for any part of the case. For nonmedically directed cases, the QZ modifier is used, which signifies that the case was done by a "CRNA without medical direction by a physician."[13] When a CRNA and anesthesiologist are working together and the anesthesiologist does not complete all 7 medical direction steps, the case should then be billed as nonmedically directed (Figure 7.4).

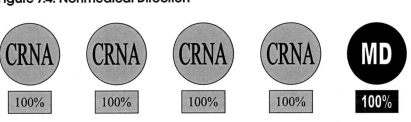

Figure 7.4. Nonmedical Direction

CRNA 100% CRNA 100% CRNA 100% CRNA 100% MD 100%

- All CRNAs are nonmedically directed.
- In nonmedical direction the anesthesiologist is personally performing the case. The anesthesiologist is not medically directing.
- A nonmedically directed CRNA can bill Medicare directly for 100% of the PFS for the CRNA's service.
- 5 concurrent cases = 500% payment
- CRNAs in all states can bill as nonmedically directed.

Personal Performance Under Medicare Part B

A *personally performed* service is one in which the anesthesiologist performed the entire anesthesia service alone. For a personally performed service, the *AA* modifier is used.[14]

Medical Supervision Under Medicare Part B

Medical supervision occurs when the physician/anesthesiologist medically supervises more than 4 concurrent anesthesia cases.[14] Medical direction occurs when the physician is medically supervising 4 or fewer concurrent anesthesia cases. A physician/anesthesiologist is paid less per case for medically supervising than for medically directing. According to Medicare regulations, if the physician medically supervises more than 4 concurrent anesthesia cases, Medicare pays the physician only up to 4 base units per case multiplied by the anesthesia conversion factor (Figure 7.5). In medically directed cases, each case is typically worth more than 4 base units. Under medical supervision, CRNAs can still bill 50% of the full PFS value of the case just as they would if the CRNAs were medically directed. The Part B medical supervision model is generally not an optimal payment model because Medicare is paying less than 100% of the PFS for a case that is medically supervised. For a medically supervised service, the *AD* modifier is used.[13]

Supervision Under Medicare Part A

Federal law states that for a hospital, a critical access hospital, or ambulatory surgical center to participate in the Medicare program, a physician must supervise CRNAs unless a state chooses to opt out of the supervision requirement.[15,16] Supervision of CRNAs falls under Medicare Part A, Conditions of Participation and is not the same as medical direction, which falls under and is defined under Medicare Part B, Conditions of Payment. Supervision is not a payment requirement. According to

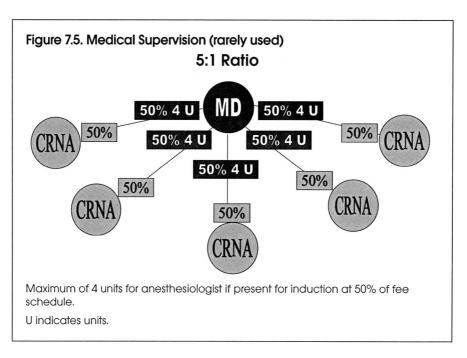

Figure 7.5. Medical Supervision (rarely used)
5:1 Ratio

Maximum of 4 units for anesthesiologist if present for induction at 50% of fee schedule.

U indicates units.

the CMS: "CRNAs may furnish the entire anesthesia service without medical direction, while still under the supervision of the operating surgeon. Payment rules for CRNAs as well as for physician anesthesiologists do not change as a result of this [supervision] rule."[17]

The Code of Federal Regulations clearly states who can provide anesthesia services and under what conditions they may provide these services.[15,16] A CRNA may provide anesthesia services when the CRNA is "under the supervision of the operating practitioner or anesthesiologist who is immediately available if needed." Therefore, supervision of CRNAs is not limited to only anesthesiologists. Under federal law, a CRNA can be supervised by either the operating practitioner or by an anesthesiologist. Operating practitioners may also include dentists or podiatrists, for example.

Currently, according to the Medicare Part A Conditions of Participation Surveyor Interpretive Guidelines,[18] effective April 2005, for hospitals and critical access hospitals, immediately available means that the supervising anesthesiologist or operating practitioner, as applicable, must be physically located within the operative suite or in the labor and delivery unit, prepared to immediately conduct hands-on intervention if needed, and not engaged in activities that could prevent the supervising practitioner from being able to immediately intervene and conduct hands-on interventions if needed. The operating practitioner is considered immediately available when he or she is conducting surgery on the patient. The CMS does not require a second operating practitioner whose function is to supervise the CRNA.

The surveyor interpretive guidelines are used by Medicare surveyors, and at varying degrees by the Joint Commission, state health departments, and other accrediting bodies, to determine whether a facility is complying with Medicare's rules and regulations. The interpretive guidelines are intended to provide clarification to healthcare professionals and facilities on how to comply with Medicare's rules and regulations. Although practice literature defines and differentiates between anesthesia and analgesia, Medicare regulations do not currently define these terms. This means that CRNAs, whether providing anesthesia services in preparation for a surgical procedure or providing an analgesic labor epidural, have to be supervised by a physician.[18]

The role of hospitals and providers in complying with Medicare Part A supervision is to demonstrate that the supervision has taken place. The hospital does this by developing a written policy customized to its facility that addresses how the hospital will comply with the supervision rules and by demonstrating that the hospital adheres to the rules it set up for itself. According to CMS staff, there are many ways for a hospital and other facilities to demonstrate compliance with Medicare's rules. For example, a hospital could develop a written policy that states that all of its surgeons can supervise CRNAs and that the hospital will demonstrate that supervision has taken place by including both the name of the surgeon and the CRNA on the patient's medical record. The key to demonstrating compliance with Medicare's rules is for the hospital to be organized in establishing and maintaining its policies and for the hospital to follow the rules that it sets for itself. The CMS, however, does not specify exactly how to comply and leaves the specifics to the hospital's discretion. A supervising operating practitioner or physician signature is not required by CMS for compliance. Lack of compliance by a hospital can lead to citations by CMS and risks the hospital's Medicare participation status, a coveted status for most hospitals.

What Is the State Supervision Opt-out?

Since the November 13, 2001 finding that a federal requirement of CRNA supervision is not necessary to ensure patient health and safety, Medicare allowed states to opt out of the operating practitioner supervision of CRNAs requirement entirely.[15,19] This regulation lists the steps a state must take for its hospitals to be exempt from complying with the supervision requirement.

To opt out, the governor must sign a letter to CMS requesting exemption from operating practitioner supervision of CRNAs. The letter must attest that he or she has consulted with the state boards of medicine and nursing about issues related to access to and the quality of anesthesia services in the state and has concluded that it is in the best interests of the state's citizens to opt out of the current physician supervision requirement, and that the opt-out is consistent with state law. The state's decision to opt out is effective upon CMS receiving the governor's letter requesting the opt-out. It is the equivalent of sending a postcard in that there are no additional appeals or approval processes once the letter stating that the state is opting out is received.

Which Are the Opt-out States?

To date, 15 states have opted out of the supervision requirement. Opt-out states include Alaska, California, Idaho, Iowa, Kansas, Minnesota, Montana, Nebraska,

New Hampshire, New Mexico, North Dakota, Oregon, South Dakota, Washington, and Wisconsin. Graduate nurse anesthetists who decided to practice in these states will not have to comply with the Medicare Part A supervision requirements.[20]

Are Surgeons Who Supervise CRNAs as Under Medicare Part A Liable for the Actions of CRNAs?

According to CMS, Medicare Part A supervision by an operating practitioner does not mean that the operating practitioner must have the same or any specific level of anesthesia training, education, and experience as CRNAs or anesthesiologists to be qualified to supervise CRNAs. Nor does supervision require that operating practitioners be specifically privileged by the hospital to supervise CRNAs.[18] Rather, supervision is a more general term. The principles that determine the liability of a surgeon for negligence associated with the anesthesia portion of a surgical case are the same whether the surgeon works with a CRNA or an anesthesiologist.[21] Certified Registered Nurse Anesthetists are required to carry malpractice insurance through their employer or individually, and CRNAs are individually responsible for the anesthesia services they provide.

Facilities, providers, and even CRNAs commonly confuse Part A supervision with Part B payment for medical direction. This confusion is apparent in the many facilities that require that the anesthesiologist play the duel but unnecessary role of Part A supervising practitioner while simultaneously attempting to bill Medicare Part B for medically directing CRNAs. These facilities have inaccurately concluded that CRNAs must be medically directed. Consequently, these facilities may incur the unnecessary costs of hiring an (or an additional) anesthesiologist whose salary is much greater than a CRNA's salary, the increased paperwork of complying with the Part B medical direction payment requirements, and the increased compliance risk of not adhering to the payment rules. Alternatively, a nonmedically directed model, which is allowed in all states and in which CRNAs or facilities can bill Medicare directly for 100% of the PFS, provides a facility with more scheduling flexibility and enhanced financial efficiency while still providing safe, high-quality anesthesia care for surgical cases at all levels of acuity. The differences between supervision and direction are highlighted in Table 7.3.

Table 7.3. Supervision vs Medical Direction

Supervision	Medical direction
Part A	**Part B**
Hospital participation	Individual practitioner payment
Physician supervision required unless state has opted out	Rules of payment
	Not safety rules
CRNAs in all states can bill as nonmedically directed.	CRNAs do **not** have to be medically directed to bill for services.

What Is the Safety Record for CRNAs?

Anesthesia patient safety outcomes are comparable among nurse anesthetists and anesthesiologists. Pine et al recently concluded: "The type of anesthesia provider does not affect inpatient surgical mortality."[22] In addition, based on recent claims data, although all provider premiums are increasing, CRNA premium increases have been the lowest in opt-out states (AANA Insurance Services staff, oral communication, January 2008).

Because premiums tend to increase when there have been claims made against a provider's malpractice insurance coverage, this suggests that anesthesia care by a CRNA who is not supervised by a physician is just as safe as the care provided by an anesthesiologist.

What Are Medicare's Anesthesia Teaching Payment Rules?

Medicare will only pay for anesthesia services that are delivered by a qualified anesthesia provider.[13,14,23] Although CRNAs and anesthesiologists are qualified providers, student nurse anesthetists, graduate nurse anesthetists, and medical anesthesiology residents are not deemed to be qualified anesthesia providers. Student nurse anesthetists, graduate nurse anesthetists, and anesthesiology residents cannot bill Medicare for providing anesthesia services; however, Medicare does pay for teaching student nurse anesthetists and residents how to provide anesthesia services. Medicare has developed anesthesia payment teaching rules for this purpose. The amount a teaching CRNA or anesthesiologist can bill Medicare for teaching a student nurse anesthetist or anesthesiology resident is likely to change in 2010 based on legislation passed in July 2008, the Medicare Improvements for Patients and Providers Act of 2008.[5]

To provide the growing number of student nurse anesthetists with ample opportunity to administer anesthesia for cases at all levels of acuity, it is important that any future changes to the anesthesia teaching rules be equitable for both teaching CRNAs and anesthesiologists, and that CRNAs play an active role in developing these rules. Nurse anesthetists, nurse anesthesia program directors, and student nurse anesthetists should continue to have a strong voice and to advocate at the federal level for equitable treatment in this and other payment and practice areas.

Medicare's Anesthesia Teaching Payment Rules

Medicare pays CRNAs and anesthesiologists for teaching student nurse anesthetists and residents how to provide anesthesia services. A CRNA can be paid for teaching student nurse anesthetists, and an anesthesiologist can be paid for teaching student nurse anesthetists and residents. Medicare does not pay student nurse anesthetists or residents for the anesthesia services they provide. Medicare does not pay graduates for the anesthesia services they provide. Not until graduate nurse anesthetists are certified and become enrolled as Medicare providers may they bill and be paid directly by Medicare for services.

Teaching CRNAs[23]

If a nonmedically directed CRNA is teaching 1 student nurse anesthetist, the CRNA can bill for 100% of the service if the CRNA remains continuously present for the entire procedure. If not continuously present, the CRNA can bill 50% of the service (Figure 7.6).

If the nonmedically directed CRNA is teaching 2 student nurse anesthetists, 1 in each of 2 rooms, the CRNA can bill for each of the 2 rooms using a discontinuous time (DCT) payment formula. Discontinous time is the time during which the CRNA was present with the student nurse anesthetist or face-to-face with the patient. The CRNA can bill only for the time in the room, and the CRNA must be present in each room with the student nurse anesthetist for preanesthesia and postanesthesia care. Discontinuous time can yield greater than 50% payment for each case. This ratio of 1 teaching CRNA to 2 student nurse anesthetists was derived by CMS from the AANA Council on Accreditation of Nurse Anesthesia Educational Programs and is referenced in CMS's regulation. This means that a teaching CRNA does not have to be in the same operating room as a student at all times. This allows students to learn to work with the autonomy and responsibility that they will have as CRNAs; however, the teaching CRNA should remain nearby and otherwise active in supervising the student (see Figure 7.6).

Payment formula: Base units + DCT × $20.25 (2008 national average anesthesia conversion factor).

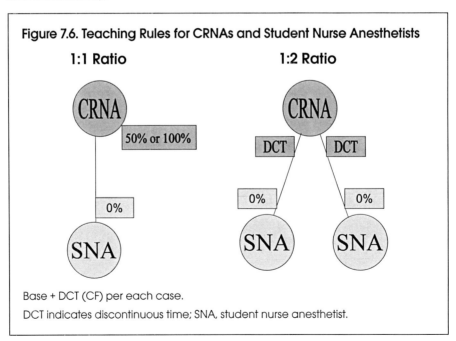

Figure 7.6. Teaching Rules for CRNAs and Student Nurse Anesthetists

Base + DCT (CF) per each case.

DCT indicates discontinuous time; SNA, student nurse anesthetist.

Teaching Anesthesiologists[14]

If an anesthesiologist is teaching 1 resident or 1 student nurse anesthetist, the anesthesiologist can bill for 100% of the service if he or she remains continuously present for the entire procedure. If not continuously present, the anesthesiologist can bill for only 50% of service (Figure 7.7 and Figure 7.8).

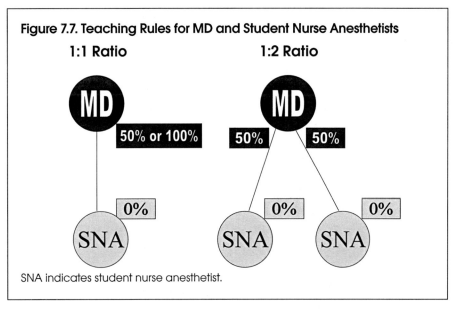

Figure 7.7. Teaching Rules for MD and Student Nurse Anesthetists

SNA indicates student nurse anesthetist.

If an anesthesiologist is teaching 2 student nurse anesthetists, 1 in each of 2 rooms, the anesthesiologist can bill 50% of each service provided in each room. This means that a teaching anesthesiologist does not have to be in the same operating room as a student at all times. This allows students to learn to work with the autonomy and responsibility that they will have as CRNAs; however, the

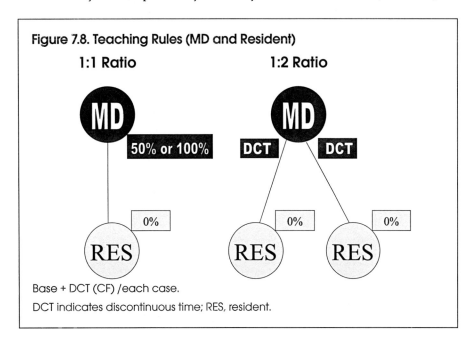

Figure 7.8. Teaching Rules (MD and Resident)

Base + DCT (CF) /each case.
DCT indicates discontinuous time; RES, resident.

teaching anesthesiologist should remain nearby and otherwise active in supervising the student. This also applies when an anesthesiologist is teaching anesthesiology residents.

If the anesthesiologist is teaching 2 residents, 1 in each of 2 rooms, the anesthesiologist can bill for each of the 2 rooms using the DCT payment formula. Discontinuous time is the time in which the anesthesiologist was present with the resident or face-to-face with the patient. The anesthesiologist can bill *only* for the time in the room, and he or she must be present in each room for preanesthesia and postanesthesia care. Discontinuous time can yield greater than 50% payment for each case (see Figure 7.7 and Figure 7.8).

Payment formula: Base units + DCT × $20.25 (2008 national average anesthesia conversion factor).

Teaching in a Medical Direction Model[14]

If the CRNA is medically directed while teaching a student nurse anesthetist, the CRNA can bill for 50% of the service and the anesthesiologist can bill for 50% of the service (medical direction) (Figure 7.9).

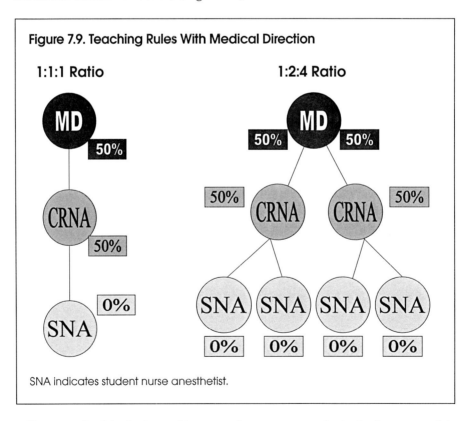

Figure 7.9. Teaching Rules With Medical Direction

SNA indicates student nurse anesthetist.

If an anesthesiologist is teaching a student nurse anesthetist in 1 room, and is supervising or medically directing a resident, intern, or CRNA in a second room, the anesthesiologist can bill 50% for teaching the student nurse anesthetist and 50% for teaching the resident or 50% for medically directing the CRNA (Figure 7.10). For all 1:2 ratio teaching rules models, see Figure 7.11.

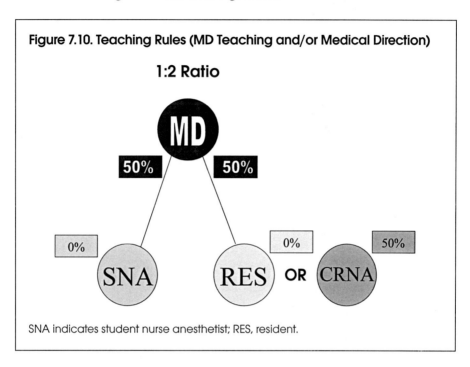

Figure 7.10. Teaching Rules (MD Teaching and/or Medical Direction)

SNA indicates student nurse anesthetist; RES, resident.

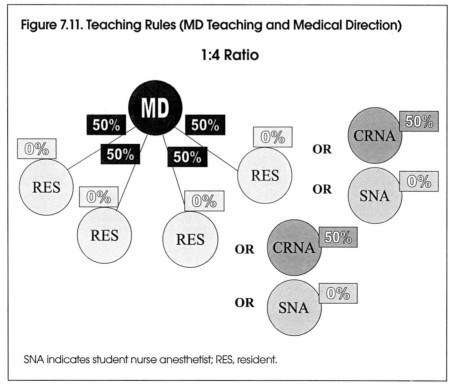

Figure 7.11. Teaching Rules (MD Teaching and Medical Direction)

SNA indicates student nurse anesthetist; RES, resident.

Billing Questions for Graduates and New CRNAs

Can a graduate nurse anesthetist bill Medicare for anesthesia services?

No.

Can anyone else (such as a CRNA, anesthesiologist, hospital, or anesthesia department) bill Medicare for the graduate's services?

No. A CRNA has billing rights and can therefore assign his or her billing rights to another entity. A graduate does not have billing rights, and therefore has no billing rights to assign to another provider. Attempting to bill Medicare for a graduate's services in this way could be considered fraudulent.

At what point can a nurse anesthetist bill Medicare directly for his or her services?

Once a new CRNA's enrollment application has been filed by Medicare, a CRNA can bill for services he or she provides 30 days prior to the enrollment application filing date.

Must a nurse anesthetist have his or her certification before receiving a Medicare national provider identifier (NPI) number?

Yes.

Is certification completion required to bill Medicare?

Yes.

A Medicare policy issued November 2008 and effective January 1, 2009 allows healthcare providers to be paid by the Medicare program for services delivered up to 30 days before the date of filing a new Medicare provider enrollment application.[24] Once a new CRNA's enrollment application has been filed by Medicare, the CRNA can bill for services he or she provided 30 days prior to the filing date. The new rule applies to both physicians and nonphysician providers such as CRNAs who would bill Medicare Part B for their services.

To file a Medicare provider enrollment application, most new CRNAs will be expected to provide the following with their applications: (1) documentation of certification from the Council on Certification of Nurse Anesthetists, (2) as applicable, a licensure certificate from the state board of nursing from the state in which the CRNA will be practicing, (3) a National Provider Identifier (NPI) (nurse anesthetists cannot obtain an NPI until they are certified),[11] (4) credentialing documents from the nurse anesthesia school from which they graduated, and (5) as applicable, employer credentialing documentation.

Certified Registered Nurse Anesthetists should be aware that although some states do not require a licensure certificate, other states and other credentialing bodies may take several weeks to provide a new CRNA with the licensing certificate or documentation that the CRNA must present to Medicare to enroll as a Medicare provider. Graduate nurse anesthetists or new CRNAs who are not yet Medicare providers can provide anesthesia services consistent with the laws and regulations of the state in which they are practicing. When working with graduates, especially for Medicare purposes, many facilities have chosen to institute separate policies for the appropriate oversight or supervision of graduates. Medicare holds facilities accountable for following the policies the facility establishes for itself. Many times private payers may have different rules that allow for graduates to bill for their services. Graduates and employers should check with the private payers to determine their payment rules.

The best advice for graduate nurse anesthetists is to take and pass the Certification Examination as soon as possible after graduation and to prepare their provider enrollment applications ahead of time, to the extent possible, so that the application is ready to send to Medicare as soon as they have their supporting application documentation. Graduate nurse anesthetists and new CRNAs are not revenue sources to their employers who bill Medicare until they are enrolled as Medicare providers.

Can CRNAs Be Paid for Inserting Lines, Pain Management, and Providing Other Medical and Surgical Services?

According to Medicare, CRNAs may bill Medicare for pain management, line insertion, and other medical and surgical services if CRNAs are allowed to furnish these services under state law.[13] The next step is to determine whether CRNAs in your state can provide these services, understanding that specific services may or may not be explicitly delineated in state law. Your state nurse anesthetists association and board of nursing may have more detailed information regarding CRNA scope of practice in your state.

Payment can be made for medical or surgical services furnished by nonmedically directed CRNAs if they are allowed to furnish these services under state law. These services may include the insertion of Swan-Ganz catheters and central venous pressure lines, pain management, emergency intubation, and the preanesthetic examination and evaluation of a patient who does not undergo surgery. Payment is determined under the PFS on the basis of the national PFS conversion factor, the geographic adjustment factor, and the resource-based relative value units for the medical or surgical service.

Can My Hospital Participate in Medicare's Rural Pass-Through Program?

Many graduate nurse anesthetists will begin and continue their careers working in a rural hospital. Rural hospitals commonly face a greater shortage of available healthcare providers to have on staff and a shortage of funding to provide surgical services to their communities. Nurse anesthetists are the sole anesthesia providers in most rural hospitals, affording these medical facilities obstetrical, surgical, trauma stabilization, and pain management capabilities that might not otherwise be available. One way critical access hospitals can better afford to provide anesthesia and surgical services is to participate in Medicare's rural pass-through program.[25]

Before 1983, a lump payment was given to hospitals by Medicare based on the diagnosis-related groups (DRGs) for all services provided to Medicare beneficiaries at the hospital. The hospital would receive the DRG payment through Medicare Part A and anesthesiologists could bill Medicare Part B individually for the anesthesia services. Nurse anesthesia services, however, were grouped into the DRG payment such that the payment for CRNA services came out of the total DRG payment provided to the hospital. Therefore, hospitals would receive less in DRG payments if they used CRNAs for anesthesia services. To resolve this inequity, Congress allowed facilities to be reimbursed for their CRNA expenses from the Medicare program over and above the DRG payment. If the hospital chooses to participate in the rural pass-through program, the CRNA and the hospital agree not to bill Medicare Part B for CRNA anesthesia services and instead include the costs of these CRNA services as they relate to the treatment of Medicare patients in the annual Medicare cost report. Medicare then pays the hospital a lump sum for CRNA services and related expenses during the next calendar year.

Currently, anesthesiologists are not eligible for pass-through funding. Therefore, anesthesiologists or the hospital must bill Medicare Part B for anesthesiologists' services.

The hospital includes provider salaries and the facility and equipment costs incurred in serving Medicare beneficiaries as a part of its Medicare cost report. The funding pass-through hospitals receive in reimbursement is calculated according to the total costs for the hospital, which are included in the Medicare cost report. Pass-through hospitals receive additional funding beyond their total costs as an incentive to continue to serve the Medicare population in rural areas. The hospitals can choose to use that funding in a variety of ways, from increasing salaries in order to keep providers at the hospital to improving facilities and equipment. The federal definition of rural vs urban areas appears in the Code of Federal Regulations.[26,27]

In addition to the lump payment from Medicare Part A, pass-through hospitals are also paid an additional amount specifically for the cost of CRNA services. The cost is calculated according to the PFS. Rather than being paid for CRNA services through Part B, the CRNA services are paid for through Part A pass-through funding. The hospital then pays the CRNA a salary (if the CRNA is a hospital employee) and/or the appropriate contracted amount for anesthesia services.

Pass-through facilities can keep their pass-through status when they bill other payers (non-Medicare payers) for CRNA services, regardless of whether the patient is a Medicare beneficiary or not, as long as neither the facility nor the CRNA bills Medicare Part B for the CRNA services.

The Code of Federal Regulations[28] lists the requirements a hospital or critical access hospital must fulfill to receive rural pass-through funding from Medicare Part A for CRNA anesthesia services. Appendix 7.1 at the end of the chapter presents the requirements as listed in the Code of Federal Regulations.[28] Nurse anesthetists should work with their hospital and local Medicare carrier to determine their hospital's eligibility to participate in the rural pass-through program.

Do Private Insurers Pay CRNAs for Anesthesia Services?

The vast majority of private health insurers do pay CRNAs the full PFS amount for their services and only a very few insurers do not pay. This, however, is not to suggest that payers will always pay CRNAs the same amount, because payers are highly motivated to cut costs.

Under federal law, private payers have wide discretion in determining which types of practitioners they will pay and how much they will pay each practitioner. A Medicare payer/carrier is required by law to pay a CRNA the same rate for the same service provided to a Medicare beneficiary as it would pay an anesthesiologist; however, private payers/insurers are not required to pay the same rate, nor are they required to include CRNAs as eligible providers for payment in all settings. The laws of the state in which CRNAs practice may say otherwise, so CRNAs should review what their state laws say about discrimination against providers who are not physicians,

At this time, the option remaining for CRNAs who find themselves being paid at a lesser rate or not being paid at all by private payers is to persuade the private payer otherwise, which can be a challenge. Arguments that demonstrate the safety, quality, and cost efficiency record of CRNAs, and Medicare's payment to CRNAs for the full PFS amount can be persuasive. Nurse anesthetists should be prepared to demonstrate to payers the value of CRNAs and their services.

Where Do I Go for Answers to Coding and Billing Questions?

What is the reimbursement and base unit amount for a certain service or procedure? Which code do I use? Does Medicare or do other payers pay for or cover a certain service or procedure? Specific coding questions such as these are typically best answered by a certified billing and coding expert or by your Medicare carrier. Some CRNAs bill for their services on their own, although most do not because of the complexity of billing and coding rules. Most CRNAs tend to assign their billing rights to their employer or to a billing and coding company.

Answers to coding questions can vary depending on the insurance carrier, whether Medicare or a private insurer. Answers to coding questions are also heavily dependent on the specific case in question and therefore are usually answered on a case-by-case basis. It is imperative that CRNAs, like all providers, bill for their services correctly. Because of the complexity and the expansive and technical nature of coding for services and procedures, as well as the importance of correct billing, these questions are best answered by certified billing and coding experts.

New CRNAs should either learn how to bill accurately for their services or hire a billing and coding expert experienced in billing for anesthesia services. Whether CRNAs are doing the billing or have hired someone to bill for them, CRNAs are ultimately responsible for the payment claims made on their behalf.

What Is a National Provider Identifier? How Do I Get My NPI?[29]

Upon passing the Certification Examination, CRNAs should apply immediately for an NPI number. Without this number, CRNAs will not be able to bill Medicare and Medicaid for their services.

Until recently, all CRNAs had to have their own universal provider identification number (UPIN) or be included in a group UPIN along with other anesthesia providers to bill the CMS for services. Many CRNAs had multiple UPINs, each number tied to a facility in which they practice or to the specific insurers they bill for anesthesia services.

To alleviate the paperwork and burden of tracking multiple UPINs, CMS replaced the UPIN with the NPI. For CRNAs who work in multiple regions and facilities, using multiple UPINs has resulted in often-delayed payments for services. The NPI is especially useful for CRNAs because it eliminates the need for multiple UPINs. Certified Registered Nurse Anesthetists keep their NPIs throughout their careers, no matter in which facility or region they practice. Although many CRNAs assign their billing rights to another entity, such as a hospital or anesthesia group employer, individual CRNAs benefit from securing individual NPIs. CRNAs apply through the NPI enumerator for their NPIs.

Nurse anesthetists are eligible to apply for and be assigned an NPI by Medicare on the date of their certification as CRNAs. To apply for the NPI, CRNAs will also need to include a taxonomy code for CRNAs on the NPI application form. The taxonomy code for CRNAs is 367500000X - Nurse Anesthetist, Certified, Registered.

Certified Registered Nurse Anesthetists who assign their billing rights to another entity should check to see if their billing entity has applied for an NPI on their behalf. If so, the CRNA may want to work with the billing entity and the NPI enumerator to list both the billing entity and the CRNA as the primary contacts for the NPI. For privacy and fraud prevention reasons, only designated persons have access to your NPI number and associated billing information.

Who Can Perform the Preanesthesia, Intraanesthesia, and Postanesthesia Evaluations?

According to Medicare, the preanesthesia, intraanesthesia, and postanesthesia evaluations "must be completed and documented by an individual qualified to administer anesthesia." The preanesthesia evaluations must be completed within 48 hours before the surgery, and postanesthesia evaluation must be completed and documented within 48 hours after surgery.[18] The person who completes the postanesthesia evaluation does not have to be the same person who provided the anesthesia service.[30] According to Medicare: "an individual qualified to administer anesthesia" includes an anesthesiologist, medical doctor or doctor of orthopedics, dentist, oral surgeon, podiatrist, CRNA, or an anesthesiologist's assistant.[18] This means that CMS has recognized that CRNAs are qualified to complete the pre-anesthesia, intraanesthesia, and postanesthesia record.

Student nurse anesthetists are not considered qualified anesthesia providers under Medicare's definition. This means that although students should learn how to complete and document preanesthesia, intraanesthesia, and postanesthesia records, they are not to document and complete these records solely on their own.

The teaching CRNA or anesthesiologist must document and complete these records and take a very real and active role in documenting and completing them.

What is Pay for Performance? Can CRNAs Participate?

Programs run by CMS and private payers, known generally as pay-for-performance or value-based purchasing, are programs in which a Medicare Part B provider's payment is made based on the quality of a provider's services. Nurse anesthetists, physicians, and other providers are now required to participate in the CMS Physician Quality Reporting Initiative (PQRI), a pay-for-performance program administered by CMS.

The movement toward pay-for-performance initiatives is fueled by the fact that the SGR and the PFS payment rules create a flat payment system in which poor or mediocre providers are reimbursed at the same rate as excellent or above-average providers. The Medicare Payment Advisory Commission, which advises Congress, has found that the increases in healthcare spending each year do not correlate as closely as they should with increased value and improved quality. Consequently, for many years, MedPAC has recommended to Congress that it support efforts to tie higher payments to increased value and quality.

The drive toward establishing pay-for-performance programs is supported by the results of the CMS Premier Hospital Quality Incentive Demonstration project.[31] This project required providers to report whether certain tasks or measures known to improve patient outcomes were done for each patient. In the program's first year, hospitals that achieved specified thresholds or significantly improved their performance with respect to a set of quality improvement measures were rewarded a total of $8.85 million in bonus payments.

In 2007, CMS established the PQRI.[32,33] Under the 2008-2009 PQRI, Medicare Part B providers who report measures applicable to their practice are eligible for a 2.0% increase in payments.[5,34] This 2.0% increase and any proposed increases in subsequent years should not necessarily be considered a bonus, however. Due to the annual SGR derived cuts, total payments to providers, including payment to those providers who earn the 2.0% bonus, will not be as high as payments would have been. Essentially it means that a provider's payment will not be cut by 2.0%.

CRNAs are eligible and are expected to report these measures. Student and graduate nurse anesthetists should be prepared to do the same. Many CRNAs have been reporting quality measures for many years through pay-for-performance programs initiated by private insurance payers and individual healthcare facilities. The reporting of quality measures is not limited to the public sector. Private insurance payers and individual facilities instituted the reporting of measures. For the 2009 PQRI program; there are 5 anesthesia-related measures: (1) perioperative care: timing and administration of prophylactic antibiotics; (2) prevention of catheter-related bloodstream infections: central venous catheter insertion protocol; (3) preventative care and screening: body mass index screening and follow-up; (4) documentation and verification of current medications in the medical record; and (5) patient codevelopment of treatment plan/plan of care.[34]

The AANA has directly contributed to the development of these and future measures as members of the American Medical Association Physician Consortium for Performance Improvement Anesthesiology Work Group, which develops measures. These measures are vetted by the National Quality Forum and the Ambulatory Quality Alliance, and many are eventually adopted by CMS and added to the list of PQRI measures.

Pay-for-performance programs are here to stay. Each year CRNAs should expect to be asked to report more measures. It is imperative that students, graduate nurse anesthetists, and CRNAs participate in the development of anesthesia measures that improve patient safety and quality and that allow CRNAs their full scope of practice. The study and development of quality measurement presents ample research opportunities for students, graduate nurse anesthetists, and CRNAs to pursue. It is important that the nurse anesthesia profession be proactive in developing and reporting quality measures. Furthermore, CRNAs should welcome the responsibility associated with reporting quality measures. This is consistent with nurse anesthesia's tradition of improving patient safety and quality.

Can CRNAs Bill Medicare for Teaching Student Nurse Anesthetists How to Insert Lines, Provide Pain Management Services, and for Providing Other Medical and Surgical Services?

According to CMS (J. Menas, written communication, December 2006), depending on the decision of your local Medicare carrier, CRNAs and anesthesiologists can bill and be paid for teaching these services to student nurse anesthetists. There is no prohibition by CMS for CRNAs and anesthesiologists to bill for teaching these services. However, because CMS national payment rules and policies do not specifically address this issue, it is up to your local Medicare carrier to decide whether to pay for teaching these services to student nurse anesthetists. Centers for Medicare and Medicaid Services staff has stated that CMS might consider establishing a national payment policy that would allow for payment under these types of clinical practice arrangements.

In the short term, this means that for CRNAs and anesthesiologists to bill for teaching these services to student nurse anesthetists, they should contact and work closely with their local Medicare carrier and their billing entity. In the immediate future, this is the best route to pursue. Any long-term strategy that the AANA might pursue will likely need more time for development and vetting among CRNA educators, AANA committees, staff, and the AANA Board of Directors.

Summary

Now that you have read through this chapter, you are well on your way to being fluent in Medicare as a second language for CRNAs. If you have to look back at this chapter to refresh your memory, that is fine. That is exactly what you should do, because learning to speak Medicare, like learning any other language, takes patience and practice. With this new fluency you will be able to better advocate for yourself, your profession, and your patients.

Appendix 7.1. Requirements for Rural Pass-Through Funding

1. For cost-reporting periods beginning on or after October 1, 1984, through any part of a cost-reporting period occurring before January 1, 1989, payment is determined on a reasonable cost basis for anesthesia services provided in the hospital or CAH by qualified nonphysician anesthetists (CRNAs and anesthesiologist's assistants), employed by the hospital or CAH or obtained under arrangements.

2. For cost-reporting periods, or any part of a cost-reporting period, beginning on or after January 1, 1989, through any part of a cost reporting period occurring before January 1, 1990, payment is determined on a reasonable cost basis for anesthesia services provided in a hospital or CAH by qualified nonphysician anesthetists employed by the hospital or CAH or obtained under arrangement if the hospital or CAH demonstrates to its intermediary before April 1, 1989, that it meets the following criteria:

   A. The hospital or CAH is located in a rural area and is not deemed by the federal government to be located in an urban area.

   B. The hospital or CAH must have employed or contracted with a qualified nonphysician anesthetist, as of January 1, 1988, to perform anesthesia services in that hospital or CAH. The hospital or CAH may employ or contract with more than 1 anesthetist; however, the total number of hours of service furnished by the anesthetists may not exceed 2,080 hours per year.

   C. The hospital or CAH must provide data for its entire patient population to demonstrate that, during calendar year 1987, its volume of surgical procedures (inpatient and outpatient) requiring anesthesia services did not exceed 250 procedures. For purposes of this section, a surgical procedure requiring anesthesia services means a surgical procedure in which the anesthesia is administered and monitored by a qualified nonphysician anesthetist, a physician other than the primary surgeon, or an intern or resident.

   D. Each qualified nonphysician anesthetist employed by or under contract with the hospital or CAH has agreed in writing not to bill on a reasonable charge basis for his or her patient care to Medicare beneficiaries in that hospital or CAH. This means that the CRNA and the hospital must each agree in writing not to bill Medicare Part B for the CRNA's services. The hospital risks losing its pass-through status and Medicare funding if the CRNA or the hospital bills Medicare Part B for the CRNA's services.

3. To maintain its eligibility for reasonable cost payment in calendar years after 1989, a qualified hospital or CAH must demonstrate before January 1 of each respective year that for the prior year its volume of surgical procedures requiring anesthesia service did not exceed 500 procedures or, effective October 1, 2002, did not exceed 800 procedures.

4. A hospital or CAH that did not qualify for reasonable cost payment for nonphysician anesthetist services furnished in calendar year 1989 can qualify in subsequent years if it meets the criteria in paragraphs C, 2, A, B, and D of this section, and demonstrates to its intermediary prior to the start of the calendar year that it met these criteria. The hospital or CAH must provide data for its entire patient population to demonstrate that, during calendar year 1987 and the year immediately preceding its election of reasonable cost payment, its volume of surgical procedures (inpatient and outpatient) requiring anesthesia services did not exceed 500 procedures or, effective October 1, 2002, did not exceed 800 procedures.

5. For administrative purposes for the calendar years after 1990, the volume of surgical procedures for the immediately preceding year is the sum of the surgical procedures for the 9-month period ending September 30, annualized for the 12-month period.

(Adapted from the Code of Federal Regulations.[28])
CAH indicates critical access hospital.

References

1. March 2006 report to the Congress: medicare payment policy. Medicare Payment Advisory Commission website. March 2006. http://www.medpac.com/document/Mar06_EntireReport.pdf. Accessed December 17, 2008.

2. Blackwell PK. Medicare latte factor formula, medicare as a second language. Presentation presented at: AANA New Nurse Anesthesia Education Program Directors Conference; March 2005; Park Ridge, IL.

3. National Healthcare Expenditures Projections 2002-2017. Centers for Medicare & Medicaid Services website. http://www.cms.hhs.gov/National HealthExpendData/Downloads/proj2007.pdf. Accessed December 18, 2008.

4. US Government Accountability Office. Medicare Physician Payments: Medicare and private payment differences for anesthesia services. In: *Report to the Subcommittee on Health, Committee on Ways and Means, US House of Representatives.* GAO Publication 07-463. Washington, DC: US Government Accountability Office; 2007:15.

5. Medicare Improvements for Patients and Providers Act of 2008 (MIPPA), H.R. 6331/P.L.110-275. http://thomas.loc.gov. Accessed February 14, 2009.

6. Proposed revisions to payment policies under the Physician Fee Schedule, and other Part B payment policies for CY 2008. *Fed Regist.* 2007;72(133):38122.

7. Medicare Payment Advisory Commission. *Report to Congress: Medicare Payment Policy.* Washington, DC: Medicare Payment and Advisory Commission; March 2008:34.

8. Payment for the services of CRNAs. *Code Fed Regul.* 42CFR §414.60.

9. Conditions for payment. *Code Fed Regul.* 42CFR §415.110.

10. Medical direction for anesthesia services. *Fed Regist.* November 2, 1998; 63(211):58842-58843.

11. Social Security Act, Sec. 1848, 42 U.S.C. 1395w-4(a)(4).

12. Gunn IP. Nurse anesthesia: a history of challenge. In: Nagelhout JJ, Zaglaniczny KL, eds. *Nurse Anesthesia.* 3rd ed. Philadelphia, PA: Elsevier Saunders; 2005:13-14.

13. Medicare claims processing manual, chapter 12 – physician/nonphysican practitioners, 2008. Sections 50 and 140. Centers for Medicare & Medicaid Services website. http://www.umsl.edu/~garziar/hipaa/Medicare_claims_ processing_manual.pdf. Accessed January 30, 2009.

14. Additional rules for payment of anesthesia services. *Code Fed Regul.* 42 CFR §414.46.

15. Conditions of participation, anesthesia services. *Code Fed Regul.* 42 CFR §482.52.

16. Conditions for coverage surgical services. *Code Fed Regul.* 42 CFR §416.42

17. Medicare and Medicaid Program; hospital conditions of participation: anesthesia services. *Fed Regist.* January 18, 2001;66(12):4674-4682.

18. Medicare state operations manual, appendix A – survey protocol, regulations and interpretive guidelines for hospitals. 2005. §482.52(Tag-A0417), Centers for Medicare & Medicaid Services website. http://www.cms.hhs.gov/manuals/downloads/som107ap_a_hospitals.pdf.

19. Medicare and Medicaid Program; hospital conditions of participation: anesthesia services. *Fed Regist.* November 13, 2001;66(219):56762.

20. Federal supervision rule opt-out information. AANA website. http://www.aana.com/Advocacy.aspx?ucNavMenu_TSMenuTargetID=49&ucNavMenu_TSMenuTargetType=4&ucNavMenu_TSMenuID=6&id=1790&terms=opt+out. Accessed October 2008.

21. Blumenreich GA. Another article on surgeon's liability for anesthesia negligence. *AANA J.* 2007;75(2):89-93.

22. Pine M, Holt KD, Lou YB. Surgical mortality and type of anesthesia provider. *AANA J.* 2003;71(2):109-116.

23. Centers for Medicare & Medicaid Services. Anesthesia services and the teaching CRNA. Medicare carriers manual, part 3 – claims process. Washington, DC: Centers for Medicare & Medicaid Services. 2002:6-11. August 29, 2008. Transmittal 1766.

24. Rules and regulations. *Fed Regist.* November 19, 2008;73(224): 69766-69774.

25. Critical access hospital fact sheet. Centers for Medicare & Medicaid Services website. June 2008. http://www.cms.hhs.gov/MLNProducts/downloads/CritAccessHospfctsht.pdf. Accessed May 2009.

26. Federal rates for inpatients operating costs. *Code Fed Regul.* 42 CFR §412.62.

27. Definitions. *Code Fed Regul.* 42 CFR §414.605.

28. Other payments. *Code Fed Regul.* 42 CFR §412.113.

29. Medicare NPI implementation. Centers for Medicare & Medicaid Services website. http://www.cms.hhs.gov/NationalProvIdentStand/06_implementation.asp. Accessed February 14, 2009.

30. Medicare and Medicaid Programs; hospital conditions of participation: requirements for history and physical examinations; authentication of verbal orders; securing medications; and postanesthesia evaluations. *Fed Regist.* November 27, 2006;71(227):68672-68690.

31. Centers for Medicare & Medicaid Services. Premier Hospital Quality Incentive demonstration project: project overview and findings from year one. Premier Inc website. http://www.premierinc.com/quality-safety/tools-services/p4p/hq/index.jsp. Accessed April 13, 2006.

32. Medicare Program. tax relief and health care act of 2006. P.L. 109-432, Division B, Title I, Sec.101

33. Rules and regulations. *Fed Regist.* November 27, 2007; 72(227):66366.

34. US Department of Health and Human Services, Centers for Medicare & Medicaid Services. Medicare Program; revisions to payment policies under the physician fee schedule and other revisions to Part B for CY 2009; and revisions to the amendment of the e-prescribing exemption for computer generated facsimile transmissions; proposed rule. *Fed Regist.* July 7, 2008;73(130):38502-38567.

Chapter 8

Generational Dynamics in Nurse Anesthesia Education

Lisa Mileto, CRNA, MS
Anne Marie Hranchook, CRNA, MSN

Key Points

- Generational differences affect anesthesia education and have an impact on both clinical and classroom pedagogy. To harmonize a diverse student population, educators should understand what motivates members of different generations and institute teaching techniques that meet their needs.

- A generation is a cohort of individuals who were born during a specified range of years and who are deeply influenced by shared experiences. The United States has a 4-generation workforce including Traditionalists, Baby Boomers, Generation X, and Generation Y.

- Cross-generational conflict in the academic environment can hinder both student achievement and faculty job satisfaction. Commonalities exist between members of Generation X and Generation Y that lend to teaching strategies that work for both groups.

- Advancements in technology have likely had the greatest impact on the learning styles of Generations X and Y. Instructors must shift from being primarily lecturers to designers of learning methods, a paradigm shift from focusing on teaching to emphasizing learning.

Introduction

The children now love luxury; they have bad manners, contempt for authority; they show disrespect for elders and love chatter in place of exercise. Children are now tyrants, not the servants of their households. They contradict their parents . . . and tyrannize their teachers.

—Socrates

Disapproval of young people's behavior is a recurring societal theme. In today's environment, educators are confronted with keeping a generationally diverse group of learners motivated. Assisting educators to navigate generational diversity, with its challenge and promise, is the focus of this chapter.

Generational differences affect anesthesia education and have an impact on both clinical and classroom pedagogy. The first steps in harmonizing a diverse student population are to understand what motivates members of different generations and to institute teaching techniques that are flexible enough to meet their needs.

A generation is a cohort of individuals who were born during a specified range of years and who are deeply influenced and bound together by shared experiences. A generation is defined not only by the parameters of age but also by the events that influenced their lives. The events people experience in their formative years can determine who they are and how they see the world. Events that capture the attention and emotions of millions of young people contribute to the development of a generational personality.[1] War, natural disaster, pop culture, public heroes, music, and technology are examples of defining events. These events shape a generation and have a profound effect on a person's development.

There is little change in a generation's values throughout the lives of its members. Generational characteristics are frequently attributed to a group's age. Statements such as: "These young people today . . . " illustrate how age is incorrectly attributed to a generational cohort's behavior. It is often the group's core values guiding the behavior.

Overview of 4 Generations

For the first time in history, the United States has transitioned from a 2-generation workforce to a 4-generation workforce, which includes Traditionalists, Baby Boomers, Generation X, and Generation Y.[2] This multigenerational workforce is due, in part, to increased longevity. In the early 1900s, the average life expectancy was 47 years, but it has increased and is now 78 years.[3]

Table 8.1 provides a depiction of generational groups delineated by birth years.[4] Current statistics in nursing education indicate that Generation X and Generation Y students are being taught mainly by Baby Boomers. The average age of nursing faculty nationwide is 45 years, and the average age of nursing students in baccalaureate programs is 27 years.[5]

Table 8.1. Comparison of 4 Generations

Generation	Birth years	Current age (2009)	Population (million)
Traditionalists	1920-1945	64-89	75
Baby Boomers	1946-1964	45-63	80
Generation X	1965-1980	29-44	46
Generation Y	1981-2000	9-28	76

Traditionalists

Maturity: Be able to stick with a job until it is finished. Be able to bear an injustice without having to get even. Be able to carry money without spending it. Do your duty without being supervised.

– Ann Landers

The Traditionalists were born between 1920 and 1945. Defining events that occurred in their formative years included the Roaring Twenties, the Great Depression, World War II, and Prohibition.[6] Families gathered to listen to the radio, children read Superman comics, and baseball brought a new hero, Babe Ruth.

The Great Depression left a permanent impression on the minds of Traditionalists. In 1933, President Franklin Delano Roosevelt promised the depression-weary people of the United States a "New Deal."[6] Roosevelt implemented banking reform laws, emergency relief, work relief, and agricultural programs. The Social Security Act provided for long-term financial protection. The Servicemen's Readjustment Act of 1944, commonly known as the GI Bill, provided college or vocational education for returning World War II veterans.[6]

The core beliefs of the Traditionalists are listed in Table 8.2. Influenced by the events of their time, the Traditionalists developed characteristics such as a strong commitment to civic duty, patience, and respect for authority.[1] Traditionalists are quiet, private, hardworking, and patriotic. They have a no-nonsense, practical approach to life that contributes to their conservative, formal behavior and dress. Traditionalists hold numerous chief executive officer positions in Fortune 500 companies and are a staunch political force.[2] Traditionalists are motivated to save their money, pay in cash rather than with credit, and buy products made in the United States of America.

Table 8.2. Core Beliefs of Traditionalists

Sacrifice

Hard work

Conformity

Law and order

Respect for authority

Patience

Duty before pleasure

Compliance with rules

Baby Boomers

They will redefine old and cool and success before they are done with the world they have sworn to make over in their own Sharper Image.

— David Stillman

The Baby Boomers (Boomers) were born between 1946 and 1964. After nearly 200 years of a declining population, the post World War II boom produced 1 baby every 17 minutes for 19 years.[2] Raising children was no longer a necessity for survival. Growing up in a time of economic expansion and prosperity, major social movements, and national optimism, Baby Boomers were cherished by their parents and represented the hope for the future that their parents fought to preserve.

Defining events that occurred during the Boomers' formative years included the Cold War, the Vietnam War, the Cuban Missile Crisis, and air raid drills.[4] Boomers were raised in an era of great change. They witnessed the civil rights movement and they were empowered by campaigns and protests. Rosa Parks, the assassinations of Martin Luther King and John F. Kennedy, the McCarthy hearings, and Woodstock all left an indelible mark.[7]

During this era, women's rights took center stage.[7] President Kennedy established the President's Commission on the Status of Women and appointed Eleanor Roosevelt as the chairperson. The commission reported substantial discrimination against women in the workplace and made recommendations for improvement in hiring practices, paid maternity leave, and affordable childcare. In 1963, *The Feminine Mystique,* written by Betty Friedan, was published, illuminating the dissatisfaction of American housewives with the narrow role imposed on them by society.[8] Soon after, new laws such as the Equal Pay Act of 1963 and Title VII of the Civil Rights Act of 1964 cleared the path for women to enter the workforce in record numbers.

The 1960s also was a time of great technological advancement. Inventions during this time included the handheld calculator, bar coding, and random access memory (RAM). Outer space captured the imaginations of the public and scientists. Some of the most dramatic advances were in the area of manned space flight.[7]

In contrast to their Traditionalist parents, Boomers embraced radical social change.[9] The Baby Boomers witnessed a cultural shift from poodle skirts and hula hoops to peace signs, rock and roll, antiwar campaigns, and love-ins.[2] An emerging drug culture and sexual freedom coincided with introspection and spiritual evaluation.

Privileged by wealth and prosperity, today's Boomers cherish anything trendy— cell phones, luxury cars, vintage wines, designer merchandise—and they are willing to work for it. They take a 60-hour workweek in stride.[4,9] Boomers focus their energy on expanding their longevity and enhancing their retirement. This is a reflection of their drive for personal gratification and wellness. The core beliefs of the Baby Boomers are outlined in Table 8.3.

Baby Boomers are concerned about their workplace environment. They value participation, fairness, and equality. Boomers are team players who believe in inclusion and collaboration. Conversely, they are fiercely competitive and will go to great lengths to get what they want.[2,4]

Table 8.3. Core Beliefs of Baby Boomers

Optimism

Teamwork

Personal gratification

Health and wellness

Personal development

Work

Spirituality

Generation X

A person should not believe in an "-ism," he should believe in himself.
I quote John Lennon, "I don't believe in the Beatles, I just believe in me."
— Ferris Bueller, *Ferris Bueller's Day Off*

Members of Generation X were born between 1965 and 1980 and comprise an estimated 46 million people. During their formative years, Gen X struggled with inflation, the energy crisis, nuclear proliferation, and corporate layoffs and corruption.[2] Many defining events led Gen X to develop a prevailing skepticism. Institutions that were previously stable and respected began to fail, leading to distrust and disappointment. Watergate, the energy crisis, inflation, the fall of the Berlin wall, Operation Desert Storm, and the Challenger disaster were all sentinel events that influenced the collective psyche of Gen X.[2]

During their formative years, the nature of the family structure began to change for Gen X. The proliferation of working mothers and rising divorce rates were influential in shaping their attitudes and beliefs.[2,9] The number of single-parent households and dual-income families led to many children being labeled "latchkey kids." Gen X developed a "survivor mentality."[9] They sensed early on that no one was going to hold their hands, and they learned to take care of themselves.

Today's members of Gen X are cautious spenders who are not influenced by trendy brand names, hype, or gimmicky marketing techniques.[2] Gen X members highly value balance in their lives; they strive for harmony between their work and personal lives. As they push to gain freedom from the clutches of Baby Boomer rules, Gen X members often face a backlash from the current dominant force in the workplace. This cohort wants to work smarter, not harder. Quite simply, Gen X wants to have fun at work.[4]

Members of Gen X are highly independent and work well alone. They have little regard for corporate life and frequently challenge or work around authority and the status quo. They are independent problem solvers, concrete thinkers, and masters of multitasking. Gen X is technologically literate, and they are global thinkers.[2,4,10]

A dominant force in college classrooms for the past 20 years, Gen X has been studied extensively in terms of learning style and values.[10] In contrast to the Boomers, Gen X scorns materialism and status seeking. Dressing casually is "now and forever" for this group. Gen X is resistant to labels or generalizations. Skeptics by nature, they feel the future is uncertain and believe they can only trust themselves.[2,9] Tough economic times during their lifespan have led Gen X to worry about Social Security, retirement, and their ability to fund their children's education. The core beliefs of Gen X are outlined in Table 8.4.

Gen X is often labeled as disloyal, uncommitted, and cynical. Some refer to them as "slackers." On the contrary, Gen X members are no less motivated to succeed than previous generations, but they choose to define success in their own terms. Seeking life balance, Gen X members do not define themselves by their work. They are voracious learners and are creative and resourceful.[11]

Table 8.4. Core Beliefs of Generation X

Balance

Technoliteracy

Fun

Casualness

Self-reliance

Pragmatism

Generation Y

They want to study, travel, make friends, make more friends, read everything (superfast), take in all the movies, listen to every hot band, and keep up with everyone they have ever known.

– Mark Edmundson

Generation Y (Gen Y) is the newest generation to enter the classroom and the workforce. Born between 1981 and 2000 and comprising nearly one-third of the current population, Generation Y is a formidable force with a clear agenda. They have been and continue to be raised in a child-focused environment. Like the Boomers, Gen Y was raised during prosperous times. It was commonplace for their Boomer parents to find the time and the money to pursue raising "exceptional" children. Parents were involved in the minutiae of their children's lives in a style of parenting coined "helicopter parenting."[12] Belted into car seats, wearing bike helmets, and having nearly constant adult supervision, Gen Ys are used to being protected and guided. They have received extensive accolades for all of their accomplishments and are the recipients of "trophy overload." As children, they often had busy, overplanned lives.[13] Frequently shuffled off to playdates and planned activities, they developed a strong sense of teamwork and commitment.

Gen Y has adapted to living with the constant threat of terrorism.[14] Sentinel events in their lifetime included the September 11 attacks the bombings in Oklahoma City and at the Atlanta Summer Olympics. During their lifetime, Gen Y has witnessed school shootings such as the one that occurred at Columbine High in 1999. Parents and teachers of Gen Y educate them about stranger danger, bullying, and avoiding cyber predators. Gen Y has developed street smarts that they use to navigate the world. Living in turbulent times, they are determined to live their best lives *now*.[2,9,14]

Television programming provided a plethora of positive, self-help strategies. Members of Gen Y were told from the time they were toddlers that they can be anything they can imagine. This contributed to Gen Y members regarding themselves as "special." This group arrived when society started revaluing children. The childbearing focus of the 1970s was contraception; "children should be seen, and not heard." In contrast, Gen Y came during an era of reproduction, fertility, and adoption.[14]

Gen Y is frequently referred to as the narcissistic generation. A study of college students across the United States revealed that narcissism has steadily increased since 1982. The Narcissistic Personality Inventory was completed by 16,475 students between 1982 and 2006. By 2006, two-thirds of the students had above-average scores on this inventory, ranking 30% higher than students did in 1982.[15] Current technology feeds narcissism. MySpace and YouTube encourage attention seeking and self-promotion.

At 76 million members strong, Gen Y is heavily marketed.[14] Their Boomer parents spend billions of dollars each year, and Gen Y is not afraid to ask for money. Cell phones with unlimited texting, i-Pods, and small, fully loaded laptops are required parental purchases before sending students off to college. Often moving home after college, they feel safe and financially protected. As a whole, Gen Y can take greater work risks, making them mobile and able to pursue better, more satisfying jobs. Changing jobs is not viewed as a stigma by Gen Y, but as an asset.[16]

Gen Y is techno-savvy and wireless, having access to information 24 hours a day, 7 days a week. The creation of the Netscape browser in 1995 made the Internet accessible to everyone, allowing Gen Y to multiply possibilities.[17] Their social network is web-based (Facebook, MySpace, and instant messaging), allowing Gen Y to become global citizens and contributing to their expectation to work and have social communication anytime and anyplace. Global positioning systems on their phones allow them to navigate traffic and locate friends across the country. Gen Y has been and continues to be on fast forward. Often stating "I'm bored," Gen Y members are accustomed to fast entertainment, fast cash, and fast relationships.

Gen Y is the most culturally diverse generation; 36% are nonwhite or Hispanic.[10,14] They value diversity, embrace collaboration, and tolerate differences of opinion. They are compliant and respectful of authority, yet they do not hesitate to challenge authority. Members of Gen Y believe respect is earned and not granted solely because of title or rank. They are exceptionally altruistic and are collectively hopeful and future oriented.[2,4,9] The core beliefs of Gen Y are outlined in Table 8.5.

Generational Conflict

Cross-generational conflict in the academic environment can hinder both student achievement and faculty job satisfaction. Bridging the gap creates a collaborative environment that stimulates learning and creates harmony. Table 8.6 depicts the

Table 8.5. Core Beliefs of Generation Y

Optimism

Confidence

Achievement

Sociability

Diversity

Civic duty

viewpoints of 4 generations. It is not uncommon for Baby Boomers and Traditionalists to have a perception that members of Gen X and Gen Y lack commitment.[4] Clinical educators and faculty complain that students arrive late, do not want to stay to finish cases, and have a casual attitude. Frequently labeled as disrespectful in the classroom, Gen X and Gen Y students are often bored by traditional lecture styles. Instructors are often offended by students' frequent use of cell phones and laptops and by their impersonal emails.

The Boomers have matured to see themselves as the be-all and end-all generation. Zemke et al[2] liken them to the older sibling who has been dethroned by a new arrival. Boomers feel displaced by Gen X, whom they believe are upsetting the world the Boomers made better. The younger Gen X is seen as cynical and lazy. On the other hand, Gen X is skeptical of the Boomers. They prefer self-reliance over the Boomer's affinity for teams and have refused to bow to the Boomer-driven work ethic. Gen X is committed to preserving their life outside of work and the classroom, and members believe that they can bring more promise and energy while doing so.[18] The Boomers are judgmental and critical of a generation they do not understand.

Both Boomers and Gen X believe that members of Gen Y lack direction and are overly reliant on frequent positive feedback. They feel that Gen Y members are needy and have an air of entitlement. Hira[18] states, referring to Gen Y: "This is the most high-maintenance workforce in the history of the world. The good news is they're also going to be the most high-performing." Viewed by Boomers

Table 8.6. Viewpoints of the 4 Generations

	Traditionalists	Boomers	Gen X	Gen Y
Future outlook	Practical	Optimistic	Skeptical	Hopeful
Turnoffs	Profanity	Political incorrectness	Cliché, hype	Techno-illiteracy, intolerance
Work ethic	Dedicated	Driven	Balanced	Determined
Relationships	Personal sacrifice	Self-gratification	Reluctance to commit	Crave community
View of authority	Respectful	Love/hate	Unimpressed	Team-oriented

and Gen X as ambitious and demanding, Gen Y members question everything. On the other hand, Gen Y members exhibit values such as honesty, caring, moral courage, patriotism, and democracy.[2] Emerging differences are found between Gen Y and their predecessors. Gen Y members believe they will do a better job of upholding these values and that the older generations have talked the talk but Gen Y will walk the walk.

The struggle that occurs between generations is being played out in hospitals across the United States. A philosophical shift is occurring in the field of medicine. Generational influences are creating marked changes in physician work schedules and resident and medical student education. A 2008 *Wall Street Journal* article by Goldstein[19] states: "US medicine is in the middle of a cultural revolution, as young physicians, intent on balancing work and family, challenge the assumption that a doctor should be available to treat patients around the clock." Physicians are searching for and finding jobs that have a predictable schedule. For example, medical residents pushed for and received limited weekly hours and time off post call in 2002.[19] Even with the limited hours, a survey of medical residents in 2006 found that lack of free time was the biggest concern for 63% of respondents.[19] Anesthesia students are pushing for a similar shift.

Educational Strategies for Generations X and Y

Anesthesia educators should be knowledgeable about generational differences when designing graduate anesthesia programs for Gen X and Gen Y students. Meeting graduate students' educational needs requires an understanding of their values and learning styles. Exponential advancements in technology have likely had the greatest impact on the learning styles of Gen X and Gen Y. Today's students are products of thousands of hours of exposure to constantly changing images via cable television and the Internet. The use of the latest technology is second nature to most; therefore, they expect technological sophistication in their graduate anesthesia program. Instructors must shift from being primarily lecturers to being designers of learning methods, a paradigm shift from focusing on teaching to emphasizing learning.[20]

Teaching Generation X Students

Gen X students are creative, self-sufficient, and easily adaptable, and are techno-literate.[2] They show a preference for self-paced, independent learning. Online learning modules with pictures and video, study questions, and case scenarios are effective teaching tools for Gen X. They often prefer online courses. When in the classroom, Gen X students identify with an instructor who effectively utilizes technology and who provides a creative presentation. They value immediacy, efficiency, and quality in educational design.[20]

In contrast, Gen X members are turned off by instructors whom they feel waste their time, micromanage, or use pressure tactics to teach. This group is not motivated by fear or long-term reward strategies.[9] For example, although appreciative of examination content clues, they do not learn from threats about passing grades or instructors who create test anxiety. Pragmatic and down-to-earth, Gen X prefers educational strategies that focus on outcomes that are clearly outlined and reflect real-world skills necessary for success.[20]

Teaching Generation Y Students

Gen Y is a cohort of students that began entering colleges in 2000. As members of the largest generation, they are packing college classrooms. The largest high school class in US history is expected to graduate in 2010.[10] Currently, much research is being conducted to determine the values, learning styles, and marketing potential of this generation.[14,16]

Although similarities exist in the teaching methods favored by both Gen X and Gen Y, Gen Y has unique educational needs. Growing up in a world of instant gratification, Gen Y members perceive that their issues or needs are not valued if there is a delay in response longer than what they consider appropriate.[20] Their expectations for rapid results for test grades, written evaluations, or course handouts can be a source of frustration for instructors. Twenty-four–hour access to university, hospital, faculty, and educational resources is a common expectation.

Generation Y is addicted to visual media.[10] It is not surprising then that 2- to 3-hour classroom lectures with handouts and minimal student interaction do not inspire or motivate Gen Y. They use the Internet, sometimes unwisely, to research a subject. Academic misconduct is on the rise and can be linked to the plethora of information available on the Internet and ease of access.

Members of Gen Y are, by nature, holistic learners, exploring with their minds and responding by doing. Gen Y learns well in a participative, positive learning environment in which they can think and investigate possibilities.[20] With the availability of high-fidelity human-patient simulation and interactive e-learning, instructors have numerous tools that meet the needs of today's students. Dramatic innovations in technology, increasingly potent pharmacologic agents, complex medical cases, and advances in surgery and anesthesia make human-patient simulation an important educational tool. Students can safely practice high-acuity, low-frequency skills in a carefully monitored environment. Simulation centers allow for team training and the development of highly effective communication across disciplines and generations.

The effective use of online courses provides opportunities for critical thinking. Online tools allow for group discussion, posting of assignments, and feedback on tests and written assignments. Online courses permit the flexibility that Gen X and Gen Y crave by allowing them to work on their own time.

Gen Y students are "better prepared, more confident and . . . more willing to do what it takes to succeed."[20] They are accustomed to devoting their time and energy toward accomplishing their goals and being rewarded for doing so. These students want more direction than their Gen X predecessors. They need encouragement to seek greater autonomy and self-reliance.[21] This group often finds the transition to graduate education difficult. As high-achieving undergraduate students who found academic success with little effort, they may have unrealistic expectations about what it takes to handle the rigors of nurse anesthesia education. Gen Y students may benefit from information on study techniques and time-management skills, the development of study groups, and other forms of collaborative learning. Table 8.7 shows the learning characteristics of Gen Y.

Gen Y students tend to be overachievers, but they have been overly managed.[14,16,22] Often rewarded for participation instead of achievement in elementary education, they will challenge a grade or an evaluation. They often expect grade inflation and instant success in the clinical setting. This group struggles with setting goals and identifying their individual strengths and weaknesses. They request more supervision and structure than Gen X.

Gen Y students aim to please, and following the rules replaces the rebellion of Gen X. They require more mentoring initially but have shown an ability to make dramatic and constructive changes in a short time.[10] Praise is high on the list of expectations from Gen Y. Zaslow[23] states: "Bosses, professors, and mates are feeling the need to lavish praise on young adults, particularly twentysomethings, or else see them wither under an unfamiliar compliment deficit."

Table 8.7. Learning Characteristics of Generation Y

Holistic learners

Based in real world tasks

Spontaneous and undirected playfulness

Kinesthetic

Graphic and visual

Strategies for Teaching Both Gen X and Gen Y

Commonalities between Gen X and Gen Y lend to teaching strategies that work for both groups. Students today need to be given high and clear expectations. Frequent student-faculty contact is one of the most important educational tools for providing expert, high-quality instruction. Recurrent and timely feedback about academic and clinical performance is essential.

Both Gen X and Gen Y prefer an interactive, energetic classroom style. Neither group is intimidated by authority. This can occasionally lead to classroom antics that Boomer instructors perceive as disinterest and even disrespect. Allowing time for active student participation is essential for maintaining an attentive, engaged group.

Making learning fun is not new, but this idea gains greater meaning when we realize that Gen X and Gen Y students have the expectation that their learning is up to the instructor. They believe that the amount and quality of learning is the teacher's responsibility, not the students.' In light of this perspective, instructors may consider the benefit of changing the way they impart information by incorporating fun into their teaching strategies. Problem-based learning and quiz bowl sessions are successful methods of instruction.

Today's students become engaged by lectures that include pictures and images vs those with only text. Current textbooks look more like web pages with numerous key points, charts, highlights, and graphs. The visual image, not the printed word, is the preferred means of communication. The old approach relied on textual directions to walk students through steps in their assignments. A more modern, effective approach uses visual aids to illustrate steps and give directions instead of a step-by-step list.

Getting faculty to embrace change in their instructional style may be challenging. Some instructors cling to the view that content not covered in class will not be understood. Faculty may deem anesthesia education to be different and believe that what has been done in the past has worked, so it should not be changed.

Summary

A generational transformation is occurring in classrooms across the United States. Baby Boomer faculty are teaching record numbers of Gen X and Gen Y students. This great generational transition has substantial implications for anesthesia educators. Instructors need to develop teaching styles and expand resources to meet the needs of a new generation of students.

Each generation has innate core values based on the events and experiences of the era in which members spent their formative years. These core values affect learning styles, work ethic, perceptions of others, and how people communicate. Gen X and Gen Y offer core values that can bring positive changes to graduate nurse anesthesia programs and the healthcare workforce. Anesthesia educators who anticipate generational differences will be equipped to meet their students' educational needs and diffuse intergenerational conflicts that can emerge when values are not aligned. Embracing generational differences, using them to refine the way we educate, and implementing educational strategies described in this chapter will help deliver success. Anesthesia educators are in for a challenge and a tremendous opportunity.

References

1. Strauss W, Howe N. *Generations: The History of America's Future, 1584 to 2069.* New York, NY: William Morrow; 1991:27-42.

2. Zemke R, Raines C, Filipczak B. *Generations at Work: Managing the Clash of Veterans, Boomers, Xers, and Nexters in Your Workplace.* New York, NY: AMACOM; 2000:1-150.

3. US Department of Health and Human Services. Centers for Disease Control and Prevention: The National Center for Health Statistics. Centers for Disease Control and Prevention website. http://www.cdc.gov/nchs/index. Accessed December 29, 2008.

4. Lancaster LC, Stillman D. *When Generations Collide.* New York, NY: Harper Collins; 2002: 3-48.

5. US Department of Health and Human Services. The registered nurse population: Findings from the 2004 National Sample Survey of Registered Nurses. US Department of Health and Human Services Health resources and services administration website. http://bhpr.hrsa.gov/healthworkforce/rnsurvey04. Accessed December 29, 2008.

6. Brokaw T. *The Greatest Generation.* New York, NY: Random House; 1998:1-18.

7. Brokaw T. *BOOM! Voices of the Sixties.* New York, NY: Random House; 2007:1-282.

8. Friedan B. *The Feminine Mystique.* New York, NY: WW Norton & Company; 1963:15-32.

9. Martin CA, Tulgan B. *Managing the Generation Mix: From Collision to Collaboration.* 2nd ed. Amherst, MA: HRD Press; 2006:1-160.

10. Elliot R, Norwood A, Mangum C, Haynie L. Generational differences in nursing students' preferences for teaching methods. *J Nurs Educ.* 2006;45(9): 371-374.

11. Tulgan B. *Managing Generation X: How to Bring Out the Best in Young Talent.* New York, NY: WW Norton & Company; 2000:17-268.

12. Cline FW, Fay J. *Parenting With Love and Logic: Teaching Children Responsibility.* Colorado Springs, CO: Pinon Press; 1990:23-25.

13. Swenson C. Next generation workforce. *Nurs Econ.* 2008;26(1):64-68.

14. The echo boomers [transcript]. *60 Minutes.* CBS television. October 3, 2004.

15. Crary D. Study finds students narcissistic. *Associated Press.* February 27, 2007.

16. The millennials are coming [transcript]. *60 Minutes.* CBS television. November 11, 2007.

17. Edmundson M. Dwelling in possibilities. *Chron Higher Educ.* 2008;54(27):B7-B11.

18. Hira NA. You raised them, now manage them. *Fortune.* 2007:155(10):38-46.

19. Goldstein J. As doctors get a life, strains show quest for free time reshapes medicine: a 'team' approach. *The Wall Street Journal.* May 8, 2008:W1,W6.

20. Coomes MD, DeBard R. *Serving the Millennial Generation.* San Francisco, CA: Jossey-Bass; 2004:5-86.

21. Twenge JM. *Generation Me.* New York, NY: Simon & Schuster; 2006:17-158.

22. Marano HE. *A Nation of Wimps: The High Cost of Invasive Parenting.* New York, NY: Broadway Books; 2008:142-241.

23. Zaslow J. The most-praised generation goes to work. *The Wall Street Journal.* April 20, 2007:W1,W7.

Chapter 9

The Importance of Effective Communication

Betty J. Horton, CRNA, PhD

Key Points

- The importance of effective communication skills has been brought to national attention by a variety of groups, such as professional membership organizations, regional and specialized accrediting agencies, private foundations, and branches of the federal government.

- The acquisition of effective communication skills can improve the work performance of program administrators, didactic faculty, and clinical faculty in the office, classroom, and clinical areas. Skill development requires knowledge of communication and opportunities to practice. Fortunately, there are many opportunities in nurse anesthesia programs to practice these skills.

- Student nurse anesthetists must develop advanced skills in communicating with their patients and with all healthcare professionals involved in patient care. Instructors must help students to expand their skills and to recognize the importance of clear and accurate communication in preventing errors and increasing patient safety.

- Evaluation of both instructors and students on communication skills is advisable. Feedback from the evaluations can help them succeed in attaining specific goals.

Introduction

Communication skills are an essential element of professionalism and a reflection of an individual's intellect, preparedness, and character. This makes advanced communication skills a desirable outcome of nurse anesthesia education. Effective communication skills are also important to professional organizations, which must relay information to and solicit feedback from their members and the public on various issues.

National Perspectives

The American Association of Nurse Anesthetists

Communication with the American Association of Nurse Anesthetists (AANA) typically begins when we are student members and continues throughout our lifetimes. The AANA shares information about its many services for nurse anesthetists and communicates other important messages to us. In return, members volunteer their services to the AANA and share their opinions with organizational leaders. Certified Registered Nurse Anesthetists (CRNAs) have found that belonging to their professional organization provides them with a common voice on matters that affect both education and practice.

The AANA also values communication with the public as exemplified by a news release on patient safety[1] that emphasized the importance of open communication between the anesthetist and patient before and after surgery. The AANA's message indicated that honest communication could help ensure a successful outcome and decrease the incidence of complications. The AANA suggested that patients ask important questions, reveal personal information, discuss anesthesia options, and ask about adverse effects and preparation for anesthesia. Questions about what would take place during and after administration of an anesthetic were also encouraged.[1]

The Council on Accreditation of Nurse Anesthesia Educational Programs

The Council on Accreditation of Nurse Anesthesia Educational Programs (COA) believes that the development of communication skills is important in the education of the nurse anesthetist as documented in its Standards for Accreditation of Nurse Anesthesia Educational Programs.[2] Accredited programs must demonstrate that graduates have knowledge, skills, and competencies in communication so they can effectively communicate with individuals influencing patient care and use appropriate verbal, nonverbal, and written communication in the delivery of perianesthetic care.[2] Graduates who have attained these skills are competent communicators in patient care situations. Instructors must help students to acquire good communication skills during classroom and clinical experiences.

The COA also has expectations for the way programs should communicate with the COA on matters of accreditation. There are several accreditation policies in place that outline this expectation, such as progress reports and deadlines for compliance with the standards and criteria of the COA.[3] The cardinal rule is that it is essential for CRNA educators to know the COA's standards and policies and to communicate with the COA in a timely manner.

The Commission on Collegiate Nursing Education

Some nurse anesthesia programs reside in schools of nursing that are accredited by the Commission on Collegiate Nursing Education (CCNE) and honor its requirements as a program within the larger institution. In early 2008, CCNE proposed revised Standards for Accreditation of Bachelors and Graduate Nursing Programs.[4] Item II-F in the standards requires that there be processes by which the evaluation of individual student performance is communicated to students by faculty. In addition, CCNE will continue to require documented use of certain professional nursing standards and guidelines. Among the standards are those delineated in The Essentials of Master's Education for Advanced Practice Nursing[5] and The Essentials of Doctoral Education for Advanced Nursing Practice,[6] as applicable to the type of degrees offered. There are multiple examples related to communication in both of these documents. An example in the master's essentials states: "Course work should provide graduates with the knowledge and skills to communicate with other healthcare professionals."[5] An example in the doctoral essentials states: "The Doctor of Nursing Practice program prepares the graduate to employ effective communication and collaborative skills in the development and implementation of practice models, peer review, practice guidelines, health policy, standards of care, and/or scholarly projects."[6]

The National League for Nursing Accrediting Commission

There are also some nurse anesthesia programs located in schools of nursing accredited by the National League for Nursing Accrediting Commission (NLNAC); therefore, they are affected by this accreditor's requirements. The accreditation standards promulgated by NLNAC for master's degree programs, NLNAC Standards and Criteria: Master's Degree/Post-Master's Certificate Programs in Nursing[7] indicate that the interchange of information between the accreditor and others is important. Standard 1.3 requires its communities of interest to have input into the program processes and decision making, and standard 6.3 requires that evaluation findings be shared with its communities. The NLNAC Standards and Criteria: Clinical Doctorate Degree Programs in Nursing identify the same requirements in Standards 1.3 and 6.4.[8]

The Institute of Medicine

Poor communication among healthcare professionals has been identified as a potential problem by the Institute of Medicine. It increases the risk of errors, patient complaints, and malpractice claims.[9] Analyses of adverse events in surgery revealed that underlying causes are often communication failures rather than technical problems.[10] These findings indicate that students need to become competent in both communication and technical skills to maximize patient safety. In fact, the relationship between communication and patient safety is so important that the Institute of Medicine strongly recommends striving for effective communication among healthcare professionals. The Institute of Medicine encourages educators to ensure that students become working professionals who are proficient in using information technology and working as part of an interdisciplinary team.[11-13]

The Institute for Safe Medication Practices

Medication errors by student nurses have been analyzed by the Institute for Safe Medication Practices. A report indicated that having 2 people, student and instructor, involved in administering medications to a patient made communication breakdowns in patient care more likely. This finding should be seriously considered by all clinical instructors who need to carefully monitor communication between themselves and students to safeguard against errors in medication administration.[14]

The Anesthesia Patient Safety Foundation

An article in the Anesthesia Patient Safety Foundation publication *APSF Newsletter* noted that team training is helpful to improve communication. Importantly, effective communication was seen as a vital link to the delivery of safe, effective healthcare. According to the article, the goal for improving communication through training was to reduce medical errors.[15]

Others

Many accreditors, in addition to those mentioned above, have established learning outcomes that are not specific to the technical aspects of a profession. Students preparing to become engineers are required to have the ability to communicate effectively; students studying to become pharmacists must learn to think critically and communicate effectively; and physician residents must be able to demonstrate effective interpersonal and communication skills. Accreditors that evaluate universities also recognize the importance of teaching students to communicate. For example, Middle States Association of Colleges and Schools has a goal that graduates will be skilled in oral and written communication.[16] It would be difficult to find an accrediting agency that did not expect students to be more proficient in communication by graduation.

The Importance of Communication in Educational Programs

During an ordinary day, a typical nurse anesthetist spends time speaking with people in a variety of situations. A CRNA talks with patients, physicians, or coworkers; a clinical instructor talks with students; or a program administrator meets and talks with didactic and clinical instructors. The CRNA also communicates frequently in writing and with nonverbal body language. Thus, effective communication abilities contribute to a CRNA's success in the office, classroom, and clinical area.

Program Administration

A program administrator who is good at written communication can develop a persuasive proposal that stands out from the competition to secure a budgetary increase or to win grant funding. According to a publication from Harvard Business School, the more readable your proposal, the better your chances of success.[17]

Classroom

Written and oral communications are intellectual and practical skills that students are expected to develop at the undergraduate level.[16] Many universities offer courses in interpersonal communication skills and public speaking to undergraduates. The goals of these courses are to prepare students to organize and express ideas clearly and appropriately; master standard use of written and oral communication; and listen, observe, interpret, and understand others.[18] Students must continue learning to write and speak clearly and effectively in graduate school. This applies to all graduate students, including nurses, who are pursuing a career in nurse anesthesia.

The educational relationship is a communicative relationship between 2 human beings that requires mutual respect, trust, and concern. Nurse anesthesia instructors do not usually have degrees in education, so they must learn as much as they can about good instructional practice. One technique is to communicate to students early in the educational experience that you have high expectations for student learning, including acquisition of knowledge about effective communication.[16]

To help students polish their communication skills, you can plan practical activities such as helping them become competent in interviewing patients, developing written anesthesia care plans, and completing medical records accurately. As an instructor, you will need to assess students' interviewing and writing techniques and give them opportunities to refine these skills before assignment in the clinical area. You can also provide other writing and speaking opportunities in the classroom, including class presentations, journal clubs, topical papers, and capstone projects involving written work.[16]

A characteristic of a quality curriculum is a culminating experience in which the students integrate the learning to produce an intellectual work such as a research project, a policy paper, or a scholarly dissertation.[16] External examiners can quiz students, allowing them to demonstrate knowledge of their subjects and test their communication skills. This activity should represent an integration of learning throughout an education program and represent a student's most advanced work.

Clinical Instruction

Evaluating performance is a major responsibility for CRNAs who are involved in clinical instruction. The goal is to provide feedback that helps students improve. To do this, you must avoid judgments and communicate criticism in a positive, constructive way during the evaluation.[17] You do not want students to become defensive when you provide feedback but instead, to listen, reflect, and be influenced by what is said. This can happen when students feel safe talking with you because past conversations have demonstrated that you have their best interests in mind. Speaking thoughtfully and respectfully creates a learning environment in which students feel safe to express agreement or respectful disagreement with you.[19]

Another responsibility of a CRNA is to be a role model. If your messages to members of the surgical team are delivered in a clear, concise manner that minimizes misunderstandings, students will learn effective communication from your example. To accomplish this, you need to be direct and honest in communicating with others.[19,20]

Effective clinical instructors use several communication strategies when interacting with students. They review care plans and offer suggestions; ask pertinent, thought-provoking questions about the case; discuss how clinical events correlate with course work; explain clinical issues clearly; and discuss evaluations by offering positive feedback or constructive criticism about performance. In addition, both didactic and clinical instructors should become familiar with the contents of the student handbook. Only by knowing the written policies can you apply them or communicate them to students.

Review of the Basics

Verbal Communication

Effective verbal communication means speaking clearly and concisely, conveying information, or articulating an opinion.[21] Educators engage in verbal communication most commonly in face-to-face meetings or during telephone conversations. Regardless of the setting, a good communicator is comfortable speaking to others in a manner that helps listeners to understand and willingly receive the message. Learning the skills necessary for good verbal communication takes time.

It takes practice to speak with a student about a problem in a way that allows the student to readily accept criticism. Some instructors advise that you write down the main points you want to make before speaking with the student. This will keep your message focused, and the student will find what you are saying easier to understand. When delivering the message, consider starting by asking a question to engage the student in conversation, so that he or she will be more receptive to what you have to say. Starting with a declarative, judgmental sentence such as "That was a stupid thing to do!" is not helpful. To label a person or action as "stupid" shows that you have made no effort to understand the student's position and cuts off any thoughtful exploration of how to correct the problem.[20] Instead, inquire about the student's performance by asking a question, such as "How did you decide to do that?" This approach is nonthreatening and engages the student in a constructive conversation in which problems can be identified and performance improved.

Nonverbal Communication

Facial expressions, body postures, gestures, and eye contact are all examples of nonverbal communication known as body language. A great deal has been written about body language. Researchers have found that the meaning of gestures depends on personal style and settings, what has gone before, and expectations for the future. Some researchers have found that facial expression and tone of voice are 90% of communication between people.[20]

Researchers have also found that the meaning of body language depends on cultural norms, and there is evidence that patterns of nonverbal communication are highly variable among cultures and among different groups. Everyone does not follow the same rules. For example, in some cultures it is polite for a speaker to look directly at the listener, while the listener is expected to watch the speaker without looking away. This behavior may be unacceptable in a culture in which direct eye contact is avoided.[20]

Body language conveys messages that support or contradict what a person says. As an example, arms crossed across the chest may mean that the person is not receptive to further information on the issue being discussed; however, body language can be easily misinterpreted. Distress signals may originate from events at home or other places rather than from work. This means that, although body language is useful, it cannot be precisely interpreted. Body language should be viewed in the context of the situation and seen as an indication of a potential problem, rather than as concrete evidence.[20] Do not ignore body language; just pay attention to all nonverbal forms of communication to see if they add meaning to the spoken words.

Listening

The effectiveness of verbal communication depends on how well people listen to you rather than what you say. According to 1 report,[20] the average person remembers only half of the content heard immediately after hearing it, no matter how carefully he or she listened. About half to one-third of the content is forgotten within 8 hours, and only 25% of what was said is remembered 2 months later.

In another study, respondents expressed more approval of those who listened more than they talked. People who talked more than they listened during a conversation met with disapproval. Those who always insisted on quiet while they were talking or dominated a conversation met with strong disapproval.[22]

A good listener is physically active and this skill can be taught. Universities and colleges now provide courses in listening, and proprietary organizations sometimes offer workshops to teach listening as part of communication training.[20] Listening skills include an attitude of curiosity and patience that promotes the acquisition of ideas rather than facts. Listening attentively is important to understanding. Effective listeners:[19,20]

- Express interest in the other person's views.
- Acknowledge the emotions that the other person appears to be feeling.

- Restate what they have heard to show that they understand.
- Express agreement when they agree.
- Build on what the other person appears to have left out.
- Compare their views with the other person's views and, if there are differences, do not suggest that the other person is wrong.

These activities are possible because we think much faster than we talk. The proper use of thinking time helps you concentrate on what is being said. Improper use of thinking time lets your mind wander away from the speaker's message.

Listening ability is affected by emotions. We tend to ignore what we do not want to hear, and we accept what we hope to be true. You can help avoid this problem by withholding any judgment until after the speaker has finished. Listen instead of judging what is said, think about each point the speaker makes, and search for evidence of beliefs you share. You will likely find that your early emotional judgment was right or wrong by listening objectively to what the speaker said.[20]

A student's listening ability is also affected by emotions when he or she receives a negative evaluation or must be disciplined. Because of this fact, it is good practice to have 2 faculty members present during a conference and create a written record of the session to verify the content if questions arise later.

Written Communication

The written word is used by instructors and their students in many ways. Being able to convey your message in writing using proper grammar[21] is important in memos, letters, emails, reports, meeting minutes, care plans, evaluations, resumes, publications, grant proposals, and curriculum vitae. The tone of your writing should be appropriate to the occasion. It may need to be formal or informal, detailed, or a summary of ideas. For example, minutes contain summaries of topics discussed at a meeting.[17]

Whether you are a program administrator or a didactic or clinical instructor, you should know how to write a report. Before beginning to write, it is necessary to have a clear goal in mind. Describe the goal in 1 or 2 sentences that explain the idea and its benefits for the reader. All ideas presented in the remainder of the report should relate to the main goal.[17]

The writing process includes 4 stages:[17]
1. The *madman* brainstorms and jots down ideas in no particular order with no judgment about their value or grammatical structure.
2. The *architect* organizes relevant ideas into an outline. The notes that were generated during brainstorming are placed into groups of related ideas. At this stage, some ideas will be discarded and others will be structured into a linear outline that makes sense.

3. The *carpenter* adds structure in the form of sentences. Once an outline and the main ideas have been developed, the carpenter begins writing to present the ideas logically, without worrying about grammar or style.
4. The *judge* rules on grammar and style. The manuscript is corrected and polished to communicate clearly what the writer wants to say.

Your language needs to convey your ideas clearly and directly. Any arguments should proceed logically and should be persuasive. If you use jargon, it must be understandable to your audience. Key points that are too long, too technical, difficult to read, or full of jargon should be edited. Do not waste the reader's time with irrelevant information.

Write a first draft and as many others as necessary. Strive for clarity, brevity, and white space on the page when you edit. To increase clarity, cut unnecessary words. Simplify your ideas by breaking long sentences with many clauses into several sentences. Read the report aloud when proofreading to help spot repetition, ambiguity, awkward phrasing, and other flaws. Credibility killers include misspellings, grammar and punctuation errors, use of the wrong name, and inconsistent formatting.[17]

Some written reports benefit from an executive summary. Its purpose is to communicate key points from the larger report. It is not a preface or introduction and does not introduce new material. The length of an executive summary ranges from 1 or 2 paragraphs to 1 or 2 pages. The executive summary can be 10% to 15% of the length of the full report.[17]

Memos

Memos are short versions of correspondence that communicate a condensed message with a central idea. They should describe the situation, the issue or problem, the question, and the answer. A description of the situation should be concise but complete and factual. The issue or problem the memo addresses should be explained clearly. Next, ask what can be done about the issue, followed by possible solutions to the question.[17]

As with any written communication, readers will find your memo compelling if the information and ideas are logically ordered. The message should be the focus of the memo. Trying to impress the reader or establish authority by expressing complex thoughts in a long narrative can make the memo hard to comprehend. Eliminate unnecessary language.

Email

Email is a popular method of communication that is widely used in nurse anesthesia programs for the interchange of information among faculty, students, and clinical sites. Remember to keep an up-to-date address book and know how to use it. This will save you considerable time in the future.

Although the value of communicating by email is well recognized, the speed with which it can be sent and its often informal composition pose real and substantial risks. Do not say anything you would not want everyone to read. Legally, email belongs to the organization that provides the system and the linkup. You do not have privacy, and the courts can obtain email records from the organization. You may want to keep printed copies of email you sent or received regarding important issues if there is a possibility of problems, appeals, or litigation.[20]

Never send email when you are angry or tired. If you are an administrator, you should never reprimand, reward, or fire someone by sending an email. It is your responsibility to inform the individual in person. It is also a good rule to refrain from reprimanding anyone by email. There is no substitute for a face-to-face meeting to communicate to an instructor or a student that a change in performance is necessary. Face-to-face meetings are particularly important with disciplinary proceedings that must be confirmed in writing.

Avoid common mistakes in email writing. For example, do not use dense blocks of uninterrupted text, and do not forget to include a descriptive subject line. Using white space and paragraphs makes it easier for the reader to identify key points and gain a more complete understanding of what you are communicating. A subject line that describes the main idea of your message gives the reader a good idea of what is to follow. Subject lines also are helpful to the reader in identifying your message among a long list of others at a later date.

Do not fail to proofread. Set the completed, spell-checked document aside for a few minutes, and then read through it again. Spell-checkers do not catch the wrong word spelled correctly. If the email must be error free, proofread it slowly forward and backward. Proofreading on a computer screen is not easy. You may even want to avoid sending an email that must be error free. Even deleted emails can be resurrected and widely read by people you never intended to see them.

Opportunities for Instructors to Increase Learning About Communication

Individuals involved in the education of nurse anesthesia students have many opportunities to increase their communication skills, such as formal courses, online classes, and books on the topic. Workshops or conferences, such as the AANA's Assembly of School Faculty, often offer topics to attendees that are related to effective communication. There are plenty of opportunities to practice your communication skills, such as written and oral delivery of student evaluations, oral communication during meetings, and programmatic self-study evaluation.

Student Evaluations

Anonymous surveys of surgical residents and attending surgeons revealed that both residents and faculty valued communication skills as important to patient care. The surveys suggested that an evaluation instrument that measured communication skills may strengthen the feedback process.[23] The findings of this survey are also applicable to the evaluations of faculty and students in nurse anesthesia programs.

Nurse anesthesia instructors play a dual role in the development of communication competencies. First, instructors should continually strive to strengthen their own ability to communicate effectively. Second, instructors should assist their students to expand upon their basic communication skills. Performance indicators can be used to measure the success of both instructors and students.

Evaluations of an instructor can include rating his or her communication skills with items such as the following:

- Demonstrates the ability to communicate ideas in a clear, concise manner.
- Views the educational process as an interactive exchange between student and teacher.
- Facilitates discussion, inquiry, and scholarship among students and faculty.
- Demonstrates excellent interpersonal communication skills with regard to students, faculty, and clinical staffs.

Evaluations of a student's communication skills can include items such as the following:

- Conducts thorough preanesthetic interviews.
- Consults with instructor regarding findings and observations.
- Seeks assistance by asking appropriate questions; counsels patients in preparation for anesthesia.
- Communicates effectively with patients, discusses plans of care, and puts the patient at ease.
- Demonstrates interpersonal skill and effectiveness in communicating with the healthcare team.

Oral Communication in Meetings

Meetings can be identified by size, and the size determines how much chance you will have to speak. An assembly consists of at least 100 people who listen to speakers. A council consists of 40 to 50 people who listen to speakers but can ask questions or make other contributions. A committee, ideally 4 to 7 people, provides a setting where members can communicate freely under the guidance of a chairperson. Regardless of the size of the meeting, an agenda is most important in speeding up the proceedings. If you are responsible for writing the agenda, be sure to give enough information to help members form some ideas or gather information before the meeting so that they will be prepared to communicate their ideas.[20]

Both program administrators and clinical instructors participate in many types and sizes of meetings. The basic purpose of a meeting is for people to gather in a group to contribute different knowledge and experiences. At times, the group uses a meeting to obtain individual ideas for solving a problem.

Educators spend an inordinate amount of time in meetings; however, in every human culture, people gather frequently in small groups and occasionally in larger groups to communicate. When there are no meetings at work, people will meet outside of work. Meetings are valuable because people who attend and get involved in discussions become committed to the decisions and goals of the group. The frequency of meetings can define the degree of group unity.[20]

A group of people can often produce better ideas, better decisions, and solve problems more efficiently than an individual; the group can also produce worse outcomes or produce nothing if the meeting is ineffective. Good communication skills are necessary for participants to use the time spent in meetings wisely. When participants listen carefully, the discussion can remain centered on the topic or problem. This is facilitated when the chairperson opens the meeting by calling attention to the importance of listening.[20]

During the meeting, the chairperson's role is to assist the group toward the best conclusion as efficiently as possible, to interpret and clarify, to move the discussion forward, and to bring it to a resolution that everyone understands and accepts. If an item is complex, the chairperson should display the main topics so that everyone can see the proposed direction for the discussion. Differing viewpoints, presented politely, should be encouraged, and difficult conversations should not be avoided. People who are skilled at communicating during meetings do not necessarily agree with every idea; they simply make it pleasant for everyone to express their ideas. When people feel comfortable communicating, more information is gained and better decisions can be made. If people don't get involved in the conversations, they will probably not be committed to the final decision.[19]

It is not uncommon for meetings to be held to discuss a draft document. Avoid allowing the group to redraft the document during the meeting. The group should agree on the document's faults and assign someone to produce a new draft later.[20] Assignments are important at the end of every meeting to avoid inaction and failure to meet expectations. The chairperson must follow up on commitments and hold people accountable.

At the end of each agenda item, the chairperson should give a brief summary of the decisions reached. These summaries can become part of the minutes. The person who records the minutes should include the time, date, location, attendees, and any absences. The date and place of the next committee meeting should be communicated at the end of the meeting and in the minutes.[20]

Writing Self-Study Evaluations

Writing a self-study evaluation is an important part of maintaining accreditation of a nurse anesthesia program. A completed self-study evaluation communicates to the accrediting agency that the program is in compliance or has plans to come into compliance with education standards. Self-study evaluations are ideally completed by a committee so that input is obtained from key institutional and program personnel as well as students. Participating in writing a self-study evaluation provides opportunities for several individuals to refine their communication skills.

If you are a new program administrator, ask for assistance from an experienced person or look at examples of previous self-study evaluations. Be careful not to blindly mimic what you find in the file cabinet or in a computer database. You could be repeating the mistakes of the past.[17]

To meet the accrediting agency's expectations, think about the accrediting agency as your audience and follow the instructions precisely. If you do not, you create more work for the on-site reviewers, accreditation staff, and COA members. Failure to follow instructions when writing a self-study evaluation could result in material being rejected or returned to you. Failure to follow instructions also raises the question of whether you will abide by future requirements.

Create a realistic plan to write the self-study evaluation by establishing a timeline, responsibilities, and a budget. Include time for writing multiple drafts, creating graphics, reviewing by the committee, obtaining approvals from superiors, and completing production activities such as copying, binding, or submitting information electronically.

Case Study

Marilyn had accepted her position as administrator of the nurse anesthesia program a short time after the previous administrator retired 1 year previously. Since she became a program administrator, she developed an informal mentoring relationship with John, a CRNA with 10 years of experience in program administration at a nearby program. She appreciated John's willingness to give her advice on any problems she encountered or to answer questions about complying with accreditation requirements.

The Problem

Marilyn's problem was her inability to obtain written evaluations from some of the clinical instructors. Furthermore, when instructors did write clinical evaluations, they frequently did not communicate in person with the students about their performance. She feared that if she did not correct the problem, it would affect the outcome of the next on-site review by the COA. After unsuccessfully trying to correct the situation herself, she telephoned John for advice.

John met with Marilyn a few days after her phone call. He asked a question about her efforts to get written evaluations from the instructors. Marilyn explained that she had met with the clinical coordinator, Sarah, and demanded that the clinical instructors be reprimanded. She said that Sarah seemed unhappy with her demand and tried to make excuses. Although Marilyn told Sarah that her door was always open and she was always available to talk with her or any of the clinical instructors, the problem continued. She emailed Sarah several times since their meeting but did not receive a reply. The previous day, a student told Marilyn that she heard a rumor that the clinical site was going to cancel its contract with the program. The student said she was worried because this was the only site that offered required obstetric and pediatric cases. Marilyn admitted to John that she was sorry that she had not listened more closely to what Sarah had to say.

Problem Solving

Instead of criticizing the way Marilyn had talked with Sarah, John questioned her about her attempts to solve the problem. This engaged Marilyn in a conversation in which they explored her interaction with Sarah, including the realization that she had not been receptive to Sarah's efforts to explain what happened. Together, Marilyn and John drafted a plan to deal with the clinical evaluation problem and to try to maintain the affiliation agreement. They also discussed ways to develop positive lines of communication between the program and clinical site. During their meeting, Marilyn learned several lessons that John shared with her from his years of experience.

Lesson #1: People need to feel free to talk to others and know they will be met with sympathetic understanding. Too many administrators fail to listen, although they announce that their doors are always open. In view of this communication failure, colleagues and subordinates do not feel free to say what they want to say. The remedy is to listen and try to understand the speaker's message. Focus full attention on the speaker, ask for clarification if needed, and follow up with appropriate action. The listener should not show displeasure through verbal response or body language. Being a good listener can help you to avoid friction between individuals and build successful relationships.[21]

Lesson #2: A key to keeping communication open is a "together we can work this out" approach. Tell the person that you have confidence in his or her ability to solve a problem and will support a reasonable solution. Demanding that a person take unequivocal action shuts off communication and generates resentment.[24]

Lesson #3: In times of uncertainty, people fill communication voids with rumors. Rumors attribute the worst possible motives to those in control. Communicating the truth will lower people's anxiety, whether the news is good or bad. To dispel rumors, the most effective way to communicate is informally, one-on-one. Honest communication will help counteract rumors.[20]

Lesson #4: Often email is not the right medium for communication, especially in a contentious situation. It is better to talk face-to-face so you can fully understand the individual's perceptions. Consider confining email to concrete requests, queries, and responses that are not controversial. For chatting or networking, use the telephone. For potentially unpleasant conversations, meeting face-to-face allows your tone of voice, gestures, and facial expressions to convey a more complete message. A face-to-face meeting also helps you to understand the other person's position more fully through observation of his or her nonverbal signals.[17,25]

Lesson #5: Efforts to change behavior and communication go hand-in-hand. First, the desired behavior should be clearly stated. Second, to make it a lasting change, there should be ongoing communication with the person or people who can tell you what is and is not working.[20]

Summary

Effective communication is an asset to nurse anesthesia program administrators, didactic instructors, clinical instructors, and their students. It is a skill that can produce better understanding of people while at work or at home, or while engaged in outside activities. It also enables you to create a supportive learning environment in which students can acquire the relevant knowledge, skills, and competencies to be excellent nurse anesthetists. Always look for opportunities to practice and improve the way you communicate and the way you teach your students to communicate. You will find that there is a great deal of truth in the saying that "Communication works for those who work at it."[19]

References

1. Anesthesia patient-provider communication essential to safe care [news release]. American Association of Nurse Anesthetists website. http://www.aana.com/news.aspx?ucNavMenu_TSMenuTargetID= 171&ucNavMenu_TSMenuTargetType=4&ucNavMenu_TSMenuID=6&id=64 04. November 28, 2007. Accessed December 13, 2007.

2. Standards for Accreditation of Nurse Anesthesia Educational Programs. Park Ridge, IL: Council on Accreditation of Nurse Anesthesia Educational Programs; 2004.

3. Accreditation Policies and Procedures. Park Ridge, IL: Council on Accreditation of Nurse Anesthesia Educational Programs; 2008.

4. Proposed Standards for Accreditation of Baccalaureate and Graduate Nursing Programs. Washington DC: Commission on Collegiate Nursing Education; 2008.

5. The Essentials of Master's Education for Advanced Practice Nursing. Washington, DC: American Association of Colleges of Nursing; 1996:10.

6. The Essentials of Doctoral Education for Advanced Nursing Practice. Washington, DC: American Association of Colleges of Nursing; 2006:14.

7. Standards and criteria: Master's Degree/Post-Master's Certificate Programs in Nursing. New York, NY: National League for Nursing Accrediting Commission; 2008.

8. Standards and criteria: Clinical Doctorate Degree Programs in Nursing. New York, NY: National League for Nursing Accrediting Commission; 2008.

9. Tamblyn R, Abrahamowicz M, Dauphinee D, et al. Physician scores on a national clinical skills examination as predictors of complaints to medical regulatory authorities. *JAMA*. 2007;298(9):993-1001.

10. Flin R, Yule S, Paterson-Brown S, Maran N, Rowley D, Youngson G. Teaching surgeons about non-technical skills. *UK Surgeon*. 2007;5(2):86-89.

11. Kohn LT, Corrigan JM, Donaldson MS; Committee on Quality of Health Care in America, Institute of Medicine. *To Err Is Human: Building Safer Health System*. Washington, DC: National Academies Press. 1999.

12. Committee on Quality of Health Care in America, Institute of Medicine. *Crossing the Quality Chasm: A New Health System for the 21st Century*. Washington, DC: National Academies Press: 2001.

13. Grenier AC, Knebel E; Committee on the Health Professions Education Summit. *Health Professions Education: A Bridge to Quality*. Washington, DC: National Academies Press; 2003.

14. Institute for Safe Medication Practices. Error-prone conditions can lead to student nurse-related medication mistakes. *AANA NewsBulletin*. 2007;61(12):10-11.

15. McQuillan RJ, King H, Salas E, Gaba D, Galt K. Teamwork and team training in the operating room: can it make a difference in patient safety? *APSF Newsletter*. 2007;22(3):53.

16. Liberal education outcomes: a preliminary report on student achievement in college. Association of American Colleges and Universities website. http://www.aacu.org/advocacy/pdfs/LEAP_Report_FINAL.pdf. Accessed March 9, 2009.

17. Harvard Business Publishing. *Written Communications That Inform and Influence: The Results-Driven Manager Series*. Boston, MA: Harvard Business School Press; 2006.

18. Speech communication portfolio: why is communication important? Department of Speech Communication at Southern Illinois University, Edwardsville website. http://www.siue.edu/SPC/SPC/_Portfolio/why.html. Accessed January 23, 2008.

19. Patterson K, Grenny J, McMillan R, Switzler A. *Crucial Conversations: Tools for Talking When the Stakes Are High*. New York, NY: McGraw-Hill. 2002.

20. Harvard Business Publishing. *Harvard Business Review on Effective Communication*. Boston, MA: Harvard Business School Press; 1999.

21. Dowling T. Career article 132: basic communication skills everyone needs. Seeking Success website. http://www.seekingsuccess.com/articles/art132.php3. Accessed January 19, 2008.

22. Glynn CJ, Huge ME. Opinions as norms: applying a return potential model to the study of communication behaviors. *Commun Res*. 2007;34(5):548-568.

23. Hutul OA, Carpenter RO, Tarpley JL, Lomis KD. Missed opportunities: a descriptive assessment of teaching and attitudes regarding communication skills in a surgical residency. *Curr Surg*. 2006;63(6):401-409.

24. Himes AC. Evaluating faculty with specific concerns: what, why, and how. *Acad Leader*. 2007:23(3):5,8.

25. You've got conflict: e-mail and conflict management. American Council on Education Department Leadership Project website. http://www.acenet.edu/resources/chairs/docs/holton_e-mail.pdf. Accessed March 9, 2008.

Section II

Clinical Education

Chapter 10

Theory and Principles of Adult Education for the Clinical Instructor

William Hartland Jr, CRNA, PhD

Key Points

- Clinical instructors are not only accountable for the clinical education of their students but also for all other aspects inherent to anesthesia clinical practice.

- The clinical instructor can enhance student learning by creating a physical and psychological environment that promotes learning.

- Student nurse anesthetists are adults coming from a variety of ethnic and social backgrounds who have a wealth of professional and nonprofessional life experiences.

- The clinical instructor must continually determine where on the clinical teaching continuum instruction should take place based on the student's knowledge base and level of performance.

- Adult learning principles can give the clinical instructor a framework from which to build and develop clinical teaching excellence.

- Twenty-two characteristics of an effective clinical instructor serve as guidelines that clinical instructors can use on their journey toward clinical teaching excellence.

Introduction

Healthcare professionals are cognizant of the crucial role that clinical experience plays in the education of their students. In nurse anesthesia education, these clinical experiences are often referred to as clinical practicums. It is during clinical practicums that the student nurse anesthetist is given the opportunity to apply classroom knowledge to actual practice. This application is conducted under the careful guidance and tutelage of a clinical instructor (CI).

Most nurse anesthetists can still remember their own experiences, as students, with the CIs to whom they were assigned. Some of these memories are pleasant while others are not. Many CIs gave their students a sense of excitement, satisfaction, and accomplishment in the clinical arena. These CIs helped their students reach new heights in their journey toward clinical proficiency. They were the instructors to whom the students eagerly awaited to be assigned. Unfortunately, there were also CIs who many anesthetists felt contributed little, if anything, to their educational experience. Some of these CIs appeared apathetic and uncaring; others appeared to teach by intimidation, humiliation, and fear. These were the instructors that students dreaded to see on their daily clinical assignment sheets.

In 1999, Gelmon[1] stated that teaching competency was an extremely important issue for nurse anesthesia instructors. Gelmon suggested that no instructor wants to be labeled as an incompetent teacher and no student wants to be subjected to the same. The problem arises when nurse anesthetists are placed in a teaching role for which they are ill prepared.[1]

Unfortunately, few CIs have been afforded formal educational opportunities concerning effective teaching in the clinical arena. Many CIs have presumed teaching effectiveness by virtue of their professional preparation and clinical expertise. They assume that expertise in their specialty automatically makes them experts in another. This reasoning is not restricted to the profession of nurse anesthesia. It is also prevalent in numerous professional occupations both in and out of the healthcare domain. In the profession of nurse anesthesia, CIs should be mindful that clinical competence does not automatically imply the ability to teach effectively in the clinical area. Some instructors presume teaching effectiveness by virtue of emulating CIs they had in school. They often rationalize this modeling by stating: "This is the way I was taught; and if it was good enough for me, it is good enough for you." Such experiences can definitely be an asset if the CIs being used as role models were effective clinical teachers. On the other hand, emulating an ineffective CI will most likely perpetuate more of the same.

Other CIs may claim that they learned how to teach in the clinical arena by trial and error. Their clinical teaching strategies were developed from their own successful and unsuccessful teaching experiences. Even though experience is a coach from which CIs will learn throughout their careers, there are more efficient learning methods available. Evidenced-based documentation is available in the literature to help the CI build a firm foundation in effective clinical instruction without exclusively relying on the process of trial and error.

As stated earlier, clinical instruction is an essential component of the student nurse anesthetist's educational experience. As a result, it is essential that CIs be well versed in effective clinical teaching methodology. But, what is this methodology? How does one become an effective CI? Before examining these and other issues, we will begin by examining this individual known as "the clinical instructor."

The Clinical Instructor

The responsibilities that are shouldered by the CI are substantial. Clinical instructors are not only accountable for the clinical education of their students, but also for all other aspects inherent to anesthesia clinical practice.

Professional Roles of the Clinical Instructor

As an anesthesia professional, the CI fulfills many roles. These roles include those of anesthesia provider, employee, and clinical teacher. As an anesthesia provider, the CI's primary responsibility is the safe anesthetic care and management of his or her patients. This includes working effectively and efficiently with coworkers and team members, delivering anesthesia management that is specific to each patient, and being a strong patient advocate. It also necessitates that the CI remains current in the latest developments and innovations in the specialty of anesthesia practice.

As an employee, the CI has a responsibility to his or her employer. This responsibility encompasses adherence to the protocols, policies, and directives of the employer. Such adherence is expected as a requirement for employment. Deviation from these established standards may result in disciplinary action or termination of employment.

As an educator, the CI plays a pivotal role in the clinical education of student nurse anesthetists. The CI functions as a teacher and mentor by helping students integrate didactic knowledge into practice. The CI serves as a role model to students during their professional development. The CI is also a student advocate who promotes and enhances a student's clinical learning experiences.

Domains of Learning and the Clinical Instructor

Webster's New World College Dictionary defines learning as the acquiring of knowledge or skill.[2] This acquisition involves change in behavior or performance. For our purposes, this knowledge or skill acquisition encompasses 3 domains of learning: (1) cognitive, (2) psychomotor, and (3) affective. The cognitive domain of learning is primarily concerned with new knowledge, understanding, and ways of thinking. The psychomotor domain focuses on new skills and behavior patterns such as new ways of acting or performing a task. The affective domain centers on attitudes, values, and ways of feeling.[3]

All of these domains can be further subdivided into a hierarchy of categories moving from the simple to the complex (Table 10.1). The cognitive domain begins with simple knowledge outcomes such as recall and proceeds through increasingly complex levels of comprehension such as applying certain information to new

Table 10.1. Taxonomy of Educational Objectives

Cognitive domain: the 6 cognitive levels (lowest to highest)

1. Knowledge	Ability to recall or recognize content the way it was initially presented
2. Comprehension	Ability to understand the meaning of material
3. Application	Ability to use material in new situations
4. Analysis	Ability to break down material into its component parts so that its organizational structure may be understood
5. Synthesis	Ability to arrange and combine content in such a way as to produce a new structure or idea
6. Evaluation	Ability to judge the value of material for a given purpose

Psychomotor domain: the 7 psychomotor levels (lowest to highest)

1. Perception	Use of senses to obtain cues that guide a motor activity
2. Set	Readiness to take a particular action
3. Guided response	Early stages (imitation/trial and error) in learning a complex skill
4. Mechanism	Performing with some confidence and proficiency
5. Proficiency	Skillful performance of motor acts that involve intricate movement patterns
6. Adaptation	Ability to modify movement patterns to fit special situations
7. Origination	Ability to create new movement patterns to fit special situations

Affective domain: the 5 affective levels (lowest to highest)

1. Receptivity	Willingness to pay attention to a particular educational activity
2. Responding	Responding or reacting to a stimulus. Showing an interest in something
3. Valuing	The worth an individual puts on a particular object, occurrence, or behavior
4. Organization	Bringing together different values to build an internally consistent system
5. Value or value complex	Value system integrated into learner's lifestyle

(Adapted with permission from Bloom et al[4])

situations and evaluating its appropriateness. The psychomotor domain begins with readiness for action and progresses to doing the skill, doing it proficiently, and finally, being able to create new movements that fit a particular situation. The affective domain commences with the learner's willingness to pay attention, progressing to active participation, simple acceptance, and finally, the incorporation of a specific value into the learner's lifestyle.[3]

All 3 domains of learning are pertinent to anesthesia clinical education. The CI teaches and reinforces new knowledge (cognitive domain), specific anesthesia skills and techniques (psychomotor domain), and professional values and attitudes (affective domain). To teach effectively in each of the 3 domains of learning, CIs must determine which domain subcategory best applies to the student they are assigned. To make this determination, CIs should determine their student's knowledge base and experience level. Various student classifications, such as junior and senior, only give the CI an estimate of where the individual student's educational level should be. Two students with equal time in a program may be functioning at very different knowledge or skill levels. This may be the result of the individual student's comprehension abilities, personal motivation, and previous critical care and clinical anesthesia experiences. Whatever the reason, the CI should make every effort to determine the student's present performance level. This can be accomplished by reviewing available program documentation concerning the student's performance, discussions with program faculty, talking with other instructors, or direct discussions with the student. Time constraints in the clinical arena often rule out documentation and discussions with program faculty as practical options. The CI can, however, gain valuable insight from discussions with other CIs or by simply asking students to evaluate themselves in terms of their present strengths and weaknesses.

Clinical instructors must remember that no matter how proactive they are in attempting to determine a student's performance level, they should always maintain a high level of vigilance during the actual anesthetic case management. Direct observation will give the CI valuable insight concerning the student's actual performance level.

Although it is not necessary to memorize all the subcategories in each domain, it is important to understand that the subcategories progress from the simple to the complex, depending on the student's needs and level of experience. Infants first learn to crawl before they walk and they walk before they run. The same principle applies to the student nurse anesthetist. For example, let's assume the CI is assigned a patient admitted for a coronary bypass surgery. The CI will be working with an advanced student who is experienced in the anesthetic management of the coronary bypass patient. In this scenario, the role of the CI will be primarily to help the student function at a higher level in each of the 3 domains of learning. In other words, the CI may challenge the student to consider the reasoning behind certain techniques to identify acceptable alternative techniques and even new ways to accomplish the same results. If the CI is assigned a student who has little experience with this type of patient, the CI's role will be substantially different. With an inexperienced student, the CI should begin at the lower levels of the 3 domains. The CI will assume a more active teaching role, beginning with the most basic knowledge and skills necessary for the anesthetic management of the coronary bypass patient.

The Learning Environment

Although the CI cannot force a student to learn, he or she can optimize the student's learning environment to enhance learning. This involves creating an environment that promotes learning. Ideally, the learning environment should include a supportive atmosphere and a climate of mutual respect. In other words, a learning environment should be physically and psychologically comfortable.

Physical Learning Environment

The physical learning environment encompasses many tangible factors such as classroom size, design, layout, decor, temperature, lighting, acoustics, and equipment. The more comfortable the physical environment, the more the learner can concentrate on the learning task at hand. It is extremely difficult for students to concentrate on material being taught when they are shivering because of low room temperatures or sweating from high temperatures. It is also difficult to concentrate when external or internal classroom noise is so loud that it is difficult to hear the instructor.

The CI's classroom is the operating room or other specialty area requiring anesthesia service. These clinical classroom areas are less than ideal physical learning environments. Specific surgical procedures, patient needs, and surgeon's requests may require extremes in temperature and lighting. Extremes in noise may be the result of loud conversations, music, or equipment such as orthopedic saws and drills. On the other hand, the surgeon may demand absolute silence in the room during critical portions of the operation. The size and design of the room has been predetermined by the institution. Specific surgical or diagnostic procedures govern the amount of equipment crowded into the operating room. It is evident that the CI has little control over the physical environment. As a result, CIs are left to teach in an area that many educators consider a hostile learning environment.

Psychological Learning Environment

The psychological learning environment of the operating room also encompasses many factors. These factors include the cohesiveness, emotional status, and experience of the operating room team. They include the physical condition of the patient and the complexity of the surgical procedure and anesthetic requirements. Operating room team members are sometimes perceived as being overbearing, ill-tempered, and difficult. Also, a patient's physical condition during surgery can change very rapidly.

Student nurse anesthetists quickly realize that they are no longer sitting safely in a classroom or in a laboratory practicing on a manikin. The student is now working in the real world with real patients. All of these factors can have a major effect on the student's stress level and learning comprehension.

A certain level of stress can be healthy, because it can help a student remain alert and motivated. Too much stress, however, can be harmful and can hinder and block learning. McClusky[5] addresses the issue of stress and learning in his Power-Load-Margin Theory. McClusky[5] states that the key factors of adult life are the loads the adult carries and the power that is available to help the adult carry the load. Margin is the ratio of load and power. The greater the power in relationship to the load, the more margin will be available for the student to cope with the stress.[5,6]

Load factors for student nurse anesthetists can be external or internal. External load factors include personal family problems, financial hardships, and a hostile operating room learning environment. Internal load factors include lack of self-confidence or self-worth. Power factors for the student nurse anesthetist may include previous healthcare experiences, good self-image, financial stability, and support groups. Margin, or the amount of control the student has to manage stress successfully, can be increased by either increasing the power factors or by decreasing the load factors. By increasing margin and thus decreasing stress, the student's ability to concentrate on learning also increases.

As with the physical environment, the CI also has limited control over factors of the psychological environment. These factors include the complexity of the procedure, the patient's physical status, and the cohesiveness of the team. There is, however, one aspect of the psychological environment over which the CI does have control. Clinical instructors have control over themselves and how they interact with their students and other team members. This provides the CI with a great influence on the student's level of margin. The CI can increase a student's margin by increasing the student's power or by decreasing the student's load. For example, the CI can increase a student's power by answering questions, explaining and reviewing techniques and procedures, demonstrating empathy and respect, and giving constructive feedback. The CI can decrease student load by being a mediator between the student and a hostile operating room environment, reassuring the student, and helping the student seek assistance if personal problems appear to be affecting clinical performance.

The clinical learning environment is probably the most complex learning environment in which a student and instructor must function. It is dynamic, demanding, stressful, and sometimes unforgiving. Clinical instructors are very limited in the control they have over specific factors in both the physical and psychological learning environment. They do, however, play a pivotal role in enhancing student learning in both of these environments. Even in the most hostile clinical environment, it is the CI who sets the final tone for student learning.

The Student Nurse Anesthetist

Who are these students the CI deals with on a daily basis? Student nurse anesthetists come from a variety of ethnic and social backgrounds. They all have a wealth of professional and nonprofessional life experiences. Although their ages may vary, they are all members of a group known as adult learners.

Theory of Adult Learning

Adult learning theory has its roots back in the days of Plato and Aristotle. Since then, many theories of learning have evolved. For the purpose of organization, these theories will be classified, in whole or part, into 1 of 4 categories. These categories are: (1) behaviorist, (2) cognitivist, (3) social learning theorist, and (4) humanist.[7,8]

According to the *behaviorist*, learning consists of a change in behavior. What one learns is determined by elements in the environment and not by the learner. As a result, the focus is on external behavior and observable behavior. It is the role of the teacher to arrange contingencies of reinforcement in the learning environment so that desired behavior will occur. Edward L. Thorndike's Stimulus-Response Theory fits this category, where the teacher provides the correct stimulus and the student is expected to respond accordingly. Another behaviorist theory is B. F. Skinner's Operant Conditioning Theory, in which desirable behaviors are reinforced and rewarded while undesirable behaviors are punished or ignored.[8]

Contrary to the behaviorist, the *cognitivist* does not focus on the environment. The cognitivist focuses on internal mental processes such as how information is processed, stored, and retrieved in the learner's mind. To the cognitivist, the human mind is not simply a passive exchange terminal where stimuli arrive and appropriate responses leave. Instead, the thinking person interprets sensations and gives meaning to the events that impinge on his or her consciousness. Cognitivists will put information together in their minds one way and then another way until a problem is solved.[8]

The *social learning theorist* focuses on the social setting in which learning occurs. Theories in this category suggest that people learn from observing other people. In other words, learning is a function of the interaction of persons, the environment, and the behavior. Theories of modeling and mentoring often fall into this category.[8]

It is my contention that aspects of each of the major learning theory categories can be applied to clinical anesthesia education. It is the humanistic approach, however, that appears to fit our nurse anesthesia learners more closely. From the *humanist* perspective, learning involves more than just cognitive processes and overt behavior. It is a function of motivation and involves choice and responsibility. The humanist's focus is on human nature, human potential, human emotions, and affect. Included in this category is the theory of human motivation based on a hierarchy of needs by Abraham Maslow and Malcolm Knowles' theory of andragogy.[7]

Historically, the term pedagogy has been used as a synonym for the general category of teaching. Under the pedagogical model, the teacher assumes responsibility for all decisions concerning what will be learned, when it will be learned, and how it will be learned.

The concepts of andragogy are grounded in humanistic assumptions. Knowles[8] states that pedagogy literally means the art and science of educating children. On the other hand, andragogy is a word derived from the Greek prefix "andr-," which means "man." Thus, andragogy is literally translated as the art and science of helping adults learn. Andragogy focuses more on the process and less on the content being taught. In other words, andragogy is learner-focused instead of teacher-focused. This comprehensive adult learning theory contends that adults require certain conditions to learn.[9]

With respect to anesthesia education, clinical teaching can be examined in terms of a teaching continuum (Figure 10.1). The pure pedagogical model can be positioned at the left end of the continuum and the pure andragogical model at the right. Between these 2 extremes lie various combinations of these 2 models as defined by Knowles et al.[9] At the pedagogical end of the continuum, instruction would be totally CI-directed. In this situation, it would be appropriate for the CI to assume a totally active teaching role while the student assumes the passive role of listening and observing. This approach to teaching may be appropriate in circumstances in which the student is new to the clinical environment or unfamiliar with particular procedures or techniques. For example, if a patient is admitted for a subarachnoid block, it would probably be inappropriate for a student with no previous training or instruction to perform the block. In this situation, the CI would most likely have the student observe while the CI explains and executes the procedure.

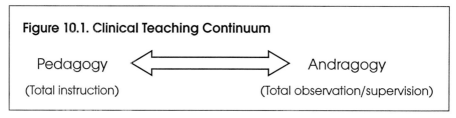

Figure 10.1. Clinical Teaching Continuum

Pedagogy ⟺ Andragogy

(Total instruction)   (Total observation/supervision)

At the right end of the continuum we find the andragogy model. In its purest sense, andragogy actually entails self-directed learning.[9] For the purpose of anesthesia clinical education, we will define the extreme andragogical end of the teaching continuum as total supervision and monitoring by the CI. At this end of the continuum, the student is totally immersed in the anesthetic management of the patient, while the CI vigilantly monitors and observes the student's performance.

For the majority of clinical experiences, it is unlikely that the CI functions totally at either of these extremes of the clinical teaching continuum. Most clinical instruction occurs somewhere between these extremes. The CI determines where on the continuum to teach, based on his or her knowledge of the student's performance, progression, and growth in the program. The CI should also be cognizant of the fact that the clinical teaching continuum is dynamic. Various situations, such as changes in the patient's condition, may necessitate right or left movement along the continuum. For example, suppose the CI is assigned to an experienced anesthesia student. The patient is basically healthy and the surgical intervention is fairly routine. The CI elects to let the student manage the case with minimal assistance. In this situation, the CI would be operating at the far right of the clinical teaching continuum. During the anesthesia induction, the student experiences problems with the laryngoscopy. The CI steps forward and assists the student by applying some cricoid pressure and making suggestions. The CI is now shifting left on the clinical teaching continuum. As difficulty with the laryngoscopy escalates, the CI now recommends an advanced difficult airway technique that the student is unfamiliar with. The CI performs the laryngoscopy successfully as the student observes the new airway technique. The CI has now shifted even further left on the continuum. Although it is the CI's goal to educate students to be independent practitioners, this is obviously not an overnight event. The process of nurturing this independence involves continuous movements and shifts along the clinical teaching continuum.

Principles of Adult Learning

Most educators agree that there is a difference between teaching adults and teaching children. There is also a great deal of agreement that the andragogical model for teaching adults is closely linked to various assumptions and principles.[7,9,10] These adult learning principles can give the CI a framework from which to build and develop clinical teaching excellence.

Principle 1: Adults Want to Learn

One thing we know about adults is that they want to learn regardless of their age. The old wives-tale that you can't teach an old dog new tricks may apply to canines but not to people. Although the capacity to learn does not diminish with age, the rate and speed of learning may vary, depending on various physiological changes such as declines in visual and audio acuity. Various pathological conditions may also have an adverse effect on learning capacity. Overall, however, adults can and want to learn. Student nurse anesthetists are no different. They are enrolled in nurse anesthesia programs for one reason: to become nurse anesthetists. It is rare that students are forced to attend anesthesia school against their will.

Principle 2: Adults Are Ready to Learn

Adults are ready to learn those things that they need to know to cope effectively with real life situations. The road to becoming a Certified Registered Nurse Anesthetist (CRNA) is long and demanding. The magnitude of information that must be learned often appears overwhelming. Despite this apparent barrier, the student is aware that mastery of this information is necessary to accomplish the goal of becoming a CRNA. Therefore, most are willing, ready, and eager to proceed with the learning process.

Principle 3: Adult Learning Is an Active Process

Adults appear to be better motivated when they are actively involved in the learning process. Adults have a desire to have some control over their lives. Many hold perceptions of themselves as independent and self-reliant individuals. They enjoy making decisions and freely offer their opinions. This especially holds true for student nurse anesthetists who come from critical care units where their decision making was valued and encouraged. In addition, many student nurse anesthetists have had various levels of supervisory experiences. Therefore, CIs must remember that one of their goals in anesthesia clinical education is to foster this independent decision-making capability in their students.

Principle 4: Adult Learning Is Goal-Directed

Adults appear to learn best when they have clear obtainable goals. In other words, before learning, adults not only need to know what they are going to learn but also why they need to know it. Therefore, one of the first tasks of the CI is to help the learners become aware of their need to know.

Children usually do not question why they are learning something in school. If they do inquire, the teachers usually respond that they are learning it because some day they will need it or that it is what they are supposed to learn in this grade in school. Although this is accepted by most children, adults are usually not satisfied with such responses. Most adults strive to accomplish a specific goal, such as becoming a CRNA. They want to stay focused on those matters that will help them reach that goal. They do not want to be sidetracked by what they perceive as unnecessary information. Obviously, the CI is a much better judge of what must be learned to become a CRNA than the student. Learning for the adult student may be hindered, however, if the student does not understand the reason why something is being taught.

It is also important that the adult learner understands exactly what the CI expects the learner to accomplish or learn during any given clinical session. This gives learners specific expectations and goals that they can focus on. In the clinical arena, this can be accomplished by the use of formal objectives or merely verbally informing the student what the clinical expectations are for the day or what the specific anesthesia experience is.

Principle 5: Adults Prefer Immediate Application of Learning

Learning that is applied immediately is retained longer and is more subject to use than learning that is not. In other words, learned material appears to be retained longer if it is applied soon after it has been taught. In anesthesia education, one of the primary purposes of the clinical practicum is to provide the student with an opportunity to apply this material or theory. Whenever possible, the CI should always strive to let the students apply what they have been taught in a timely manner. Obviously, this is dependent on the CI's judgment concerning the appropriateness of the task to the particular clinical situation.

Principle 6: Subject Matter Should Be Presented in a Logical Sequence

Learning is facilitated when there is logic to the subject matter and the logic makes sense in relation to the adult learner's repertoire of experiences. Whether teaching in the classroom or clinical arena, the CI must always strive to present new material in a logical, progressive sequence. For example, when first teaching an individual how to drive an automobile, the instructor would not tell the student to get in the car and drive around the block. There are obviously a number of issues that must be dealt with first, such as knowing state laws concerning operating a motor vehicle and understanding the basic operation of the vehicle (including how to operate controls and use instrumentation and safety devices). Once these issues have been covered, the student can then proceed to behind-the-wheel training.

The same scenario is applicable to clinical instruction. Whenever a CI is planning to teach a new skill, he or she should first break the skill into its individual essential components. Once these components are identified, they should be organized into a logical sequence of events so that each builds on the other, ultimately resulting in the accomplishment of the desired skill. For example, obviously student nurse anesthetists must learn how to intubate a patient. The technique of intubation can be broken into many components. These components include but are not limited to: equipment, preparation of equipment, patient positioning, insertion of the larynoscope, airway exposure, and insertion of the endotracheal tube. The CI should present these components as a logical sequence of events that will facilitate the student's learning of that skill. If the CI is not sure about an appropriate logical sequence of material, he or she should not hesitate to seek guidance from a colleague. If the proposed sequence of events makes sense to the colleague, it will most likely make sense to the student as well.

Principle 7: Adults Need to Be Aware of Their Progress

Learning is facilitated and reinforced when the learners are made aware of their progress. The CI cannot expect students to change or improve their performance if the students are not aware what they are doing right or wrong. Student learning can be facilitated and reinforced by the use of constructive feedback.

Constructive feedback should not be belittling or degrading. When giving feedback to a student, the CI should always focus on the desired performance, behavior, or outcome. The CI should never focus on or attack the individual as a person. For example, if you observe that your student is not holding the laryngoscope properly while performing a laryngoscopy, the student obviously must be corrected. Such corrections are best accomplished by first noting those things the student is doing correctly and then addressing the areas needing improvement. The CI should focus on the incorrect technique and behavior and not on the individual. In the above example, the CI could explain to students that success with laryngoscopy will dramatically increase if they change their grip on the laryngoscope. In this way the CI is addressing the incorrect behavior. Calling the student a "stupid, clumsy idiot" may give the CI some type of satisfaction but will do little to promote learning.

Feedback should also be specific and relevant. Early in my teaching career, I remember a student telling me that his CI had commented that he was "performing OK, for a large male student." He stated that he was not sure what to do about the "large" and "male" comment. We both laughed, but the question still remained as to the purpose and value of the feedback he was given. Vague or irrelevant feedback serves little value in helping a student improve performance.

Principle 8: Adult Learners Often Reach Learning Plateaus

The existence of periodic plateaus in the rate of learning necessitates frequent changes in the nature of the learning task to ensure continuous progress. It is well-known that some students appear to grasp concepts faster than others. It is also known that adult learners periodically encounter temporary learning plateaus or obstacles that inhibit learning progression. In other words, they appear to have difficulty understanding a concept or procedure that is necessary for further learning to progress. Learning plateaus are very common and should be expected. The CI can be instrumental in assisting a student to work through and overcome these learning plateaus.

How does the CI know when these learning plateaus surface? When such plateaus occur, students will often admit they are having trouble understanding a concept or procedure. Some students, however, may feel that such an admission could be perceived as a sign of weakness. Whether a student actively seeks help or not, the CI should be watching the student constantly for evidence of a learning plateau. The CI can accomplish this by becoming a "reflective clinical instructor."

Reflective Clinical Instructor

Donald Schön, Professor of Urban Studies and Education at Massachusetts Institute of Technology, Cambridge, Massachusetts, proposed that the most effective teachers live a life of reflection about their teaching practice. Schön labeled this kind of teacher as a "reflective practitioner."[11,12] The nurse anesthesia CI should also be a reflective practitioner. Clinical instructors should continually evaluate and reevaluate their teaching strategies, techniques, and outcomes. They should be constantly pulling in information from their environment to determine the effectiveness of their teaching. This information may be gleaned from the types of questions their students ask. It may come from observing the students affect and behavior. For example, does the student look or act confused? Are you met with a blank stare? Has the student become suddenly quiet? These signs and others may alert the CI of a present or imminent learning problem. This reflection is a dynamic process occurring before, during, and after each clinical experience.

Once the CI has identified that the student is having difficulty in learning or is experiencing a plateau in learning, strategies to assist the student can be formulated. If a student is having trouble understanding certain material, often all that is required is a further explanation. The CI should be aware, however, that if students did not understand the first explanation, they most likely will not understand a verbatim repetition of the same explanation. The CI should rephrase the explanation or use additional examples for clarification. It is also possible that a new teaching strategy would facilitate the student's learning. For example, instead of trying to reiterate how to perform a particular technique, it may be helpful to demonstrate how it is done. Once the barrier to the student's learning progression has been identified, the CI can proceed with an appropriate plan of action.

Principle 9: Adults Possess a Large Amount of Prior Knowledge and Experience

Learning new material is facilitated when it is related to what is already known. Adults accumulate a vast amount of knowledge and experiences throughout their lives. Adult learning appears to be facilitated when the instructor can present new concepts by building on information the learner has already mastered. For example, let's say a patient requires an arterial line. The student tells the CI that he or she has never started an arterial line before. The CI learns that the student has had an assortment of experiences starting intravenous lines in the critical care area. The student also claims vast experience in managing arterial lines already in vitro. Learning how to start an arterial line will be facilitated if the CI builds on the student's intravenous and arterial line management experiences as opposed to starting completely new. In this situation, the CI might first have the student recall his or her other experiences with managing arterial lines to include the purpose of the line, care, and so on. Next, the CI may have the student review the basic procedure for starting an intravenous line. At this point, the CI might point out the differences in technique in starting an intravenous line as compared to an arterial line.

The CI must be aware that past experiences can also be a detriment to learning. This is especially true when these experiences were weak or flawed. In this situation, life experiences may form patterns of behavior that may require unlearning before new learning can proceed. In the above arterial line example, it is possible that the student developed some undesirable shortcuts or techniques while starting intravenous lines. The CI must first correct these undesirable behaviors before proceeding to arterial cannulation. Before using a student's past experiences, the CI must be sure such experiences are sound and form a good foundation from which to build.

Principle 10: Adults Have a Strong Sense of Self-Esteem

Adults want to be treated as adults. Self-esteem can be defined as pride in oneself, the quality of being worthy of respect, or the belief and confidence in one's own ability and value.[2] A student's self-esteem and ego are on the line whenever he or she is asked to risk trying a new behavior in front of peers or cohorts.

When an adult's self-esteem, self-image, or psychological well-being is attacked, the adult often moves into survival mode. Whenever adult students are belittled, humiliated, embarrassed, or criticized in front of others, their primary focus switches from learning to self-preservation and survival. As a student advisor, I have had many students come to me with a common theme. During a particular clinical experience, these students felt that their CI had belittled or humiliated them in front of the operating room staff or others. During the course of these discussions, it was obvious that, following the incident, student learning had been impaired and in some instances was destroyed for the remainder of the experience.

This does not mean that students should not be corrected. As stated earlier, feedback should be constructive and not destructive. The CI should focus on the problem and never attack the individual. The CI should also make every effort to correct or counsel the student quietly and in private. Corrections should never be broadcast throughout the operating room. Once we attack a student's self-esteem we seriously damage the learning environment.

Characteristics of an Effective Clinical Instructor

In 1982, Katz[13] identified 22 of the best and worst CI characteristics as perceived by a national sampling of program administrators, CIs, and students. In 1993, Hartland and Londoner[12] conducted a follow-up study that identified and ranked

Table 10.2. Characteristics Perceived as Indicative of Effective Clinical Instructors and Their Operational Definition

Rank	Characteristic	Operational definition
1	Has clinical competence/ judgment	The CI is technically skilled, demonstrating sound application of theory and knowledge to practice.
2	Is Calm	The CI is poised and composed in the clinical area and reacts to stress in a very professional and skillful manner.
3	Has a strong ego and is self-assured	The CI demonstrates confidence in his or her own abilities and recognizes his or her own limitations.
4	Is flexible	The CI encourages his or her students to become familiar with various anesthesia techniques appropriate to the patient's needs.
5	Appropriately encourages independence	The CI assigns responsibilities to students and encourages them to act and think for themselves according to their level of education and competence.
6	Engenders confidence	The CI helps students develop self-confidence in their own ability to perform appropriately.
7	Motivates students	The CI expects students to assume an active role in the discussion and problem-solving process while encouraging them to perform and communicate at their level of knowledge.
8	Has empathy/ respect	The CI demonstrates sensitivity toward students, understands their needs, supports their self-esteem, and relates to them in a nonthreatening manner.
9	Evaluates/counsels	The CI evaluates and counsels students systematically and objectively with appropriate, constructive, and timely feedback.
10	Enjoys teaching	The CI conveys interest, motivation, and satisfaction in clinical teaching.
11	Stimulates student involvement	The CI encourages his or her students to participate actively in all aspects of anesthesia care.
12	Is a positive role model	The CI serves as an appropriate model of the type of anesthetist students want to emulate.
13	Is open-minded	The CI discusses different views relating to anesthesia care and encourages students to develop their own sound viewpoints.
14	Is sensitivity	The CI demonstrates understanding of others' feelings and supports students' self esteem.

Rank	Characteristic	Operational definition
15	Engages in scholarly teaching/has broad knowledge base	The CI demonstrates a broad reading and knowledge base, referring and applying pertinent articles and research to patient care, and explains the basis for his or her clinical actions.
16	Is accessible	The CI is available and devotes appropriate time to his or her students.
17	Has communication skills	The clinical instructor demonstrates a variety of effective verbal and nonverbal communication patterns.
18	Individualizes teaching	The CI sets objectives and adjusts teaching methods specific to the level and learning needs of each student.
19	Engages in timely feedback	The CI evaluates students' performance as close to the performance as appropriate.
20	Actively teaches	The CI interacts with the students throughout the clinical period.
21	Stimulates effective discussions	The CI skillfully encourages and facilitates discussions.
22	Uses student care plan	The CI analyzes, evaluates, and allows students to implement the care plan whenever possible.

(Adapted with permission from Hartland and Londoner.[13])

the importance of these characteristics as perceived by 354 anesthesia program administrators, CIs, and students nationwide (Table 10.2). The respondents in this second study perceived all 22 characteristics of effective CIs to be important. Mean scores indicated that all 22 characteristics were perceived to be either *very important* or *highly important*. When the researchers rank ordered the mean scores of the characteristics for all respondents, some characteristics had moderately higher mean scores than others. When the mean scores of the characteristics for each group (administrators, instructors, students) were arranged in descending order by the researcher, no significant difference was found among respondent groups. The researchers concluded that it appeared that all 4 professional groups valued the 22 characteristics and perceived them as critically important to clinical instruction. The results of these studies give the CI insight into what colleagues and students perceive to be the desirable characteristics of an effective CI. They serve as guidelines that nurse anesthesia CIs can use on their journey toward clinical teaching excellence.[14]

Summary

Progressing toward the goal of becoming an effective CI requires effort, patience, and dedication. As CIs, we must remember that our students are adult learners and that various principles of adult learning apply. We should use the perceived characteristics of effective CIs to help us identify those areas in our own clinical teaching that need improvement. We must also remember the importance of maintaining the learning environment and the power we possess to accomplish that end.

Becoming an effective CI is a journey that some believe never really ends. The CI should strive consistently for clinical teaching excellence, cognizant that the future of the nurse anesthesia profession will be in the hands of the students that are taught today.

References

1. Gelmon SB. Promoting teaching competency and effectiveness for the 21st century. *AANA J*. 1999;67(5):409-416.

2. *Webster's New World College Dictionary*. 4th ed. Cleveland, OH: Wiley Publishing, Inc; 2004.

3. Ramsborg GC. *Objectives to Outcomes: Your Contract With the Learner*. Birmingham, AL: Professional Convention Management Association; 1993:21-37.

4. Bloom BS, Mesia BB, Mesia DR. *Taxonomy of Educational Objectives*. New York, NY: David McKay; 1964.

5. Lorge J, McClusky HY, Jenson GE, Hallenbeck NC. *Psychology of Adults: Adult Education Theory and Method*. Washington, DC: Adult Education Association of USA; 1993.

6. McClusky HY. An approach to a differential psychology of the adult potential. In: Knowles MS, ed. *The Adult Learner: A Neglected Species*. 4th ed. Houston, TX: Gulf Publishing Co; 1990:149-162.

7. Merriam SB, Caffarella RS. *Learning in Adulthood: A Comprehensive Guide*. San Francisco, CA: Jossey-Bass; 1991.

8. Robinson RD. *An Introduction to Helping Adults Learn and Change*. 3rd ed. West Bend, WI: Omnibook Co; 1996.

9. Knowles MS, Holton EF III, Swanson RA. *The Adult Learner: The Definitive Classic in Adult Education and Human Resource Development*. 6th ed. Burlington, MA: Elsevier Inc; 2005.

10. Brookfield SD. *Understanding and Facilitating Adult Learning: A Comprehensive Analysis of Principles and Effective Practice*. San Francisco, CA: Jossey-Bass; 1986.

11. Schön DA. *Educating the Reflective Practitioner: Toward a New Design for Teaching and Learning in the Professions*. San Francisco, CA: Jossey-Bass; 1987.

12. Brookfield SD. *Becoming a Critically Reflective Teacher*. San Francisco, CA: Jossey-Bass; 1995.

13. Hartland W, Londoner C. Perceived importance of clinical teaching characteristics for nurse anesthesia clinical faculty. *AANA J*. 1997;65:547-551.

14. Katz LE. Characteristics of clinical teachers in nurse anesthesia. *AANA J*. 1984;52:192-197.

Chapter 11

Learning Styles and Their Effects on Clinical Instruction

John P. McDonough, CRNA, EdD, ARNP
Lillia Loriz, PhD, ARNP, BC
Kiran Macha, MBBS, MPH

Key Points

- A learning style is a particular strategy a student adopts that arises from myriad psychological, behavioral, cognitive, and affective factors.

- In an attempt to classify the divergent learning styles of individuals, many tests and assessment tools have been devised.

- Learners can be classified as 1 of the following: diverger, assimilator, converger, or accommodator.

- Each style is associated with a preference for certain types of learning activities.

- Learners may seek areas of study that are influenced by their preferred learning styles and their personality traits.

- Learning style also may be affected by the situations to which the student is subjected and the experiences the student has found brings him or her success.

- No particular learning style is more associated with academic success than another.

- Healthcare education is much more formal and rank-driven than other disciplines.

- Teaching methods that include personalization are superior for students with a variety of learning styles.

Introduction

In 2008, there were 109 programs preparing Certified Registered Nurse Anesthetists (CRNAs) in the United States.[1] Because of the increase in accredited programs and student nurse anesthetists in the past decade, the number of clinical sites has increased by more than a factor of 4: from less than 400 sites to a current total exceeding 1,800 sites.[1] This increase in nurse anesthesia clinical educational sites has brought about a role change for many CRNAs.

Certified Registered Nurse Anesthetists who were primarily responsible for the provision of anesthesia care in the past now find themselves in the role of clinical preceptor for student nurse anesthetists.[2] The knowledge, skills, and abilities required to administer anesthesia to patients differ from those required to teach others how to administer anesthesia. Clinicians who have found themselves in this position have expressed concerns regarding their lack of preparation in the theoretical concepts of the teaching process.[3]

Learning Style Concepts

As practitioners have become more involved in the clinical teaching process, they have noted that not all students seem to learn in the same way. Herbert Thelen, in 1954, was the first to use the term "learning style" in the literature.[4,5] Why is it important to consider the learning styles of students? In doing so, the preceptor becomes more able to design experiences and methodologies in accordance with the way students actually acquire knowledge.[6] A learning style is a particular strategy a student adopts that arises from myriad psychological, behavioral, cognitive, and affective factors.[7] These factors combine to create a "distinct and habitual manner of acquiring knowledge, skills, or attitudes through study or experience."[8] Although one might surmise that thinking and learning are similar, and individuals carry out the process in the same ways, this is not the case. Diagnostic tools have been created to assess cognitive styles (the way a person thinks), and they frequently show a difference between cognitive style and learning style in the same individual.[9,10] Therefore, the terms *cognitive style* and *learning style* are not interchangeable.[11-13]

In an attempt to classify the divergent learning styles of individuals, many tests and assessment tools have been devised. A frequently used assessment tool, the Learning Style Inventory (LSI), classifies learners as 1 of the following: diverger, assimilator, converger, or accommodator.[14] David Kolb's concept of learning styles was based on the personality theories of Karl Jung. Kolb's work was also influenced by the writings of John Dewey, who recognized the need for learning to be grounded in experience, and by Kurt Lewin, who claimed that for learning to be effective, people must be actively involved.[15]

Another view of learning styles that is popular with some postsecondary educators was expressed by Gordon Pask. Pask describes 3 conceptual styles: holistic, serialist, and versatile, and he describes learning as being deep, surface, or strategic.[16,17] Kolb and Pask are not the only contributors to the debate in the field of learning styles. Peter Honey and Alan Mumford created an instrument called the Learning Style Questionnaire.[18] The instruments developed by Kolb and Honey are still used today. Some believe that the LSI developed by Kolb has a firmer grounding in psychometrics than the available alternatives.[18,19] Others have expressed doubts concerning the model upon which Honey and Mumford's instrument is based.[20] Although it remains in common use today, the LSI devised by Kolb, is not accepted by all[21]; however, the Kolb LSI remains one of the most commonly used instruments today and will be explored here. Those taking the LSI are presented with 12 sentences and are asked to rank order a set of potential endings offered for each sentence.[14] The response chosen to complete each sentence is associated with 1 of the 4 types of learning styles listed in Table 11.1.

Table 11.1. Learning Approaches Associated With Specific Learning Orientations

Learning orientation	Characterized by
Concrete experience	An experience-based, involved approach to learning
Abstract conceptualization	A conceptually based, analytical approach to learning
Active experimentation	An action-based, active approach to learning
Reflective observation	An observation-based, impartial approach to learning

---

The 4 learning orientations described by Kolb can be seen as the X and Y axes of a graph. On the vertical Y axis, *concrete* and *abstract* are at the opposite ends. On the horizontal X axis, *active* and *reflective* are the opposing poles. If these 2 lines cross at their midpoint, 4 quadrants are created, as shown in Figure 11.1. The score achieved on the LSI places a learner somewhere on each axis. This score will also place the learner somewhere in 1 of these 4 quadrants. Each quadrant is identified by a word that describes the style of learning. Each style is associated with a preference for certain types of learning activities.

Learning Style Inventory

Those classified as convergers are pragmatic and prefer to learn through activities that involve abstract conceptualization and active experimentation. Convergers tend to seek the single best answer to a question or a single solution to a problem. Convergers have been found to be less emotional than other types of learners, and they would rather deal with things than people.[14]

Those classified as divergers are reflective and favor observation and concrete experiences. Divergers tend to have learning strengths opposite to those classified as convergers. Divergers are interested in people and have been described as emotional and imaginative.[14]

Those classified as assimilators tend to be theoretical and often favor abstract conceptualization and reflective observation. They do well at inductive reasoning

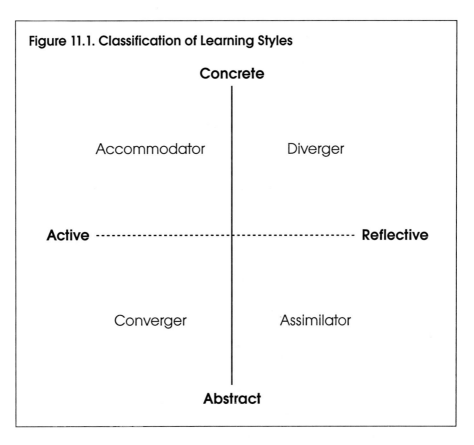

Figure 11.1. Classification of Learning Styles

Concrete

| Accommodator | Diverger |

Active — — — — — — — — — — — — — — Reflective

| Converger | Assimilator |

Abstract

and tend to pose integrated explanations for observations that others may not appreciate.[14]

Those classified as accommodators are activists who have a preference for learning activities that involve concrete experience and experimentation. They prefer to *do* things. These learners take more risks than those with other styles. When presented with a situation that does not seem to fall clearly within the parameters of a particular theoretical concept or predetermined plan, accommodators tend to resort to a process of trial and error. These learners are at ease with people but can be viewed as impatient.[14]

Individuals with different learning styles value different types of learning activities. Table 11.2 describes the activities from which learners of various styles might best benefit in an exercise designed to teach endotracheal intubation.

Differences in Learning Styles

Learning styles are not carved in stone. Learners may have a variety of learning styles, but these styles are not usually all present in the same person to the same degree.[19,22] There are data to support the concept that learners vary their preferred styles depending on their stage in the learning process.[23] Furthermore, there are also indications that learners seek certain areas of study that are influenced by their preferred learning styles and personality traits.[24,25]

Table 11.2. Preferred Learning Activities Associated With Specific Learning Styles

Learning style	Activities preferred
Converger	Receiving practical tips from an expert laryngoscopist
	Using the help feature on software used to teach intubation
Diverger	Observing how other people intubate
	Thinking about the intubation just performed by the student
	Recording thoughts about experiences with attempted intubations
Assimilator	Understanding the theory and being clear on the concept of intubation
	Reading to discover the pros and cons of different intubation techniques
	Reading a text to get a clearer grasp of what was performed
Accommodator	Picking up a laryngoscope and attempting the procedure
	Practicing intubation procedure repeatedly
	Using people skills to induce experts to help the student to develop a personal style

Learners being educated for various professions have demonstrated different learning styles when examined as groups.[26] For example, in a study that compared the learning styles of radiographers and nurses, 66% of radiographers were classified as either convergers or assimilators, whereas the nurses were primarily divergers and accommodators.[27,28] A group that contains a majority of divergers and accommodators more closely mimics the distribution of learning styles commonly seen in physicians. Those classified as convergers prefer to receive information as a symbolic representation of experience. They are more comfortable dealing with concepts and ideas than dealing with people, and they tend to be oriented toward technology.[27,28]

Preferred learning styles may change as a result of teaching methods to which a particular student is exposed during the educational process.[29] Learning style may also be affected by the types of situations to which the student is subjected and the experiences the student has found to bring success. When we examine the learning styles of student nurse anesthetists, we can see the effect of experience and exposure to a set of educational strategies. When the Kolb LSI was given to a group of student nurse anesthetists who completed less than 12 months in a nurse anesthesia program, no dominant learning style preference was noted. When the LSI was administered to a group of student nurse anesthetists who had completed more than 12 months of their programs, 80% of the students were classified as convergers or assimilators.[30] No learning style is more associated with academic success than another. Accordingly, it is important for students to know that a particular style will not guarantee success. It might be helpful to encourage students to develop their least preferred style in an effort to maximize their chances of success in varying learning situations.[26]

Although it may seem counterintuitive, there is no consensus regarding the need to align student learning styles with the teaching methods used in an educational setting. Some data show that, when teaching styles do not match learning styles of students, less than optimal results are achieved.[13,31] Studies also demonstrate a decreased failure rate and improved instructional effectiveness when there is alignment of teaching and learning styles.[32] Other studies have documented that the matching of teaching and learning styles did not have a demonstrable effect on academic performance.[33] Because the results are inconsistent and inconclusive, there is not universal acceptance of the benefits of matching teaching and learning styles.[34] Rather than matching styles, it may be more important to consider the needs of the teacher and learner in the process. When curricula are designed to facilitate the meeting of these needs, an increase of self-reflective learning behavior is reported in students.[35]

Because student nurse anesthetists are all adult learners, the question of matching teaching and learning styles may be less important than for other university-level students. When compared with younger students, adult learners tend to have more flexibility with regard to learning styles. They may be more able to adapt and be successful when teaching styles do not match their own learning styles.[36] Because there is no correlation between age and gender with any specific learning style, it is not possible to predict the preferred learning style of a student beginning the study of nurse anesthesia.[37]

Educational Differences in the Clinical Setting

Although an understanding of learning styles may be helpful, nurse anesthesia clinical education is fundamentally different from teaching chemistry or biology in a classroom. Clinical learning experiences are essential to prepare nurse anesthetists.[38] As in basic sciences, the clinical site is the "laboratory experience" where skills based on concepts introduced in the classroom are demonstrated and mastered.[39] The difference is that this laboratory setting involves patients rather than reagents and specimens. The student is under the guidance of a credentialed practitioner who remains responsible for patient care, but this is a laboratory setting in which decisions involving life and death are made.[40]

Patients do not come to hospitals to meet the educational needs of our profession. The patients with whom we interact are there for anesthesia care for a surgical or diagnostic therapeutic procedure. We are there to administer anesthesia to these patients safely. Sometimes the anesthesia provider works independently. As the only person present who is licensed by the government and credentialed by the facility to provide anesthesia care, the clinical preceptor is responsible for the quality and outcome of that care while directing the student.[41] In the clinical area, learning is experiential.[42] Patient safety must remain our highest priority. With such high stakes, a mismatch of learner preference and teaching style requires the student to adjust expectations and amend desires.

Healthcare education is much more formal and rank-driven than other disciplines. In academic medicine there are deans, department chairpersons, service chiefs, attending physicians, fellows, residents, and undergraduate medical students. In nursing, we often find deans, chairpersons, program directors, faculty, doctoral students, master's degree students, and undergraduate nursing students. In the clinical departments, respect must be shown to all members of the healthcare team, including students.[43] In some departments, clinical preceptors do not see learners as deserving of respect or in need of mentorship. Although there is conflicting evidence on the effect of matching learning and teaching styles to improve outcomes, studies show that a teaching method that includes personalization is superior for students with a variety of learning styles. Personalization of instructions may be associated with a higher degree of success than an attempt to match teaching and learning styles.[44]

Multiple Learning Styles in Clinical Education

Students should be actively involved in the process of experiential learning.[43,45] The level of involvement in the educational process is not merely a function of teacher-student interaction. In the clinical area, much learning can also come from student-student interaction as well.[46] Positive levels of teacher-student and student-student interactions are more likely to occur in clinical departments where these interactions are viewed as valuable. In earlier times, CRNA educational programs and registered nurse programs granted diplomas and were based in hospitals. It was not uncommon at that time for nursing students and student nurse anesthetists to receive all of their clinical instruction within the walls of the hospital that conducted their educational program.

As general nursing, followed by nurse anesthesia, evolved and moved away from the hospital-based educational model to a university-based academic system, the practice of having all student clinical educational experiences at a single institution became much less common. Students are now educated in programs that are based within institutions of higher learning that contract, through affiliation agreements, with multiple clinical facilities to provide educational experiences for their students.[47] In such an arrangement, students are exposed to clinical experiences in sites that may have different philosophies, staffing patterns, personnel expectations, and organizational structures. To be effective as clinical sites, these diverse departments must establish a climate in which various forms of educational interaction (eg, student-teacher, student-student, and teacher-teacher) are seen as valuable and supported.[48] It has been commonly noted that "what is valued is what gets attended to."[49] This is as true in education as in other areas of life.

Nurse Anesthesia Education

Unlike students of many other disciplines, student nurse anesthetists begin as fully licensed professionals with years of experience behind them. Depending on their previous level of professional experience and educational background, students may conceivably possess theoretical and clinical expertise exceeding that of the clinical preceptors to whom they are assigned. In such situations, it is important for teachers and learners to remember that the CRNA clinical preceptor is the individual who is most knowledgeable about the anesthesia management of the patient.

It is also important for clinical preceptors to understand that, in many cases, substantial and dramatic changes have occurred in the process of nurse anesthesia education since they were students.[47] As opposed to looking back with a combination of dread and nostalgia, it is more productive for clinical preceptors to seek the most effective and safety-driven methods to support the transition of our current student nurse anesthetists into CRNA colleagues. Our students need and deserve effective coaching and mentoring in the clinical area. That certainly does not mean that effective anesthesia professionals are created through a process of "spoon-feeding" information and not holding students responsible for their own learning success. Preceptors should ask questions that require critical thinking skills while encouraging students to present an evidence-based rationale for the decisions that they make.

Some students have low expectations for their clinical performance and are willing to see themselves as successful if they meet their expectations. Success in nurse anesthesia requires more than merely showing up. Our profession is not in the habit of awarding trophies for mere participation, which may be the experience of our current students. Asking difficult questions, expecting thoughtful and accurate responses, and helping students to become critical questioners themselves produces the best results when done in an atmosphere of mutual respect.[50]

A good clinical preceptor will set a goal of excellence and will encourage students to reach that goal. Students progress at different rates and there is no timeline or mold that fits all students.[51] By adapting the educational process to the needs of the situation, clinical preceptors can be a crucially important component in the metamorphosis of students into the expert anesthesia providers of the future.

Summary

Several distinct learning styles have been identified, and instructors may wish to become familiar with these styles and their effects on learner preferences. In the clinical area, it is more appropriate to expect students to adapt their learning styles to the teaching styles of clinical instructors than vice versa. As the individuals who are responsible for providing patient care, the clinical instructors must be comfortable coordinating the process of teaching with the process of patient care. If clinical instructors can incorporate specific teaching techniques that match the learning preferences of the students, all the better. However, data indicate that learners are capable of adjusting their preferences to match the teaching styles of instructors.

References

1. American Association of Nurse Anesthetists. Council on Accreditation of Nurse Anesthesia Educational Programs website. http://www.aana.com/Default.aspx. Accessed September 1, 2008.

2. Frels L, Horton B. Faculty positions as a career choice for professionals: part II. *AANA J.* 1991;59(4):329-337.

3. Starnes-Ott K, Kremer MJ. Recruitment and retention of nurse anesthesia faculty: issues and strategies. *AANA J.* 2007;75(1):13-16.

4. Fatt JPT. Understanding the learning styles of students: implications for educators. *Int J Sociol Soc Policy.* 2000;20(11):31-35.

5. Ehrman EM, Leaver BL, Oxford RL. A brief overview of individual differences in second language learning. *System.* 2003;31(3):313-330.

6. Lauder W. Constructing meaning in the learning experience: the role of alternative theoretical frameworks. *J Adv Nurs.* 1996;24(1):91-97.

7. Fatt JPT. Innovative teaching: teaching at its best. *Education.* 1998;118:616-625.

8. Sadler-Smith E. Learning styles: a holistic approach. *J Eur Ind Training.* 1996;20(7):29-36.

9. Peacock M. Match or mismatch? learning styles and teaching styles in EFL. *Int J Appl Linguistics.* 2001;11:1-20.

10. Suliman WA. Critical thinking and learning styles of students in conventional and accelerated programmes. *Int Nurs Rev.* 2006;53(1):73-79.

11. Nortridge JA, Bell ML. Recognizing RNs' cognitive style preferences. *Nurs Manage.* 1996;27(8):40-44.

12. Cook DA, Smith AJ. Validity of index of learning styles scores: multitrait-multimethod comparision with three cognitive/learning style instruments. *Med Educ.* 2006;40(9):900-907.

13. Sadler-Smith E. The relationship between learning style and cognitive style. *Pers Individual Differences.* 2001;30(4):609-616.

14. Kolb D. *User's Guide for the Learning-Style Inventory.* Boston, MA: McBer & Company; 1986.

15. Hoelker J. Classroom ideas: writing stories for one another. *Modern English Teacher.* 2002;11:33-36.

16. Entwistle N. Styles of learning and approaches to studying in higher education. *Kybernetes.* 2001;30(5/6):593-602.

17. Tickle S. What have we learnt about student learning? a review of the research on study approach and style. *Kybernetes.* 2001;30(7/8):955-969.

18. Duff A, Duffy T. Psychometric properties of Honey and Mumford's Learning Styles Questionnaire (LSQ). *Pers Individual Differences.* 2003;33(1):147-163.

19. Hauer P, Straub C, Wolf S. Learning styles of allied health students using Kolb's LSI-IIa. *J Allied Health.* 2005;34(3):177-182.

20. De Ciantis S, Kirton M. A psychometric reexamination of Kolb's experiential learning cycle construct: a separation of level, style, and process. *Educ Psychol Meas.* 1996;56(5):809-820.

21. Koob J, Funk J. Kolb's Learning Style Inventory: issues of reliability and validity. *Res Soc Work Pract.* 2002;12(2):293-308.

22. Grasha A, Yangarber-Hicks N. Integrating teaching styles and learning styles with instructional technology. *Coll Teaching.* 2000;48(1):2-12.

23. Mumford A. Putting learning styles to work: an integrated approach. *Ind Commercial Training.* 1995;27(8):28-35.

24. McDonough J. Personality, addiction and anesthesia. *AANA J.* 1990;58(3):193 200.

25. Heinström J. The impact of personality and approaches to learning on information behavior. Information Resources website. http://informationr.net/ir/5-3/paper78.html. Accessed March 25, 2009.

26. Linares A. Learning styles of students and faculty in selected health care professions. *J Nurs Educ.* 1999;38(9):407-414.

27. Fowler P. Learning styles of radiographers. *Radiogr.* 2002;8:3-11.

28. DiBartola LM. The Learning Style Inventory challenge: teaching about teaching by learning about learning. *J Allied Health.* 2006;35(4):238-245.

29. Kolb AY, Kolb DA. Learning styles and learning spaces: enhancing experiential learning in higher education. *Acad Manage Learning Educ.* 2005;193-212.

30. Sherbinski L. Learning styles of nurse anesthesia students related to level in a master of science in nursing program. *AANA J.* 1994;62(1):39-45.

31. Rassool GH, Rawaf S. Learning style preferences of undergraduate nursing students. *Nurs Stand.* 2007;21(32):35-41.

32. Ford N, Chen S. Matching/mismatching revisited: an empirical study of learning and teaching styles. *Br J Educ Technol.* 2001;32(1):5-22.

33. Joyce-Nagata B. Students' academic performance in nursing as a function of student and faculty learning style congruency. *J Nurs Educ.* 1996;35(2):69-73.

34. Thompson C, Crutchlow E. Learning style research: a critical review of the literature and implications for nursing education. *J Prof Nurs.* 1993;9(1):34-40.

35. Wagner F, Osterbrink J. *Integrierte Unterrichtseinheiten: Ein Modell für die Ausbildung in der Pflege.* Bern, Switzerland: Huber; 2001:213-217.

36. Spoon JC, Schell JW. Aligning student learning styles with instructor teaching styles. *J Ind Teacher Educ.* 1995;35(2):41-56.

37. Heffler B. Individual learning style and the Learning Style Inventory. *Educ Stud.* 2001;27(3):309-316.

38. Papp I, Markkanen M, von Bonsdorff M. Clinical environment as a learning environment: student nurses' perceptions concerning clinical learning experiences. *Nurse Educ Today.* 2003;23(4):262-268.

39. Beirer A, Osterbrink J. Qualitätssicherung in der praktischen ausbildung. *Pflegemanagement.* 1997;6(1):19-26.

40. Shen J, Spouse J. Learning to nurse in China—structural factors influencing professional development in practice settings: a phenomenological study. *Nurse Educ Pract.* 2007;7(5):323-331.

41. Abenstein JP, Warner MA. Anesthesia providers, patient outcomes, and costs. *Anesth Analg.* 1996;82(6):1273-1283.

42. Fallacaro MD. Untoward pathophysiological events: simulation as an experiential learning option to prepare anesthesia providers. *CRNA.* 2000;11(3):138-143.

43. Kalb KA, O'Conner-Von S. Ethics education in advanced practice nursing: respect for human dignity. *Nurs Educ Perspect.* 2007;28(4):196-202.

44. Horton CB, Oakland T. Temperament-based learning styles as moderators of academic achievement. *Adolescence.* 1997;32(125):131-141.

45. Gilmartin J. Teachers' understanding of facilitation styles with student nurses. *Int J Nurs Stud.* 2001;38(4):481-488.

46. Görres S, Keuchel R, Roes M, Scheffel F, Beermann H, Krol M. *Auf dem Weg Zueinerneuen Lernkultur: Wissenstransfer in der Pflege.* Bern, Switzerland: Huber; 2002:179-182.

47. Horton BJ. Upgrading nurse anesthesia educational requirements (1993-2006)—part 1: setting standards. *AANA J.* 2007;75(3):167-170.

48. Gillespie M. Student-teacher connection: a place of possibility. *J Adv Nurs.* 2005; 52(2):211-219.

49. Williamson R. Designing diverse learning styles. *Schools in the Middle.* 1998;7(4):28-31.

50. Myrick F, Tamlyn D. Teaching can never be innocent: fostering an enlightening educational experience. *J Nurs Educ.* 2007;46(7):299-303.

51. Raschick M, Maypole D, Day P. Field education: improving field education through Kolb Learning Theory. *J Soc Work Educ.* 1998;34(1):31-43.

Chapter 12

Ethics of Clinical Instruction

Kathleen R. Wren, CRNA, PhD, MS
Timothy L. Wren, RN, DNP

Key Points

- Ethics, a discipline concerned with determining what is right and wrong, is about moral duties and obligations.

- Professional organizations influence what is ethical through accepted standards of conduct expected of members.

- The Council on Accreditation of Nurse Anesthesia Educational Programs requires nurse anesthesia programs to be governed by ethical and moral standards.

- The National Task Force on Ethics in Health Education 2000 has issued a code of ethics based on core principles underlying healthcare services.

- In addition to their professional roles as a caregivers, clinical preceptors also have the obligation to inform patients that they, as preceptors and licensed personnel, are responsible for patient care and to specify the activities students will be performing.

- Clinical preceptors are responsible for providing adequate student supervision based on the student's level of knowledge and skill, the clinical situation, and patient healthcare demands.

Introduction

Clinical instruction of student nurse anesthetists is rewarding and, at times, overwhelming. Training students to think critically and solve problems in the fast-paced and fluid environment of the operating room is challenging. In some circumstances, the Certified Registered Nurse Anesthetist (CRNA) clinical instructor will find there is not enough time to teach—only to act. During these times, the CRNA instructor will most likely need to suspend teaching duties to meet the demands of the clinical situation and then return to student instruction when the situation allows. Also, clinical experiences are not structured activities. Instruction in a classroom setting can be standardized and packaged so that students receive similar information. This is not the case with clinical experiences. Clinical experiences may vary widely among students based on clinical sites, patient population, operating room schedules, clinical preceptors, and a host of other uncontrollable factors. This means that clinical teaching will also vary widely. Because of the variability in clinical practice and clinical teaching, CRNA instructors will face many ethical dilemmas during clinical instruction of students, and it is extremely difficult to determine the right thing to do in individual circumstances. Nurse anesthesia clinical instructors must understand issues of ethical decision making in education so that they may be better prepared to deal with ethical problems that are sure to arise during clinical instruction of students.

Ethics

Ethics, a discipline concerned with determining what is right and wrong, is about moral duties and obligations. Determining what is right and wrong involves cultural, societal, and social norms. For example, autonomy is highly valued in North American culture but not in middle Asian society. Likewise, professional organizations influence what is ethical through accepted standards of conduct expected of their members. Most professional codes of ethics deal with issues such as competence, conflict of interest, confidentiality, responsibility to the profession, diversity, scholarship and research, and safety for patients.[1] For instance, the American Association of Nurse Anesthetists (AANA) publishes the Code of Ethics[2] and Professional Practice Standards[3] outlining responsibilities of its professional members (Table 12.1).

Table 12.1. AANA Code of Ethics for Professional Members

Protect the patient from harm.

Be a patient advocate.

Maintain patient confidentiality.

Refuse to engage in deception.

Participate in lifelong, professional educational activities.

Contribute to the body of knowledge.

Maintain the dignity and integrity of the profession.

Evaluate research findings and incorporate them into practice.

Ethical codes are designed to help individuals determine how to best fulfill their ethical obligations in a particular situation. However, a recent study found that 76% of faculty members believe ethical codes are not helpful in discouraging unethical practices.[4]

Ethics in Clinical Education

Because of the complex nature of clinical training and the number of individuals (patients, students, colleagues, and healthcare professionals) and interests (societal, professional, community, and family) involved, clinical instructors will frequently encounter ethical dilemmas in the clinical area. Preceptors should be aware of ethical guidelines established to assist in the resolution of ethical dilemmas.

Standards for Accreditation of Nurse Anesthesia Educational Programs

The Council on Accreditation of Nurse Anesthesia Educational Programs (COA) is recognized by the US Department of Education as an accreditation body for nurse anesthesia programs. To achieve and maintain accreditation, nurse anesthesia programs must demonstrate compliance with 5 education standards and 53 associated criteria. Standard 5 is of note because it requires nurse anesthesia programs to demonstrate accountability and integrity to students and to the public.[5] Criteria that have an impact on student nurse anesthetists are summarized in Table 12.2.

In fulfilling the requirements of the COA, clinical faculty should take an active role in monitoring students' clinical workload to ensure that learning is achieved and patient safety is maintained. This may involve monitoring and providing adequately spaced breaks and mealtimes on the clinical unit as well as end-of-shift

---

Table 12.2. Ethical Responsibilities of Nurse Anesthesia Programs of Significance to Student Relationships

Help ensure the graduate's ability to interact on a professional level with integrity.

Identify, publish, and distribute the rights and responsibilities of patients, applicants, faculty, students, conducting and affiliating institutions, and the accrediting agency.

Maintain a reasonable student time commitment to studies and clinical responsibilities to ensure patient safety and promote effective student learning.

Forbid students to obtain employment as nurse anesthetists.

Prevent educational entities from falsifying their accreditation status.

Develop and implement fair grievance and appellate policies.

Develop and implement appropriate mechanisms for dealing with complaints against the program.

Provide information to students concerning ethical responsibilities in loan repayments.

Develop and implement nondiscriminatory policies.

(Adapted with permission from the Council on Accreditation of Nurse Anesthesia Educational Programs.[6])

relief. Although service is an integral part of their training, students should not be used as a cheap or captive source of anesthesia coverage. Likewise, students should never be allowed to present themselves as nurse anesthetists to patients or other healthcare personnel. Clinical faculty should also become actively involved in application, acceptance, and grievance processes of the anesthesia program. This will aid programs to develop and implement ethical policies and monitor compliance with their ethical responsibilities to their communities of interest.

National Task Force on Ethics in Health Education

To assist members of the healthcare education profession, the National Task Force on Ethics in Health Education 2000 has issued a code of ethics based on core principles underlying healthcare services. These principles include: "[a] respect for autonomy, [b] promotion of social justice, [c] active promotion of good, and [d] avoidance of harm."[6] Within the code, the task force delineates responsibilities to the public, the profession, and the employers, as well as responsibilities in the delivery of health education, research and evaluation, and professional preparation. The task force lists ethical principles to guide education of healthcare professionals in the section on professional preparation. Specifically, in their relationships with learners, educators are to:

- Treat learners with respect.
- Treat all learners the same.
- Provide a quality education as defined by the profession and the community.
- Select students based on "academic performance, abilities, and potential contribution to the profession."[6]
- Create a safe educational environment.
- Create an educational environment that helps students to learn.
- Adequately prepare for the training of students.
- Use accurate and timely information.
- Give appropriate rationales.
- Conduct evaluations that are fair, consistent, and equitable.
- Provide objective and honest student counseling.
- Provide adequate supervision based on the performance level of the learner.

Guidelines for Ethics in Clinical Teaching

The University of Toronto further defined the role of the clinical preceptor in regard to ethics in clinical teaching. In their Guidelines for Ethics in Clinical Teaching document, the University of Toronto School of Medicine faculty discuss professional responsibilities to the patient, consulting on and reporting ethical concerns, supervision of trainees, exchange of information, and confidentiality (Appendix 12.1).[7] Although written by faculty in Canada, these guidelines are also applicable to healthcare training institutions in the United States.

In addition to their professional roles as caregivers, clinical preceptors also have the obligation to inform patients that they, as preceptors and licensed personnel, are responsible for patient care and to specify the activities students will be performing.

Preceptors must allow patients to refuse student involvement in their healthcare and inform patients that their healthcare information will be shared with the student.

Clinical preceptors are also responsible for providing adequate student supervision based on the student's level of knowledge, the clinical situation, and the patient's healthcare demands. Preceptors must be active participants in the design and implementation of the anesthesia plan so that patient and learner outcomes are optimized. Preceptors must also provide accurate and timely feedback concerning student performance, critical thinking abilities, and anesthesia planning.

Clinical preceptors should be honest and ethical in their own dealings with patients and students. They should expect and demand the same high level of ethical behavior from learners. Clinical preceptors should create an atmosphere of mutual trust and acceptance so that students will be able to discuss and report ethical concerns. This also implies that preceptors be available to consult on ethical issues and concerns and to help report and resolve ethical problems and violations.

Ethical Decision Making

Ethical dilemmas occur when there is an inconsistency of values, morals, opinions, and responsibilities between stakeholders. Stakeholders are those individuals or entities that hold a vested interest in the situation. Stakeholders in an anesthesia clinical arena include the clinical instructor, the student, the patient, the patient's family, the hospital, the nurse anesthesia program, the community, and the nurse anesthesia profession.

Most ethical decision-making models advocate following a process comparable to the traditional 4-step model of nursing process (Figure 12.1) in resolution of ethical dilemmas.[8] The first step in dealing with an ethical dilemma is to fully identify and define the problem. Many times, the issue first identified is not really the problem. If the real problem is not defined, energy will be wasted in dealing with side issues while the actual problem is not dealt with and left unresolved. In looking at the underlying purpose of the ethical dilemma, the clinical instructor needs to explore the big picture view of the problem. The instructor should explore issues surrounding the problem and try to get to the heart of the problem. The instructor should ask: "What is the real problem here?" The second step in resolving an ethical dilemma is to determine possible interventions for resolving the issues.[9] This is the time to brainstorm. All ideas should be recorded and no idea should be discarded. Once interventions are delineated, the best interventions are selected and implemented. When evaluating interventions, preceptors should look at available policies, procedures, rules, and regulations related to the problem. The AANA Code of Ethics (2001), AANA Practice Standards, and National Task Force on Ethics in Health Education 2000 report publish standards of care concerning anesthesia and education practice that will provide guidance in ethical dilemmas. The clinical instructor should ask: "What principles from the code of

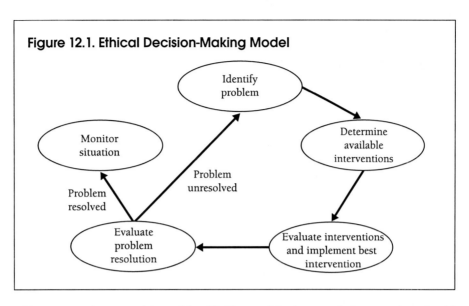

Figure 12.1. Ethical Decision-Making Model

Identify problem

Monitor situation

Determine available interventions

Problem resolved

Problem unresolved

Evaluate problem resolution

Evaluate interventions and implement best intervention

ethics are pertinent to this problem?" Also at this time, each intervention should be evaluated in terms of: (1) resources needed, (2) time commitment, (3) monetary costs, (4) learner engagement, and (5) congruence with the mission and the culture of the institution. Issues of practicality and feasibility of each option will aid in determining the likelihood of success and selection of the best intervention. After implementation of the intervention, the clinical instructor should evaluate the success or failure of the intervention in resolving the dilemma.

If the dilemma has been successfully resolved, all that may be needed is further monitoring to ensure continued resolution of the matter. If the intervention is unsuccessful, then the clinical instructor should return to the first step of ethical decision making and redefine the problem. Further data collection and collegial assistance may aid in redefining the problem more completely and exploring other potential interventions, which should increase the likelihood of successful intervention and resolution of the problem. At times, one may have to accept that complete resolution of the problem is not possible. In difficult situations or unresolved ethical dilemmas, the clinical instructor may wish to seek out the assistance of the university's ethics or bioethics department.

Ethical Dilemmas in Clinical Performance Evaluation of Student Nurse Anesthetists

Using preceptors to provide clinical instruction for healthcare professional students is not new. The training of medical students has, for many decades, relied on clinical preceptors to assist with student education. Typically, medical students undergo 2 years of didactic training and 2 years of training with monthly preceptorships, rotating among different hospital units and physician instructors.

Students in healthcare professions must not only master scientific and profession-specific content but also must be able to synthesize this knowledge and apply it in the healthcare setting. Students must acquire and practice clinical skills in the clinical setting. In turn, student performance must be evaluated in the clinical setting. The clinical preceptor often is the person who must provide feedback for the performance evaluation.

In anesthesia training, schools often have full-time faculty members who are responsible for didactic content, but it would be impossible for didactic faculty to provide all the needed clinical supervision and performance evaluations. Hence, clinical preceptors have an important role in nurse anesthesia education.

The use of clinical preceptors to provide feedback on student performance in the clinical arena is well documented.[10-14] Problems associated with clinical performance evaluation have also been discussed.[15,16] Issues in the evaluation of student clinical performance arise from a number of areas. Some of these issues include: (1) little or no training of clinical preceptors in the process of student clinical performance evaluation; (2) relative inexperience of clinical preceptors in professional clinical practice and clinical preceptorship; (3) student intimidation strategies targeted to influence preceptor evaluation and feedback; (4) cumbersome, inadequate, poorly designed student performance evaluation processes and tools; and (5) preceptors' fears of litigious actions related to student education, evaluation, and grading. Many times it is difficult for clinical preceptors "to look beyond the student's well-being, to the well-being of the patient and the profession."[16] As a consequence, clinical preceptors often do not address performance inadequacies with students or document their concerns and observations on the student evaluation tool. In these situations, an ethical dilemma arises from the incongruity of students' needs and the needs of patients, the profession, and society.

In the performance of student clinical evaluations, clinical preceptors have an ethical responsibility to create an educational environment that will help students to learn. They also have an ethical responsibility to conduct evaluations that are fair, consistent, and equitable.[1] When a clinical preceptor is reluctant to discuss and document inadequacies in a student's performance, an ethical dilemma arises. The first step in dealing with an ethical dilemma is to fully identify and define the problem. In this situation, the problem is reluctance to evaluate and document inadequate student clinical performance and may be due to little or no training of clinical preceptors in the process of student clinical performance evaluation.

Once the problem has been identified and defined, possible interventions can be generated. In our example of inadequate student clinical performance evaluation and documentation due to lack of clinical preceptor training, possible interventions may include: (1) review of the clinical evaluation tool, (2) role-playing exercises, (3) sample video vignettes of clinical performance followed by a discussion and a question-and-answer session, (4) lecture series on student clinical performance documentation, or (5) one-on-one preceptor instruction on student clinical performance documentation.

Next, the pros and cons of each intervention should be assessed. For example, reviewing the clinical evaluation tool will ensure that everyone in attendance has mastered the same content; however, preceptors should be able to accomplish this basic task before meeting as a group. This will allow meeting time for higher-level learning, such as training in the use of the evaluation tool in sample clinical situations.

After each possible intervention is assessed, the best intervention should be selected based on the likelihood of success using available resources, such as associated costs, timeliness, support personnel, and space requirements. Once the intervention is implemented, the adequacy of the problem resolution should be evaluated. If the problem has not been resolved adequately, the process should be reinitiated. Implementation of the Ethical Dilemma Intervention Evaluation is summarized in Table 12.3.

One of the most common reasons for failing to achieve resolution is when an ethical dilemma arises from an incomplete delineation of the problem. For example, inadequate student clinical performance evaluations may result from preceptors' fears of litigious actions related to student education, evaluation, and grading, instead of a lack of preceptor training. Indicated interventions in this situation would be different than those identified (above) for lack of preceptor training. In this scenario, interventions may possibly include: (1) a review of the legal basis for student clinical evaluations, (2) a lecture series on writing nonjudgmental, performance-based student clinical evaluations, (3) a lecture series on the purpose of student clinical evaluations, or (4) a journal club series on writing student clinical evaluations. When resolution to an ethical dilemma fails to occur despite appropriate intervention, the first consideration should be an incomplete definition of the problem.

Table 12.3. Ethical Dilemma Intervention Evaluation

Intervention	Pros	Cons
Review of clinical evaluation tool	All preceptors start with same information. Able to receive preceptor feedback on tool.	Very basic information. Activity lacks engagement for those who have reviewed tool.
Role-playing exercises	Engaging learning activity. Brings emotional component to context.	Need volunteers willing to role-play. Limited to face-to-face classes.
Sample video vignette	Useful in face-to-face and distance learning situations. Video may be used several times. Video may be stopped at key discussion points.	Costly. Requires production equipment and crew.
Lecture series	Cost effective. Learner is familiar and thus comfortable with this learning format.	Not engaging to learner. Limited to scheduled time periods, limiting attendance.
Preceptor instruction	Individualized instruction. Face-to-face interaction.	Costly. Time-consuming. Limited to clinical situations as they present.

Summary

Ethics, a discipline that determines right and wrong, is useful to people in many professions. In the healthcare industry, hospitals have ethics committees that review, discuss, and evaluate the morality of healthcare decisions and interventions; however, there are no ethics committees to assist clinical preceptors in the day-to-day decisions required in student learning environments. Schools have clinical objectives, and accrediting bodies, such as the COA, have recommendations for dealing with students in the clinical environment. Nevertheless, clinical preceptors must rely on their own ethical judgment when determining what is appropriate for each student, patient, and clinical experience.

   In this chapter, an ethical dilemma from the clinical perspective was discussed to demonstrate the process of ethical decision making. A model was presented, providing a visual representation of the ethical decision-making process. Interventions aimed at resolving the ethical dilemma were presented and evaluated to promote an improved understanding of the process.

   In regard to ethics, the famous British author D. H. Lawrence stated: "Ethics and equity and the principles of justice do not change with the calendar." What is ethical, what is right, does not change with the passage of time. Clinical preceptors have ethical responsibilities and moral duties to patients under their care as well as to the students they are mentoring. These responsibilities remain despite the context or concerns about relationship variables, grades, or threats of legal action.

References

1. Nickols SY, Belliston LM. Professional ethics: caught and taught. *J Fam Consumer Sci.* 2001;93(2):20-25.

2. Code of ethics. American Association of Nurse Anesthetists website. www.aana.com/crna/prof/codeofethics.asp. Accessed January 16, 2008.

3. Professional or practice information. American Association of Nurse Anesthetists website. http://www.aana.com/crna/default.asp#Professional. Accessed January 16, 2008.

4. Telljohann SK, Price JH, Dake JA. Selected ethical issues in the teaching for health: perceptions of health education faculty. *J Health Educ.* 2001;32(2):66-74.

5. Standards for Accreditation of Nurse Anesthesia Educational Programs. Park Ridge, IL: Council on Accreditation of Nurse Anesthesia Educational Programs; 2007.

6. National Task Force on Ethics in Health Education 2000. Code of ethics for the health education profession. *Health Promotion Practice.* 2000;1:200-203.

7. Guidelines for ethics in clinical training. University of Toronto website. http://www.facmed.utoronto.ca/Assets/staff/ethics.pdf?method=1. Accessed May 23, 2008.

8. Bosek M. Ethical decision making in anesthesia. In: Foster SD, Faut-Callahan M, eds. *A Professional Study and Resource Guide for the CRNA.* Park Ridge, IL: AANA Publishing; 2001:407-423.

9. Husa J. Thinking things through: coming to grips with philosophical and prudential perspectives in teachers' educational practice. Paper presented at: Biennial Meeting of the International Study Association on Teachers and Teaching; September 21-25, 2001; Fars, Portugal.

10. Bujack L, McMillan M, Dwyer J, Hazelton M. Assessing comprehensive nursing performance: the objective structured clinical assessment (OSCA) Part 1 – development of the assessment strategy. *Nurse Educ Today.* 1991;11(4):179-184.

11. Bujack L, McMillan M, Dwyer J, Hazelton M. Assessing comprehensive nursing performance: the objective structured clinical assessment (OSCA) part 2 – report of the evaluation project. *Nurse Educ Today.* 1991;11(4):248-255

12. Higgins B, Oscher S. Two approaches to clinical evaluation. *Nurse Educ.* 1989;14(2):8-11.

13. Karns P, Nowotny M. Clinical structure and evaluation in baccalaureate schools of nursing. *J Nurs Educ.* 1991;30(5):207-211.

14. Malek CJ. Clinical evaluation: challenging tradition. *Nurse Educ.* 1988;13(6):34-37.

15. Woolley AS. The long and tortured history of clinical evaluation. *Nurs Outlook.* 1977;25(5):308-315.

16. Duke M. Clinical evaluation—difficulties experienced by sessional clinical teachers of nursing: a qualitative study. *J Adv Nurs.* 1996;23(2):408-414.

Appendix 12.1. Guidelines for Ethics in Clinical Teaching

University of Toronto
May 16, 2005

Purpose

To provide guidance for patients, healthcare professional trainees, and clinical faculty or supervising clinicians in determining their rights and responsibilities when participating in clinical education in the hospital setting.

Preamble

At the 8 teaching hospitals that are fully affiliated with the University of Toronto, facilitating the education of healthcare professional trainees is consistent with the hospitals' mission statements. Healthcare professional trainees at all levels of experience encounter learning opportunities in a wide variety of clinical settings. It is the aim of the University and hospitals to provide healthcare professional trainees and clinical faculty and supervising clinicians with a welcoming learning environment and a strong positive role model for professional behavior and professional practice. In doing so, the following guidelines for the conduct of clinical teaching in the hospital environment are suggested for use across the 8 teaching institutions. Teaching is not only defined as "specific acts" but includes all activities when someone in training is providing care to patients on a day-to-day basis.

University healthcare professional trainees and clinical faculty and supervising clinicians participating in clinical teaching at the 8 fully affiliated hospitals and the hospitals' designated teaching locations (ie, community settings) are expected to adhere to the Regulated Health Professions Act (RHPA), the policies and procedures outlined by the host hospital and the policies and procedures of the University. These guidelines and policies should be used by all clinical faculty and supervising clinicians and healthcare professional trainees for ethical situations that arise in the general course of healthcare activities. In addition, healthcare professionals should make use of any ethical guidelines provided by their professional colleges or organizations.

The University and hospitals are committed to:

Their role in teaching healthcare professionals

The University and hospitals:

1. Are committed to excellence in patient care, teaching, and research.

2. Are committed to the education and training of healthcare professional trainees.

3. Agree that clinical teaching is an essential component in the development of healthcare professional trainees.

4. Agree to communicate to patients that their institutions are learning environments and that therefore healthcare professional trainees are involved in patient care on an ongoing basis.

Their responsibility for patient care

The University and hospitals:

5. Agree that clear communication with patients is essential to facilitate clinical teaching in a hospital environment.

6. Agree that patients must be informed as to whom is responsible for their care and that the physician in charge is responsible for informing the patient.

Informed consent and clear communication among patients, healthcare providers and healthcare professional trainees

The University and hospitals:

7. Affirm that the mission of a teaching hospital includes the delivery of patient care by different healthcare professionals and learners in all professions (eg, physicians, nurses, allied health professionals). As such, continued excellence in the quality of patient care is expected, and healthcare professional trainees will be involved in patient care activities.

8. Agree that patients have a right to know that healthcare professional trainees may be involved directly in their care under the supervision of clinical faculty/supervising clinicians. It is the responsibility of the clinical faculty/supervising clinician to inform the patient that healthcare professional trainees may provide patient care.

9. Agree that a patient has the right to be explicitly informed about the specific teaching activity in which the patient will be participating.

10. Agree that the clinical faculty or supervising clinician is responsible for informing the patient about teaching activities and obtaining verbal consent from a patient before proceeding with teaching activities that involve the patient.

11. Will implement procedures to ensure that information is provided to a patient on procedures in which a healthcare professional trainee will participate.

12. Will ensure that the relevant university faculties and their affiliated teaching hospitals will define the profession-specific invasive procedures that require a patient's written consent before a healthcare professional trainee's participation in the defined invasive procedure.

13. Will define other teaching activity circumstances under which a patient's written consent is required (eg, recording interviews and examinations).

14. Agree that patients have the right to refuse to participate in teaching activities that are purely educational in nature (eg, teaching sessions with healthcare professional trainees bringing patients into seminars or lectures).

15. Agree that patient information is invaluable for the education of healthcare professional trainees.

16. Agree that healthcare professional trainees will have access to patient information and that patients will be informed that healthcare professional trainees have access to the patient's information.

17. Agree that patients have the right to refuse the use of their information for conferences and seminars when the identity of the patient is provided.

Consulting on and reporting ethical concerns

The University and hospitals:

18. Are committed to the highest standards of ethical conduct in teaching activities, including integrity and honesty.

19. Agree that it is the responsibility of the clinical faculty or supervising clinician to provide not only instruction in clinical reasoning and technical skills, but also to recognize the importance of providing a role model to trainees for ethical practice, including maintaining confidentiality and affording the patient dignity and respect, and to be open to questions trainees may have pertaining to what constitutes ethical practice.

20. Agree that the clinical faculty or supervising clinician must provide the healthcare professional trainee with an opportunity to discuss an ethical or difficult situation.

21. Agree that a healthcare professional trainee has the obligation to refuse to participate in patient care or clinical teaching if the healthcare professional trainee has ethical concerns about the activities; is concerned regarding his or her own competency, or lack of knowledge, lack of understanding of the duties, tasks, and responsibilities; or believes there is a lack of explanation or supervision.

22. Agree that the clinical faculty or supervising clinician must accept the learner's refusal to participate in patient care activities or clinical teaching.

23. Will ensure that healthcare professional trainees and clinical faculty or supervising clinicians are aware of individuals to approach with ethical concerns.

24. Agree that healthcare professional trainees and clinical faculty or supervising clinicians have the right to consultation with a bioethicist, clinical ethics consultant, or other individuals specifically trained in the management of ethical issues.

25. Will implement a procedure for healthcare professional trainees and clinical faculty or supervising clinicians to report ethical concerns.

26. Agree that in situations when a healthcare professional trainee expresses concern about ethical issues, refuses to participate in patient care activities or clinical teaching based on ethical grounds, or seeks consultation on an ethical issue, there will be no repercussions to the healthcare professional trainee.

Appropriate supervision and exchange of information relating to healthcare professional trainees and patient care

The University and hospitals:

27. Agree that the responsibility for the supervision of healthcare professional trainees lies with the clinical faculty or supervising clinician.

28. Agree that the clinical faculty or supervising clinician is responsible for the ongoing evaluation of the healthcare professional trainee's competence to determine the degree of supervision that the healthcare professional trainee requires and the degree of delegation of controlled acts that the healthcare professional trainee is able to accept.

29. Agree that the regular exchange of information between a healthcare professional trainee and clinical faculty or supervising clinician is essential for the healthcare professional trainee's learning experience and for the optimum care of the patient.

30. Agree that healthcare professional trainees are required to document patient care information and are required to notify the clinical faculty or supervising clinician of their actions.

31. Agree that the clinical faculty or supervising clinician is responsible for receiving healthcare professional trainee's communications on patient care activities, validating the healthcare professional trainee's findings in a timely way, and determining an appropriate patient management plan.

Confidentiality

The University and hospitals:

32. Agree that confidentiality agreements between hospitals and clinical faculty or supervising clinicians and healthcare professional trainees are a necessity in the hospital setting and must be adhered to in the general course of patient care and during teaching activities.

33. Agree that clinical faculty/supervising clinicians and healthcare professional trainees are required to maintain the confidentiality of patient information—including written, verbal, and electronic information—at all times.

(Adapted with permission from the University of Toronto, Toronto, Canada.)

Chapter 13

Clinical Faculty Development

Judy Thompson, CRNA, MS, APRN

Faculty are one of our greatest assets. A program of faculty development is therefore dedicated to aggressively supporting the ongoing personal and professional growth of faculty. By providing information, training, forums, connections, and activities, the program vitalizes the faculties, strengthens the program, improves the quality of instruction, and helps the school better serve the community.

—www.hcc.hawaii.edu

Key Points

- Faculty development for the Certified Registered Nurse Anesthetist educator has been around for many years, but the need for it is greater and more diverse than ever.

- The standards and guidelines of the Council on Accreditation of Nurse Anesthesia Educational Programs mandate faculty development as a requirement for accreditation of nurse anesthesia educational programs.

- Program administrators and clinical school faculty have reported what faculty development programs they have available and what they would like to see offered in the future.

- Faculty development programs can and should be brought to more educators if we are to encourage our new colleagues to become the educators of the future.

- Clinical faculty often have many roles within their programs. Faculty development may be desired to cover a wide variety of subjects.

- One region has brought faculty development to more clinical faculty through cooperation and creativity.

- Creative and stimulating programs are needed to promote faculty development among Certified Registered Nurse Anesthetist educators.

In the World of Education

What is faculty development? Educators in academic institutions seem to know. If you check the Internet or call any elementary or secondary school or institution of higher learning, you will find a wealth of information on faculty development for educators.

Faculty development holds a very important place in these institutions. Many school systems throughout the country, both public and private, mandate faculty development, linking it to certification requirements. I spoke with Ann Keene, PhD, staff development coordinator for Guilford Public Schools, Guilford, Connecticut, the small town where I reside (September 2005). According to Keene, teachers are required to attend 90 hours of faculty development workshops for 5 years to remain certified and to be considered for promotion in her school system. Boards of education look at student test scores and student evaluations to plan the content of the faculty development workshops for their staff. They also consider district and personal goals of individual faculty members when organizing available options. The objectives must answer the following question: How will student improvement and/or achievement occur? Staff development days are written into most academic calendars in the school systems across the country. Many elementary and secondary schools give their students days off so their educators can make the most of their schools' staff development courses.

Cheryl Watson, PhD, associate professor of Biological Sciences at Central Connecticut State University (CCSU), New Britain, Connecticut, described the faculty development program at her university (September 2005). Faculty development for educators at CCSU includes learning new clinical techniques, contextual material (ie, new information, updates, and recent discoveries), technological skills (eg, Microsoft PowerPoint, multimedia, and presentations or simulations that could be used in teaching), educational techniques (eg, how students learn most effectively and how to alter teaching or examination style to maximize learning), and personal management skills (eg, conflict resolution, communication, stress management).

In the World of the CRNA Educator

There exists in the world of education a wide variety of offerings to expand on and teach academic educators to be better teachers, but what about us, the nurse anesthesia educators? Many of us are placed into the position of teacher when we are assigned to precept a student from one of the ever-expanding nurse anesthesia programs. As more and more programs adopt clinical sites of all types to broaden the opportunities for their students, more nurse anesthetists and anesthesiologists are expected to take on roles as educators, which are new and different from their roles as clinicians.

To many of us, precepting is a new experience. How many of us were ever prepared to communicate our knowledge as practitioners, deal with learning styles, and challenge, motivate, reinforce, and evaluate one another? Many of us not only become clinical instructors within nurse anesthesia programs but also take on roles as clinical coordinators, didactic instructors, and members of academic committees dealing with curriculum, evaluation, advertisement, due process, and admissions. With ever-expanding and challenging roles for the nurse anesthetist, where do we learn to be educators? When given these roles, where do we learn to do them well?

Our Standards

The Standards for Accreditation of Nurse Anesthesia Educational Programs address faculty development. Standard III criterion VI states: "The educational environment provides opportunities for faculty development."[1] This is a requirement for all nurse anesthesia programs, but what areas specifically should this cover? This is widely interpreted and leaves much open for our programs. In 1999, the American Association of Nurse Anesthetists Education Committee surveyed the administrators of nurse anesthesia programs and compiled a list of offerings within the various schools for faculty development (Table 13.1) and a list of offerings that the administrators of the schools would like to see made available for their faculties (Table 13.2).

According to the survey, faculty development often consists of anesthesia department staff meetings in which the nurse anesthetists get continuing education credits. The meetings may be in-services on new equipment, drugs, techniques, or

---

Table 13.1. Faculty Development Activities Available

Annual report preparation

Self-study workshops

Management

Leadership

Computer competency/technology training
- Microsoft PowerPoint
- Microsoft Excel
- Word processing
- Microsoft Access
- Adobe Photoshop
- Scanning
- Internet usage

Grant writing

Mentoring

Guiding research

Simulator training

Statistics workshops

Evaluation in-services

Crisis resource management training

Journal clubs

(Adapted from the AANA Education Committee Survey of Program Directors, 2003.)

Table 13.2. Activities Program Directors Would Like to See Available for Faculty

Teaching techniques and strategies

Internet forums for sharing

Workshops for administrators, associate administrators, and faculty

The adult learner

Styles in learning

Testing and item writing

Research methods and protocol

Hands-on regional teaching techniques

Public speaking and communication

Objective writing

Evaluation (This is the most requested topic by faculty.)

Counseling

Creation of a faculty pertinent video on educational/teaching "how to's"

Dealing with the difficult student and conflict resolution

Legal and ethical issues

(Adapted from the AANA Education Committee Survey of Program Directors, 2003.)

clinical updates. They may consist of clinical case study presentations by students or faculty or a morbidity and mortality conference. They may also consist of school updates from the administrator or senior student research projects. Some programs occasionally fund some faculty to attend seminars or meetings specifically geared toward educational issues.

Clinical affiliation sites are sometimes left to fend for themselves in developing their faculty and improving the skills of those who find themselves in the role of teacher. These sites may not be able to send faculty to attend programs at the parent facility because of geographic, economic, or time constraints. Clinical sites and the training that they provide to our students are the backbone of our students' education. The anesthesia providers who teach the students in the clinical area are our role models, mentors, and the primary educators for the clinicians our students will become.

Evolution of Faculty Development

The standard relating to faculty development has undergone substantive changes throughout the years. In the late 1960s, the standard required that all faculty members of nurse anesthesia programs receive preparation in evaluation and instruction. The AANA organized an intensive workshop lasting several days in Chicago, Illinois. Classes were taught by an expert in the field of education. Following the course, attendees were required to spend several weeks as interns in anesthesia programs other than their own. They returned to Chicago after their internships, participated in more didactic instruction, and took a written examination. The AANA awarded a teacher's certificate following successful completion of this course. This course was an optional offering but helped participants develop ideas to reach more faculty members. This program, although considered a valuable experience to those who were able to attend, did not reach the clinical CRNAs who were precepting and educating the students in an anesthesia program. The impracticality of this approach was eventually its demise.

The I CARE workshops were also early attempts to reach more faculty members. Instituted in the 1970s, they were scheduled to include as many program faculty as possible. Linda Brogan, CRNA, MHS, APRN, former program administrator at the Hospital of St Raphael, School of Nurse Anesthesia, New Haven, Connecticut, (September 2005) said that schools were required to either send their faculty members to these workshops or to have them participate within their own programs. The content included instruction, curriculum, testing, and measurement. Non-CRNA educators were contracted to put together and administer the I CARE program. Participants who chose to seek approval with a university accepting the coursework could obtain college credit. The lectures were recorded on cassette tapes and played to sequestered clinical faculty for a 2-day period.

In the early 1990s, the revision of the standards broadened the language regarding faculty development. Coursework specific to evaluation and instruction was no longer mandated. In an attempt to be less prescriptive, the revised standards left it up to the schools to develop their faculty in ways of their own choosing. Faculty development could include a wider variety of topics such as those of a clinical, technological, and scientific nature. Methodology of education was eliminated as a requirement.

With the mandate in the late 1990s that the teaching of regional anesthesia administration be included in all curriculums, the AANA promoted a new faculty development offering, Teaching the Teachers. In an interview (October 2005), Betty Horton, CRNA, DNSc, former AANA director of Accreditation and Education, described the program, which was held at an army base and was designed to instruct nurse anesthesia educators to teach regional anesthesia in their programs. A manual was written to accompany the course. Unfortunately, attendance was less than expected and the program was not repeated.

Teaching Us to Be Teachers Today

So, why do we need faculty development and what do we need now? Unless one came from a nurse anesthesia program that offers a master's degree in education (and at present there is only 1 program that does), program faculty need education to be the best and most effective teachers they can be. Our clinical faculty are role models for our students. They give students the "pearls" of administering a safe anesthetic and allow students to make decisions, try techniques, correlate didactic knowledge in the clinical arena, and gain autonomy through their preceptorship. Some day we hope this experience with a CRNA preceptor will lead the new clinician to teach other student nurse anesthetists as a preceptor.

Some university programs offer education courses as part of their master's degree coursework. Although these courses are important additions to our students' academic preparations, student nurse anesthetists at CCSU, say that these courses are sometimes too generic to feel relevant to the role in the clinical area (September 2005). Many times these courses, if offered, are the new nurse anesthetists' first introduction to educational preparation. If the courses are relevant, they are often very well received and can spark an interest in teaching.

Members of the New England Assembly of School Faculty stated that clinical faculty members often have dual roles within their anesthesia programs (September, 2005). Many prepare and deliver individual didactic presentations or teach entire courses within the curriculum of an anesthesia program. These faculty members often seek information on communication, preparation, and evaluation among other offerings related to faculty development. Administrators of programs, clinical coordinators, and clinical faculty who serve on the schools' committees may seek expanded types of faculty development. These might include curriculum design, examination preparation and item writing, interviews, public speaking, objective writing, the use of technology in research and delivery of information, and evaluations.

What's Out There in the World of "Teach Us to Be Teachers"?

In 1997, the members of the New England Assembly of School Faculty examined this question. Programs were expanding and new programs were opening, and the structures of some of the existing programs were changing as they signed on affiliates, both academic and clinical. With these changes came many clinical practitioners who assumed the role of faculty. These new faculty and many of the existing faculty looked to the program administrators for guidance to best serve the students and the school. The AANA, in particular the Assembly of School Faculty and the AANA Education Committee organizers, provided the leaders with the ideas for this type of faculty development. Many program administrators who were members of this New England group regularly attended the Assembly of School Faculty meeting and benefited from the programs and speakers. The program administrators wondered how they could get this valuable information back to share with the clinical faculty at home.

The administrators decided to organize a workshop with an educational theme. It was called the New England Assembly Faculty Development Workshop. To fund this project, they petitioned the schools, whether university or hospital based, to contribute a modest amount of money to the project. A few pharmaceutical representatives also contributed after they were convinced that this was far more worthwhile than buying morning bagels for the department. The administrators chose a speaker many of them had heard at the Assembly of School Faculty. The speaker was positive, energetic, and motivated, and she shared some pertinent information on effective communication, student motivation, and conflict resolution. Her presentation was relevant to faculty interaction with students and colleagues.

Those participating in the workshop were granted continuing education credits for the all-day program, and lunch was provided free of charge in the hospital cafeteria for all who came. Attendees wore name tags stating their affiliation site and school to encourage networking among all those in attendance. It was truly a faculty appreciation seminar.

"If you build it (right), they will come" had become the new philosophy of this group. The organizers sat back and waited and they *did* come. The objective of the New England Assembly of School Faculty then was to provide a free workshop in educational issues, provide an opportunity for all faculty members at both the academic and clinical sites to network and share concerns, and to provide a thank-you to their colleagues.

The objectives have not changed, and the workshop has been held every year since 1997. It has been expanded to a much larger and nicer location, better food is provided, and it is now open, for a modest fee, to those outside the geographical area of New England. This workshop even won the Crystal Apple award in 2002 for innovation in education from the AANA. Continuing education credit is still granted and the workshop continues to be held for the faculty at the affiliating institutions without charge.

The evaluations of this program have been enlightening. Attendees have told us what they need and want. The organizers have taken the lead of the educators in attendance and continue to design workshops in the areas where the need for knowledge is greatest.

Thus far, the program has included topics on legal issues, dealing with the difficult student, conflict resolution, effective teaching methods, public speaking, management styles, evaluation, generational differences in learning, mentoring, simulation, teaching evidence-based research, and using trigger films as an aid to developing and assessing clinical instructors.[2] Lectures, interactive presentations, role play, videos, and discussion formats also have been used.

Thoughts on Faculty Development in the Future

The model is simple and it works well. Plans are being made to expand on this program in the future by offering more of these educationally themed workshops. Those involved continue to seek input from faculty members on what they need and want. Program administrators can correlate much that they learn from other programs, residencies, and universities to this teaching situation.

Historically, the AANA has been involved in promoting faculty development and the AANA should continue to provide this support and opportunity to nurse anesthesia programs and their faculty members. Offerings held at the Assembly of School Faculty meeting have been beneficial to the educators in attendance. Several years ago, a formal faculty development program was held with much praise and support from those who participated.

In the future, clinical CRNAs and students need to be encouraged to become involved in education and to be comfortable in this role. Many students are now sponsored financially to attend the Assembly of School Faculty meeting and encouraged to adopt the role of a CRNA educator. Attendance at this meeting has steadily increased. The National Board of Certification and Recertification of Nurse Anesthetists (NBCRNA) could encourage or require CRNAs to obtain a portion of their recertification continuing education credits in educational offerings (eg, evaluation, mentoring, and conflict resolution) if they are involved in the teaching of students. Teaching of technology as it relates to education (eg, Microsoft PowerPoint presentations and use of the Internet to obtain educational information) should be considered for continuing education credits. Nurse anesthesia faculty who prepare and deliver lectures and/or coursework to students should be eligible to receive continuing education credits, because many of them do this on their own time and without compensation from the schools.

Educational offerings should continue to be presented at the AANA Annual Meeting in addition to those at the Assembly of School Faculty meeting. The offerings selected each year by the AANA Education Committee have been excellent and diverse. Some of the speakers used in the past should be encouraged to regionalize their presentations to reach a wider audience. Funding should be a combined effort within specific areas through contributions and support from the anesthesia programs, whether they are university, hospital-based, freestanding, or combined programs. Regions could be encouraged to promote programs such as the Assembly of School Faculty or faculty development workshops to provide a better opportunity to reach more CRNA educators. Individual state associations could become involved in providing support as well.

Summary

Nurse anesthetists are trained to be clinicians first and foremost. The role of the educator seems to have fallen on our shoulders. Some CRNAs are natural-born teachers with the gift of patience, the knowledge to precept, and the ability to motivate, but the majority of preceptors and educators need the tools for "teaching us to be teachers" that good faculty development programs can provide. With the shortage of educators that programs are facing, we need faculty development today more than ever. Nurse anesthetists must be taught to be educators as well as clinicians and take advantage of the educational training available to help us be comfortable in this much-needed role.

References:

1. Standards for Accreditation of Nurse Anesthesia Educational Programs. Park Ridge, IL: Council on Accreditation of Nurse Anesthesia Educational Programs; 2008.

2. Hartland W, Biddle C, Fallacaro M. Accessing the living laboratory; trigger films as an aid to developing, enabling, and assessing anesthesia clinical instructors. *AANA J.* 2003;71(4)287-291.

3. Simpson DJ, Jackson MJB. *Educational Reform: A Deweyan Prespective.* New York, NY: Garland Publishing Inc; 1997:153-227.

Suggested Websites for Faculty Development Information

1. This site has an overwhelming number of resources on computers and technology created for healthcare professions.
Medical Computing Review website. www.medicalcomputing.org/mcr/. Accessed March 4, 2009.

2. This site is helpful in writing behavioral objectives.
Ad Prima Education Information for New and Future Teachers. http://www.adprima.com/objectives.htm. Accessed March 4, 2009.

3. Problem based learning: a paradigm shift or a passing fad? Camp G. http://www.med-ed-online.org/f0000003.htm. Accessed March 4, 2009.

4. Program for faculty development. McMaster University website. http://www.fhs.mcmaster.ca/facdev/workshops.html. Accessed March 4, 2009.

5. Bonwell C. Active Learning website. http://www.active-learning-site.com. Accessed March 4, 2009.

6. The Carnegie Foundation for the Advancement of Teaching website. http://www.carnegiefoundation.org/. Accessed March 4, 2009.

7. UW Madison classroom media support presentation tips. University of Wisconsin, Madison website. http://www2.fpm.wisc.edu/support/PresentationTips.htm. Accessed March 4, 2009.

8. The critical thinking community. Foundation for Critical Thinking website. www.criticalthinking.org. Accessed March 4, 2009.

9. Distance education clearinghouse. University of Wisconsin-Extension website. http://www.uwex.edu/disted/index.cfm. Accessed March 4, 2009.

10. Developing effective lectures: eight steps to active lecturing. Ferris State University Center for Teaching, Learning & Faculty Development website. http://www.ferris.edu/htmls/academics/center/Teaching_and_Learning_Tips/Developing%20Effective%20Lectures/8stepstoactive.htm. Accessed March 4, 2009.

11. Tips for effective PowerPoint presentations. http://www.cheney268.com/training/PowerPoint/PowerPointTips.htm. Accessed March 4, 2009.

12. PowerPoint in the classroom. Actden website. http://www.actden.com/pp/. Accessed March 4, 2009.

13. Problem-based learning. University of Delaware website. http://www.udel.edu/pbl/. Accessed March 4, 2009.

14. Learn the Net: the Internet owner's manual. Michael Lerner Productions website. www.learnthenet.com. Accessed March 4, 2009.

15. King RM. Managing teaching loads and finding time for reflection and renewal. Association for Psychological Science. http://www.psychologicalscience.org/teaching/tips/tips_0102.cfm. Accessed March 4, 2009.

Chapter 14

Simulation in Nurse Anesthesia Education

Alfred E. Lupien, CRNA, PhD, FAAN

Key Points

- Simulation is the representation of an object, situation, procedure, or environment through the use of another.

- Simulators used in nurse anesthesia education can be broadly classified as computer screen-based simulators, task trainers, or high-fidelity, full-body simulators.

- Advantages of using simulation include controlled exposure to rare and critical events; expansion, compression, or reiteration of time; consistency of educational opportunities for all students; and the opportunity to explore the consequences of clinical decision making without compromising patient care or safety.

- Simulation can be used to reinforce concepts of basic science, help students prepare for entry into clinical practice, or augment actual clinical experiences.

- Simulation sessions should build on each student's existing knowledge. The level of difficulty and extent of faculty participation should be adjusted to promote goal achievement.

- Active participation by students is essential for effective learning through simulation. Student verbalization of observations and thought processes during the simulation enables the faculty to have a more complete appreciation for learner performance.

- Postsimulation debriefing, either oral or augmented with video recordings, is essential, particularly when the simulation's objective includes nontechnical skills.

Introduction

Simulation is defined as the representation of an object, situation, procedure, or environment through the use of another.[1,2] In anesthesia education, simulation can be as simple as using a banana to teach epidural needle insertion[3] or as complex as a realistic, life-sized manikin with functioning physiological systems. Advantages of using simulation as an instructional modality include:

- Controlled exposure to rare and critical events not consistently available to all students in actual clinical practice
- The ability to isolate events and match the educational session's level of difficulty with the learner's expertise
- Expansion, compression, or reiteration of time as desired based on educational objectives and the learner's expertise
- Opportunity to explore the consequences of clinical decision making without compromising patient care or safety
- Consistency of educational opportunities for all students
- Reduction or elimination of production pressure
- Potential to develop enhanced situation awareness
- Enhanced clinical ethics by reducing requirements for patient involvement in learning

Although simulation has been characterized as one of the latest trends in the field of anesthesiology, in reality, the method has been used to teach nurse anesthetists for more than 40 years. Early milestones included the development of the cardiopulmonary resuscitation (CPR) training manikin Resusci Anne (Laerdal Medical Corporation, Wappingers Falls, New York) in 1960 and the first computer-controlled patient simulator in 1969.[4] The modern era of simulation began in 1990 with Anesthesia Simulator Consultant, the first software-based anesthesia simulator and the development of commercially available computer-controlled, high-fidelity patient simulators. These simulators included CAE-Link (also called MedSim-Eagle, no longer produced), Sophus (Laerdal Sophus, Kent, United Kingdom), and Medical Education and Technologies Inc (METI, Sarasota, Florida).[4,5] Use of high-fidelity patient simulators in nurse anesthesia education was first documented by Fletcher[6] at Pennsylvania's University of Pittsburgh in 1995. Later that year, the first simulation center in a school of nursing was opened at the Medical College of Georgia, Augusta.

Types of Simulators

Simulators can be classified into 3 categories: computer screen-based, task trainers, and full-body, high-fidelity simulators. A fourth type of simulator, the standardized patient, is often overlooked in discussions of simulation.

Computer Screen-Based Simulators

Computer screen-based simulators are interactive computer software products modeling specific elements of basic science or applied anesthesia care. Software is available to illustrate complex concepts or dynamic interactions, enhance decision making, and provide experience with infrequent or life-threatening events (Table 14.1). Computer screen-based simulations can be used as freestanding educational modules, to augment traditional teaching methods, or to complement task trainers and full-body simulation.

Task Trainers

Task trainers are used to teach specific skills or processes. Typical examples include anatomically correct heads for practicing airway management, necks for teaching the technique of cricothyroidotomy, chests for central line insertion, and lumbar spines for subarachnoid or epidural needle placement.

Table 14.1. Examples of Computer Screen–Based Simulation Software

Product	Manufacturer	Description
Anesthesia simulator	Anesoft Corp Issaquah, Washington www.anesoft.com	Clinical management of routine and complex anesthetics with or without critical incidents. Anesoft also distributes screen-based simulations for advanced cardiac life support, bioterrorism, critical care, hemodynamics, and sedation.
Body simulation	Advanced Simulation Corp Point Roberts, Washington www.advsim.com	Based on 45-compartment, multiple-transport enhanced Fukui-Smith model. Scenarios include applied science (eg, physiology of preoxygenation, second gas effect, and pharmacokinetics of both volatile and intravenous anesthetic agents) and clinical practice with and without critical incidents.
Gas man	H. M. Franklin Associates San Ramon, California www.gasmanweb.com	Interactive software focusing on uptake and distribution of volatile anesthetic agents.
Virtual anesthesia machine	University of Florida Gainesville, Florida http://vam.anest.ufl.edu	Internet-based simulation promoting understanding and safe use of anesthesia machine. Includes workbook and supplemental materials for additional study. Development of and access to the simulation is supported by corporate sponsorships and donations.

(A more extensive list of simulators with potential applicability in anesthesia education was compiled in 2007 by Cumin and Merry.[5])

More recently, virtual reality devices have been introduced by Immersion Medical (Gaithersburg, Maryland) and Medic Vision, Ltd (Melbourne, Australia) for venous cannulation, bronchoscopy, and lumbar epidural needle placement. These devices use sensors to determine the location of the needle or bronchoscope in 3-dimensional space. As the instrument is manipulated by the student, accurate haptic (tactile) feedback is provided and realistic corresponding anatomical images can be displayed on a computer monitor. Task trainers can be used alone to teach technical skills or in combination with computer screen-based simulators.

Full-Body Simulators

Life-sized, full-body patient simulators typically include 3 components: an anatomically correct manikin, a computer that controls multiple devices to generate physiological responses, and a user interface. Full-body simulators commercially available in the United States include SimMan (Laerdal Medical Corp, Wappingers Falls, New York) and the METI family of infant, pediatric, and adult simulators, including the Emergency Care Simulator (ECS), Human Patient Simulator (HPS), and completely tetherless iStan. Simulator characteristics vary by manufacturer and product. A full-featured device may include heart and lung sounds, palpable pulses, synchronized cardiovascular waveforms (electrocardiogram, pulmonary artery pressure, and central venous pressure), plethysmogram and hemoglobin saturation values, exhaled respiratory gases detectable with a standard respiratory gas analyzer, eyes that open and close, pupils that respond to light, and a thumb that responds to peripheral nerve stimulation. Simulators accept a variety of endotracheal and transtracheal airway devices and may respond as physiologically appropriate to defibrillation, chest tube insertion, pericardiocentesis, and needle decompression of a pneumothorax.

Sophisticated high-fidelity simulators, such as the METI HPS, include a library of preconfigured patients and allow the user to modify or create new patients. The user can also adjust individual physiological parameters such as systemic vascular resistance, venous return, ventricular contractility, baroreceptor response, pulmonary shunt fraction, oxygen consumption, bronchial resistance, functional residual capacity, lung compliance, and chest wall compliance. Simulators may also include a library of scenarios that can be superimposed to create common events, such as hypotension with tachycardia, or less common problems, including anaphylaxis and malignant hyperthermia. Once a simulation has been implemented, physiological information is communicated back to the trainer through the user interface, which includes real-time heart rate and respiratory rate, temperature, oxygen saturation, pulmonary and arterial respiratory gas concentrations, blood pressure, central venous pressure, and pulmonary artery pressures. The simulator will automatically recognize volatile anesthetics or injected medications and respond appropriately. The instructor has the options of allowing the simulation to progress based on the underlying physiological and pharmacological models, making manual adjustments through the user interface, or using preprogrammed transitions to modify progression of the simulation. Log files record events (eg, medications administered and modifications to the patient or scenario) and physiological data for retrospective review. Simulators with fewer features than the HPS may require the user to identify medications administered and/or lack a library of preprogrammed patients and scenarios.

Standardized Patients

The standardized patient is an individual who has been trained to portray the history, physical findings, body language, and personality of an actual patient.[7] The standardized patient can be either an individual with a clinical condition who has been coached to present the condition consistently or an actor who has practiced presenting a patient's condition consistently. Audio recordings (eg, heart and lung sounds), photographs of physical findings, and short videos (eg, range of motion or gait) can be used to augment the presentation of simulated patients. Advantages of using well-prepared standardized patients include accuracy in representation of a clinical condition, consistent presentation of patient history and physical findings, the ability to illustrate the progression of an illness over time, potential for customization of the situation to match specific educational goals, the ability to match the difficulty of the scenario with the learner's ability level, and the opportunity to provide feedback to the learner, including from the patient's perspective.[8] Although standardized patients are used more commonly in primary care education, they can be invaluable in teaching preanesthetic and postanesthetic assessment.

A Conceptual Strategy for Simulation

The learning process may be considered a continuum of experiences that are initially externally regulated and shared between a student and teacher, then become progressively personalized and regulated by the student as learning occurs.[9] According to Vygotsky,[9] learning is most likely to occur within a unique and evolving zone of proximal development (ZPD), which exists between what can be done alone and what the student can do only with instructor assistance. The teacher's role is to move the student through the ZPD, from guided to independent practice. Simulation provides the opportunity to individualize instruction based on each student's ZPD by adjusting scenario complexity and the degree of faculty participation, as necessary, to promote learning.

Learning in the ZPD can be subdivided into 4 stages.[10] During the first stage, the faculty member guides the student as performance transitions from external direction to self-regulation. Modeling is essential during first-stage learning. Demonstrations of expert practice serve as templates for student performance, feedback, and interactive coaching. By thinking aloud during demonstrations, the faculty member can make thought processes involved in expert anesthesia practice visible to the student. Expertly modeled behaviors and verbal cues also create essential mental references for the student facing challenging situations during subsequent stages of learning.

Direct instruction during the first stage of learning is very specific. For instance, when teaching the technical skills for direct laryngoscopy, the faculty might guide the student to: "Place the head into the 'sniffing' position, open the mouth, insert the laryngoscope blade into the right side of the mouth. While sweeping the tongue to the left, gradually advance the blade and identify the anatomical structures as they come into view . . . ." As the student's skills develop, teaching can be accomplished through other means such as prompting, questioning, or feedback on performance.

The student begins to self-regulate performance during the second stage of learning. Less instructor assistance is needed as the student uses self-developed prompts in the learning sequence. Early in stage 2, the student may recite the prompts aloud. For example, it is not uncommon for a beginning clinical student to verbalize a checklist of preparations before inducing general anesthesia: "OK . . . my anesthesia machine is turned on. Suction is available. My endotracheal tube is ready . . . ." Self-guidance becomes internalized and silent as the student progresses; however, the student may once again speak the prompts aloud under particularly difficult circumstances.

All outward evidence of self-regulation vanishes during the third stage of learning as competent performance develops. Tasks are integrated and executed smoothly. Vygotsky[9] described skills in this stage as relatively fixed and immune from both external and internal forces of change. The student feels confident of task success and wishes to be left alone to perform. Assistance may be perceived as irritating or even disruptive. In an actual clinical environment, an instructor may be obligated to intervene when a student's actions or decisions become potentially dangerous; however, simulation creates the context in which a situation can continue to unfold and allow the student to evaluate consequences of decisions and actions.

In the final stage of learning, the student reexamines task performance. This reexploration may occur during a particularly challenging or stressful situation. Externalizing self-speech, or further reversion through previous stages of learning, such as remembering the voice or actions of a teacher, are often effective in restoring competence. Reflecting after a fourth-stage learning experience, the student may recount to the instructor: "I couldn't figure out why the patient's O_2 saturation was falling, or what to do about it, but then I remembered how you and I had the same thing happen before. You started by assessing the patient and working backward from the patient toward the anesthesia machine." The outcome of the final stage of the ZPD is an enhanced understanding of the learning task.

The stages of progression through the ZPD suggest a strategy for teaching through simulation. After assessment of a student's proficiencies, simulation exercises are customized based on specific ZPDs for each task. When starting from the first stage in the ZPD, learning experiences may include significant instructor involvement. The provision of verbal or visual cues that the student will be able to reference mentally during subsequent learning experiences is particularly important during this stage. More independence will be desired as the student progresses through learning stages and begins to feel confident. During periods of independence, the instructor can allow the student freedom, yet remain available and prepared to resume teaching as the student's understanding moves out of inflexible performance during stage 3 and into the reexploration that occurs during stage 4.

General Plan for Using Simulation

Learning Objectives and Pilot Testing

Before implementing a scenario, the faculty member identifies specific learning objectives. These objectives should be understood by both the faculty and students. Ideally, simulation sessions should be based on realistic clinical events to enhance their accuracy, be matched with the learner's ability, and include opportunities for decision making.[11]

Each session should use and build on the student's existing knowledge with the level of difficulty adjusted to promote successful progression toward a goal.[12] For example, Plummer and Owen[13] studied the process of learning endotracheal intubation and noted that trainees learned intubation skills more efficiently when their intubation attempts were successful, rather than when they failed.

The simulation should be pilot tested to identify its strengths and weaknesses. Strategies should be developed to minimize limitations of the simulation. When implementing an overall plan for simulation, the following questions should be considered:

- Is the activity oriented toward the development of technical skills, cognitive skills, or the integration of both?
- Is the activity intended for faculty to model technical or cognitive skills or to encourage the student to develop the skills?
- Will feedback be provided in real time or after the session?
- Should the session be allowed to progress in whatever direction it flows or kept focused on a specific activity?
- Should learners be encouraged to focus their thinking or to explore and test ideas?

Faculty and Student Roles

Once the simulation has begun, the faculty member's attention should be directed toward determining what the student knows and is observing,[14] maintaining a productive educational environment, and protecting learner integrity.

Active student participation is essential for effective learning through simulation. The student is responsible for understanding the session's objectives and preparing thoroughly before engaging in the exercise. The learner should approach the simulation earnestly, be inquisitive, and be receptive to instructor feedback. Encouraging the student to verbalize observations and thought processes during the simulation enables the faculty to more completely evaluate performance. Once the session is complete, and unless directed otherwise, participating students should protect the confidentiality of the scenario so that incoming students can experience the session without predisposition.

Simulation can be used in all phases of the nurse anesthesia curriculum to reinforce concepts of basic science, help students prepare for entry into clinical practice, and augment real clinical experiences (through rare-event training and crisis resource management). Depending on the types of simulators used, the focus can be psychomotor or cognitive.

Psychomotor skill development encompasses activities ranging from teaching isolated technical skills (eg, correcting an obstructed airway or performing direct laryngoscopy) to combining the skills into complex production sets, such as sequences for the induction of general endotracheal anesthesia. When teaching technical skills, Greaves[15] suggested a 5-step process for effective instruction:

1. The faculty member demonstrates the technique in real time as the student observes.
2. The faculty member repeats the demonstration at a slower speed, adding an explanation of each step.
3. The faculty member repeats the technique a third time while the student explains each step.
4. The student repeats the technique as the faculty member observes.
5. The student continues to practice with decreasing supervision.

Cognitively focused simulation includes the introduction of new concepts through reinforcement of knowledge, critical thinking, situation awareness, decision making, and teamwork in a dynamic environment. At its highest level, simulations combine both the cognitive and psychomotor domains. For example, successful management of a difficult airway requires both a comprehensive set of technical skills and the abilities to think critically and act decisively. Postsimulation debriefing, either oral or augmented with video recordings, is essential, particularly when the objective of the simulation includes development of nontechnical skills. Savoldelli et al[16] demonstrated that performance of nontechnical skills improved by 11% (video-assisted oral) to 15% (oral) after debriefing, whereas performance scores did not change without debriefing.

The extent to which simulation can be integrated into nurse anesthesia education depends on factors such as the types of simulators available, frequency of access to simulators, overall number of students, number of students for each simulation session, sequencing within the curriculum, and faculty availability. The time commitment for individual faculty members to participate in small-group instruction for large classes of students can be substantial.

The following examples illustrate strategies to leverage resources by designing simulation sessions with varying levels of faculty involvement.

Types of Simulation by Level of Faculty Involvement

Continuous Instruction: Teaching technical skills (such as effective airway management) using simulation requires closely supervised personal instruction. Following large-group, classroom-based instruction on the basic principles of establishing and maintaining the airway, technical considerations are reinforced by instructor-led demonstrations for small groups of up to 8 students, using task trainers and full-body simulators. Smaller groups may be more appropriate for student return demonstrations and refining technical skills. Student dyads can be effective, with 1 student receiving direct instruction while another student is observing and learning vicariously. The instructor can use the observer to point out nuances of technique and to monitor correct performance. To supplement faculty involvement, each student might be encouraged to maintain a journal noting areas needing improvement and strategies for success.

A high-fidelity simulator, by itself, can be used to provide meaningful feedback for 1 dyad of students while the instructor is working with another. For example, to develop mask ventilation skills, the simulator can be programmed to desaturate quickly by increasing oxygen consumption and intrapulmonary shunt. Clinically meaningful feedback is provided to the student who has been instructed to maintain adequate ventilation for a period of 5 to 10 minutes. Over time, each student develops techniques for correct placement of the face mask and for manually augmenting ventilation.

Guided Instruction: Continuous faculty participation may not be required as students' technical skills improve and their familiarity with simulators and anesthesia equipment increases. In fact, for some students, independence and confidence may increase when clarification with a faculty member is not an immediate option. For guided simulation exercises, the instructor prepares a set of learning activities and objectives, meets with the students for a brief demonstration and clarification of session expectations, and then encourages the students to work in small groups (depending on the nature of the activity) to complete the assigned tasks or objectives. At a designated time, the faculty member meets with each small group of students to discuss their findings and add clarification. For some exercises, students may also be expected to compile a group report.

Unsupervised Instruction: Only limited faculty participation may be necessary for completion of some basic science laboratory exercises or continued practice in the development of production sets, such as sequences for induction of general anesthesia. Small groups of students may work toward completion of specific project objectives without the immediate availability of faculty once the students have demonstrated fundamental skills and their ability to operate the simulator.

As with guided instruction sessions, clearly stated exercise objectives with measurable monitored outcomes are essential for maximum effectiveness. The following practical strategies are suggested for successful facilitation of unsupervised simulation sessions:

- Encourage the students to work in pairs or small groups when refining technical skills and sequences, so that an observing student can monitor and provide feedback for the student who is practicing skills.
- Maximize simulator availability and student productivity by requiring students to reserve times to work on specific skills or exercises.

- Increase accessibility to the simulation laboratory by hiring and training a student assistant to extend the laboratory's hours of operation.
- Monitor the progress of each student to ensure that he or she is successfully meeting faculty expectations for cognitive and psychomotor skill development.

Examples of Simulation Exercises

The following exercises are examples of various uses of simulation, including standardized patients and screen-based and full-body simulators. Topics include cardiovascular physiology and principles of anesthesia care.

Basic Anesthesia Skill: Preanesthetic Assessment of Student "Personae"

Goal: To provide experience evaluating patients and developing plans for anesthesia care.

Description: Realistic patient scenarios that can be consistently re-created are developed during the preliminary phase of this 2-phase exercise. As an alternative to actual standardized patients, the faculty members develop a comprehensive matrix of patients of both sexes and of various ages and weights, with conditions that students are likely to encounter during the early phases of their clinical education. The matrix includes common surgical procedures, pathophysiological processes, medications, allergies, and concerns about anesthesia. Each student selects or is assigned a patient case from the matrix, then develops a persona complete with unique history and physical findings. Visual and audio media (eg, photographs of a patient's airway or recording of lung sounds) can be used to illustrate physical characteristics. Each student documents the persona's preanesthetic assessment and submits it to the faculty for review. Once the faculty member accepts the assessment, the student adopts the persona's characteristics for the remainder of the exercise.

During the second phase of the exercise, students interview their classmates' personae and document the findings. Based on the goals of the exercise, the assignment either can be limited to preanesthesia assessment or can be extended to include the development of a plan for anesthesia care, presentation and defense of the plan to faculty, or implementation of the plan on a full-body or screen-based simulator.

Required Equipment: Visual or audio media as desired, anesthesia assessment forms (or formats), and simulation scenarios (if desired).

Learner Instructions: Conduct a thorough preanesthetic patient evaluation on a persona you have not interviewed previously. Address any concerns of the "patient," counsel the patient, and document your assessment to include preparation of preanesthetic orders for diagnostic tests, fluids, and medications as indicated. Submit your findings and documentation to the persona for peer review before forwarding them to the faculty advisor for critique. Be prepared to present and defend your plan.

Unanticipated Event: Contaminated Oxygen Supply*

Goal: To explore how contamination of the oxygen supply is manifested by a patient and monitoring systems.

*Adapted with permission from a demonstration by Anthony Bryant, CRNA, MN, and Matthew Kervin, CRNA, MN.

Description: Contamination of the oxygen supply of an anesthesia machine will present differently based on the nature and timing of the contamination. For this exercise, contamination is introduced by completely "crossing over" the oxygen and nitrous oxide (N_2O) hoses between the gas source and anesthesia machine (Figure 14.1). Patient signs and symptoms will vary during induction of general anesthesia based on technique (eg, standard or rapid sequence or duration and efficiency of preoxygenation). The scenario can be implemented as a controlled exercise (focusing on monitoring systems) for novice students or as an unknown event for more experienced students.

Required Equipment: METI HPS, respiratory gas monitor, anesthesia machine with standard patient monitors, induction supplies, and modified gas supply hoses.

Learner Instructions: Novice students should select "standard man" from the list of available patients. Record baseline vital signs and monitoring data before administering any medications or oxygen. Induce general anesthesia using different techniques (eg, standard induction with and without preoxygenation, rapid sequence induction, and slow inhalation induction) and observe how and when hypoxia or hypoxemia is detected. Describe how the presentation differs based on the technique selected. Be prepared to discuss the strengths and limitations of various respiratory gas monitors and how a patient's oxygen reserve is affected by techniques for induction of general anesthesia.

Figure 14.1. Modified Gas Supply Hoses Used to Create Contaminated Oxygen (O_2) Supply.

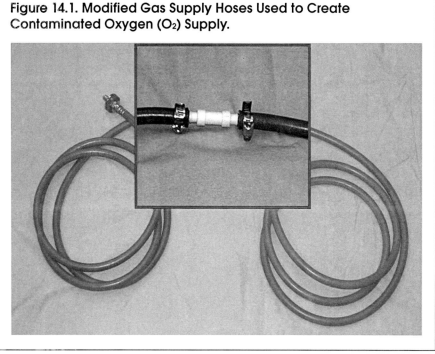

Source end of O_2 hose has been attached to the machine end of the nitrous oxide (N_2O) hose and vice versa.

As an unplanned event for more advanced students, the scenario begins with any spontaneously breathing patient, as desired. The learner is directed to initiate general anesthesia based on the clinical context provided. Contamination should be detected during the equipment check or during preoxygenation.

Anesthesia Principles: Fluid Management of a Patient With Valvular Heart Disease*

The purpose of this exercise is to illustrate the relationship between theoretical knowledge of cardiovascular pathophysiology and daily clinical practice. The student is able to observe effects of clinical decision-making on cardiac preload, afterload, and contractility by manipulating the intravascular volume of a patient with valvular heart disease (eg, aortic stenosis). Optimal fluid volume is determined as the student plots a Starling curve (Figure 14.2) from data collected during the exercise.

Required Equipment: METI HPS with cardiovascular monitor, or a computer screen-based simulator.

Learner Instructions For METI HPS: Select the patient "standard man" or another patient as directed from the list of available patients. If necessary, modify the patient's physiology to match the intended pathophysiological condition. For each valvular condition to be studied, predict how cardiovascular parameters will respond to changes in fluid volume. Starting with baseline values, construct a comprehensive table of cardiovascular measurements by incrementally increasing (or decreasing) fluid volume. Plot cardiovascular (pressure/volume) performance and be prepared to discuss the congruence between your predictions and findings.

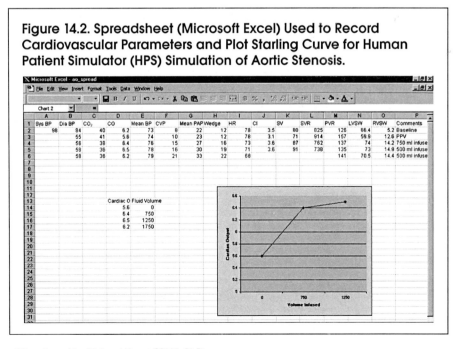

Figure 14.2. Spreadsheet (Microsoft Excel) Used to Record Cardiovascular Parameters and Plot Starling Curve for Human Patient Simulator (HPS) Simulation of Aortic Stenosis.

*Developed by Richard Haas, CRNA, PhD.

Caveats to Simulation

The use of simulation can greatly enhance the education of student nurse anesthetists; however, there are also cautions and risks associated with the instructional modality. First and foremost, although patient simulators are becoming increasing realistic, they are incomplete generalized representations of human physical (surface) appearance, anatomy, physiology, and responses to pharmaceuticals. The simulator's intended use should be one of the first considerations when developing an educational session using simulation. In most circumstances, the simulator is used either as a surrogate for an actual human patient or as an educational vehicle, for example, to teach psychomotor skills.

Accuracy of the underlying physiological and/or pharmacological models is essential when simulation is used to teach physiology or pharmacology. Reference documentation describing model development is available for simulation products; however, it may be difficult for the end user to independently and completely validate the scenarios. Before implementation of a simulation, the faculty should determine whether simulator response is consistent with literature reports and personal experience. If not, simulator responses should be adjusted or inconsistencies noted for the students.

As an educational vehicle, the absolute validity of surface features or underlying models *may* be less critical. When provider performance is the focus of a simulation, facets to be considered are whether the simulator promotes the development of the intended correct technical skills, decisions, and actions. Instructors should also consider whether any characteristics of the simulator, or lack thereof, would induce the learner to either defer action or implement a course of action other than intended in the scenario.

Zull[12] uses the term the *teaching trap* to caution educators that learning is a continuous sensory experience and that *any* educator action, intended or unintended, may induce learning. This trap is similarly applicable with simulation. Although one of the fundamental goals of simulation is to provide experiences that the student can transfer to the clinical environment, the faculty should be constantly attentive to the correctness of generalizations that may be formed through simulation. For example, students practicing with one particular airway simulator may observe that an endotracheal tube has been placed to the correct depth when the tube's 18-cm mark aligns with the simulator's lip line. Over time, students practicing direct laryngoscopy and intubation can be observed adjusting a newly inserted tracheal tube's depth to 18 cm even before chest auscultation (or examination of a capnographic waveform). If the learner prioritizes aligning external markings over clinical evidence, then an inappropriate generalization has been made.

Finally, faculty should constantly be reminded of the adage "practice doesn't make perfect; perfect practice makes perfect." The development of fundamental clinical skills is one of the primary reasons for encouraging students to practice using part-task trainers and high-fidelity patient simulators; however, unintended and/or poor habits can also be reinforced when practicing without formative evaluation. Alternatively, simulation can be used to nurture positive clinical habits beyond technical skills. For example, requiring students to use a precordial stethoscope when practicing with a high-fidelity simulator can signal the importance of this monitor and promote continuous auscultation in clinical practice.

Simulation: A Broader Perspective

The scope of this chapter has focused narrowly on the use of simulation as an instructional technique for nurse anesthesia education. Applications of simulation continue to broaden as simulators become more sophisticated, realistic, and accessible. Simulation is being used to teach team performance and resource management.[17-21] As accepted by the Council on Certification of Nurse Anesthetists, simulation also is emerging as an alternative to actual clinical experience for some procedural skills such as central venous cannulation and fiberscopically assisted tracheal intubation. Simulation is also being used to enhance the instructional skills of clinical faculty through techniques such as the use of trigger films, which provide opportunities for faculty to explore how they might respond to situations encountered in the operating room with students.[22]

Although full-body simulation sessions can be quite realistic, limitations have been identified. Hotchkiss et al[23] reported that simulation participants were distracted by the recording cameras and demonstrated exaggerated vigilance. Participant actions were characterized as "rapid, mechanical, and anxious."[23(p473)] The investigators suggested that the simulations were unable to completely capture the operating room culture and that scenarios based on substandard care contributed to a sense of improbability. By contrast, anesthesiology residents participating in a multisite evaluation of full-body simulation described the sessions as realistic.[24]

Perhaps the emerging trend generating the most attention is the use of simulation in performance evaluation. Before it can achieve widespread adoption, the validity and reliability of evaluation methods must be documented thoroughly. Educators at the Canadian Simulation Centre for Human Performance and Crisis Management Training have developed a system to score performance of anesthesia providers managing clinical scenarios with imbedded clinical problems. They reported strong scorer interrater reliability ($\kappa = .96$, $P < .001$)[25] and moderate internal consistency ($\alpha = .66$).[26] The scoring method also effectively discriminated performance among varying categories of students, residents, and anesthesiologists.[26,27] Beyond the assessment of technical skills, the assessment of behavioral performance is also essential for evaluating provider actions and decision making during crisis situations.[28] Focusing on the nontechnical skills of task management, teamwork, situation awareness, and decision making, Fletcher et al[29] reported on a successful pilot study of the Anaesthetists' Non-Technical Skills (ANTS) behavioral evaluation system, with the intention of additional testing.

In their reviews of performance assessment through simulation, both Byrne and Greaves[30] and Wong[31] concluded that additional evidence of reliability and validity is needed before the widespread adoption of simulation for formalized clinical performance evaluation. To date, the existing evidence is inconclusive. In 2006, Scavone et al[32] reported on the use of high-fidelity simulation to evaluate performance of anesthesia residents in the administration of general anesthesia for cesarean delivery. They concluded that their system successfully differentiated between third-year (CA-3) residents with "extensive obstetric anesthesia experience"[32(p261)] and first-year (CA-1) residents with "little or no obstetric anesthesia experience."[32(p262)] In 2007, Murray et al[33] reported success using a testing strategy in which participants completed simulations of 8 clinical scenarios to differentiate between the performance of CA-1 residents with approximately 1 month of anesthesia experience and more experienced clinicians including "advanced" CA-1 residents with an additional 7 months of anesthesia experience, CA-2/CA-3 residents, and practicing anesthesiologists. Performance scores among the advanced CA-1 residents, CA-2/CA-3 residents, and practitioners could not be differentiated. These 2 reports illustrate the potential of simulation as a testing strategy, but neither investigation achieved the level of sensitivity that would be necessary to finely discriminate levels of provider performance. Statistical analysis of the variance in participants' scores suggests that a 3-hour to 4-hour examination, including 8 and 15 scenarios, would be required to reliably quantify clinician competency.[34,35]

Summary

A comprehensive simulation program can be used to reinforce concepts of basic science and help students develop the mental models, decision-making strategies, and experiences required for competent clinical practice. Techniques include the use of computer programs; task trainers; high-fidelity, full-body simulators; and standardized patients.

Teaching strategies with beginning students may include demonstrations of expert practice and interactive coaching. Direct faculty involvement decreases as students' confidence and abilities progress.

Challenges associated with simulation include high cost (for some models), limited availability, increased faculty workload, and the potential for unintended learning. The use of simulation for competency assessment is a developing trend; however, evidence supporting simulation as the sole method for performance evaluation is inconclusive at this time.

References

1. *American Heritage Dictionary of the English Language.* 4th ed. Boston, MA: Houghton Mifflin; 2006.

2. Gardner R, Raemer DB. Simulation in obstetrics and gynecology. *Obstet Gynecol Clin North Am.* 2008;35(1):97-127.

3. Leighton BL. A greengrocer's model of the epidural space. *Anesthesiology.* 1989;70(2):368-369.

4. Rosen RK. The history of medical simulation. In: Loyd GE, Lake CL, Greenberg RB, eds. *Practical Health Care Simulations.* Philadelphia, PA: Elsevier Mosby; 2004:3-26.

5. Cumin D, Merry AF. Simulators for use in anaesthesia. *Anaesthesia.* 2007;62(2):151-162.

6. Fletcher JL. AANA Journal course: update for nurse anesthetists—anesthesia simulation: a tool for learning and research. *AANA J.* 1995;63(1):61-67.

7. Barrows HS. *Simulated (Standardized) Patients and Other Human Simulations.* Chapel Hill, NC: Health Sciences Consortium; 1987.

8. Barrows HS. An overview of the uses of standardized patients for teaching and evaluating clinical skills. *Acad Med.* 1993;68(6):443-453.

9. Vygotsky LS. *Mind in Society: The Development of Higher Psychological Processes.* Cambridge, MA: Harvard University Press; 1978.

10. Tharp RG, Gallimore R. *Rousing Minds to Life.* Cambridge, England: Cambridge University Press; 1988.

11. Glavin R, Maran N. An introduction to simulation in anaesthesia. In: Greaves D, Dodds C, Kumar CM, Mets B, eds. *Clinical Teaching: A Guide to Teaching Practical Anaesthesia.* Lisse, Netherlands: Swets & Zeitlinger; 2003:197-205.

12. Zull JE. *The Art of Changing the Brain.* Sterling, VA: Stylus; 2002.

13. Plummer JL, Owen H. Learning endotracheal intubation in a clinical skills learning center: a quantitative study. *Anesth Analg.* 2001;93(3):656-662.

14. Greaves D, Olympio M. Helping trainees to develop decision-making skills. In: Greaves D, Dodds C, Kumar CM, Mets B, eds. *Clinical Teaching: A Guide to Teaching Practical Anaesthesia.* Lisse, Netherlands: Swets & Zeitlinger; 2003:109-119.

15. Greaves D. Teaching practical procedures. In: Greaves D, Dodds C, Kumar CM, Mets B, eds. *Clinical Teaching: A Guide to Teaching Practical Anaesthesia.* Lisse, Netherlands: Swets & Zeitlinger; 2003:121-132.

16. Savoldelli GL, Naik VN, Park J, Joo HS, Chow R, Hamstra SJ. Value of debriefing during simulated crisis management: oral versus video-assisted oral feedback. *Anesthesiology.* 2006;105(2):279-285.

17. Fletcher JL. AANA Journal course: update for nurse anesthetists—ERR WATCH: anesthesia crisis resource management from the nurse anesthetist's perspective. *AANA J.* 1998;66(6):595-602.

18. France DJ, Leming-Lee S, Jackson T, Feistritzer NR, Higgins MS. An observational analysis of surgical team compliance with perioperative safety practices after crew resource management training. *Am J Surg.* 2008;195(4):546-553.

19. O'Donnell J, Fletcher J, Dixon B, Palmer L. Planning and implementing an anesthesia crisis resource management course for student nurse anesthetists. *CRNA.* 1998;9(2):50-58.

20. Undre S, Koutantji M, Sevdalis N, et al. Multidisciplinary crisis simulations: the way forward for training surgical teams. *World J Surg.* 2007;31(9):1843-1853.

21. Wayne DB, Didwania A, Feinglass J, Fudala MJ, Barsuk JH, McGahie WC. Simulation-based education improves quality of care during cardiac arrest team responses at an academic teaching hospital: a case-control study. *Chest*. 2008;133(1):56-61.

22. Hartland W, Biddle C, Fallacaro M. Assessing the living laboratory: trigger films as an aid to developing, enabling, and assessing anesthesia clinical instructors. *AANA J*. 2003;71(4):287-291.

23. Hotchkiss MA, Biddle C, Fallacaro M. Assessing the authenticity of the human simulation experience in anesthesiology. *AANA J*. 2002;70(6):470-473.

24. Schwid HA, Rooke GA, Carline J, et al. Evaluation of anesthesia residents using mannequin-based simulation: a multiinstitutional study. *Anesthesiology*. 2002;97(6):1434-1444.

25. Devitt JH, Kurrek MM, Cohen MM, et al. Testing the raters: inter-rater reliability of standardized anaesthesia simulator performance. *Can J Anaesth*. 1997;44(9):924-928.

26. Devitt JH, Kurrek MM, Cohen MM, et al. Testing internal consistency and construct validity during evaluation of performance in a patient simulator. *Anesth Analg*. 1998;86(6):1160-1164.

27. Devitt JH, Kurrek MM, Cohen MM, Cleave-Hogg D. The validity of performance assessments using simulation. *Anesthesiology*. 2001;95(1):36-42.

28. Gaba DM, Howard SK, Flanagan B, Smith BE, Fish KJ, Botney R. Assessment of clinical performance during simulated crises using both technical and behavioral ratings. *Anesthesiology*. 1998;89(1):8-18.

29. Fletcher G, Flin R, McGeorge P, Glavin R, Maran N, Patey R. Anaesthetists' Non-Technical Skills (ANTS): evaluation of a behavioural marker system. *Br J Anaesth*. 2003;90(5):580-588.

30. Byrne AJ, Greaves JD. Assessment instruments used during anaesthetic simulation: review of published articles. *Br J Anaesth*. 2001;86(3):445-450.

31. Wong AK. Full scale computer simulators in anesthesia training and evaluation. *Can J Anaesth*. 2004;51(5):455-464.

32. Scavone BM, Sproviero MT, McCarthy RJ, et al. Development of an objective scoring system for measurement of resident performance on the human patient simulator. *Anesthesiology*. 2006;105(2):260-266.

33. Murray DJ, Boulet JR, Avidan M, et al. Performance of residents and anesthesiologists in a simulation-based skill assessment. *Anesthesiology*. 2007;107(5):705-713.

34. Savoldelli GL, Naik VN, Joo HS, et al. Evaluation of patient simulator performance as an adjunct to the oral examination for senior anesthesia residents. *Anesthesiology*. 2006;104(3):475-481.

35. Weller JM, Robinson BJ, Jolly B, et al. Psychometric characteristics of simulation-based assessment in anaesthesia and accuracy of self-assessed scores. *Anaesthesia*. 2005;60(3):245-250.

Chapter 15

Teaching Psychomotor Skills and the Administration of Regional Anesthesia

Charles A. Reese, CRNA, PhD

Key Points

- Training in regional anesthesia requires mastery of both cognitive and technical skills.

- The number of regional anesthetics performed for surgery and pain control continues to increase.

- Student competence in the clinical environment does not correlate with performance on standard paper tests and assignment work.

- Educational taxonomies may be used to develop improved methods to train and assess anesthetists in regional anesthesia techniques. They provide guidance for the design, delivery, and evaluation of learning experiences as well as a simple, quick, and easy checklist for planning and executing learning episodes.

- It may be reasonable to expect students to achieve a high level of proficiency with common blocks (eg, spinal, epidural) for average patients during training; however, achieving the same proficiency with blocks in patients with significant surgical comorbidities or anatomical anomalies (eg, scoliosis, ankylosing spondylitis) may be beyond the scope of basic clinical training. It is unlikely that students will have the opportunity to become proficient in the intermediate and more advanced techniques during basic training.

- A regional anesthesia-specific adaptation of the psychomotor domain is offered for consideration.

Introduction

The role of graduate-level education in nurse anesthesia is to provide graduates a degree of proficiency and comfort in the profession. In this sense, proficiency can be defined as "advancement in knowledge." When learning to perform regional anesthesia techniques, the student must develop specific and often unique skills working with the tangible materials and tools of the techniques.

Training in regional anesthesia requires mastery of both cognitive and technical skills. The student must perform the work to develop the necessary psychomotor skills and to be able to recognize and handle the components and equipment used to perform the techniques appropriately and in the correct order. The student must also learn to understand the potential difficulties and dangers associated with the performance of the tasks.

This chapter presents a general discussion of learning taxonomy, offers a unique hierarchical taxonomy of psychomotor skills for the practice of regional anesthesia, and discusses these skills in the training of student nurse anesthetists (SNAs).

The number of regional anesthetics performed for surgery and pain control has increased substantially in the past several decades. Regional anesthesia techniques provide excellent analgesia or anesthesia and are cost-effective. There is an ever-increasing demand for regional anesthesia by both surgeons and patients. The use of these techniques allows practitioners to avoid the manipulation of the airway as well as the hemodynamic consequences often associated with general anesthesia. Although serious poor outcomes are rare, they are possible. When they do occur they may be catastrophic.

As with all clinical procedures, proper training is paramount to safe practice. Most complications appear to be related to poor fundamental technique and lack of essential precautions that should have been inculcated during the clinician's primary training. Although peripheral nerve blocks have been greatly refined by the adaptation of the peripheral nerve stimulator and ultrasound, they still require a great understanding of anatomy and substantial dexterity.

During more than 3 decades of mentoring students, I have observed that student competence in the clinical environment does not correlate with performance in standard paper tests and assignment work. There is little guidance for clinical instructors as to how to safely and effectively teach regional anesthesia techniques. There is a paucity of research on educational methods for such training; thus, the genesis of this attempt to offer thoughts regarding teaching the psychomotor components of regional anesthesia.

Regardless of the formal structure of the curriculum, SNA learners have already been exposed to the first 2 elements of learning taxonomy (ie, affective and cognitive domains) by the time they are introduced into the clinical learning environment (ie, psychomotor domain). During initial clinical practicums, most special equipment and processes, including regional anesthesia, are unfamiliar to students.

Nurse anesthesia educational programs have adapted to the graduate education framework. In most programs, time committed to didactic endeavors has reduced the time dedicated to clinical experience. Perhaps the movement toward doctoral-level preparation will further erode the critical clinical component. In addition, access to clinical resources, particularly regional anesthesia cases, is often highly competitive. This may be especially evident in programs that coexist with anesthesiology residency programs. Therefore, it is imperative to develop a clear, substantial educational justification of the clinical activities students are required to perform in order to justify the amount of clinical material and associated resources provided students as part of nurse anesthesia education. Despite pressure for enhanced revenues from increased enrollments, it is inappropriate to matriculate more students than clinical material can support. Employers and consumers have the right to expect graduates to have a full range of experiences and basic competencies while in training. This raises the concern of just what clinical experiences should be expected of students and what they should be expected to learn (ie, learning objectives) as a result of those experiences. A clear understanding of learning objectives makes it possible to design an activity that best focuses on the learning of a particular outcome or combination of outcomes.

Consumers and government regulatory organizations are becoming more focused on competency among healthcare providers. Although the definition of competency in regional anesthesia is unclear, educators and accreditation organizations need to establish ways to identify, measure, and evaluate cognitive and psychomotor skills that are less defined but necessary for the safe and efficient practice of regional anesthesia.

Anesthesiology Resident Training

Because of a lack of extensive, evidence-based data for SNAs, we must extrapolate available anesthesiology residency data. If anesthesiology residents are not performing regional techniques, it is reasonable to assume that SNAs are not performing them either.

In 1986, anesthesiology residencies were increased from 2 years' to 3 years' duration. In 1989, the length was again increased from 3 years to 4 years, including internship. Concurrently, numerous extended specialty-specific, postgraduate fellowship programs emerged, including several in regional anesthesia.

Several studies of anesthesia residencies in the United States revealed interesting, albeit disappointing, information regarding the use of regional anesthesia. In 1980, among responding training programs, regional anesthesia was used in only 21% of all cases (2.8%-55.7%).[1] This data also suggested that some residency programs failed to provide even a minimal exposure in the most basic regional techniques and that there was wide interprogram variability.

A follow-up survey in 1990 showed an increase in regional anesthesia cases (30%) attributed mostly to an increase in the use of epidurals in obstetrics and pain management. However, interprogram variability persisted (2.8%-58.5%).[2] A most extreme example cited was spinal anesthetics. Depending on the program, a resident in even well-respected programs could complete a 4-year education having performed as few as 3 or as many as 387 techniques. Interestingly, the Residency Review Committee (RRC) for anesthesiology of the Accreditation Council for Graduate Medical Education is considering increasing the number of blocks that residents must perform during their residency programs. Given current case statistics, doing so will no doubt further reduce the availability of clinical material for other students.

In 1996, the RRC began requiring a graduate to have performed a minimum of 40 spinal anesthetics and 50 epidural anesthetics (type not specified) to qualify for the board examination. The RRC also suggested, but did not require, performance of 40 peripheral nerve blocks for surgery and 25 for pain management to achieve competency; however, the types of these blocks were not specified. This lack of specificity may contribute to the disparity in training statistics. Performing 40 of the same technique may satisfy the RRC requirements, but it fails to encourage competency in the other techniques.

The most recent data (2000) showed that resident experiences in spinal and epidural anesthetics increased slightly and that interprogram variability was narrowing; however, resident experiences with peripheral nerve blocks continued to be problematic because 40% of residents still did not attain the suggested minimum experiences for peripheral nerve blocks.[3]

The RRC's requirement of only 40 unspecified peripheral nerve blocks has been questioned. Rosenblatt et al[4] reported that only 50% of residents were able to perform an interscalene block autonomously after experience with 7 to 9 cases. When the residents' experience exceeded 15 cases, 87.5% reported autonomous success. Of these, 96.3% of blocks were reported as adequate for surgery. In another survey, many graduating residents did not feel confident in performing interscalene blocks (51%), femoral blocks (62%), and sciatic (75%) blocks.[5] Interestingly, these were techniques that they had performed for fewer than 10 cases during residency. Practitioners are not likely to use a block with which they are not confident in future practice. Worse yet, they may attempt to provide blocks without the necessary skills and experience. Indeed, one survey found that 50% of practicing anesthesiologists perform fewer than 5 peripheral nerve blocks per month.[6] This data is not encouraging because it suggests that current requirements may be insufficient for graduates to approach competency. This is not only a concern for educators but also a patient safety issue.

Studies addressing clinical competence in regional anesthesia suggest it may take 60 to 90 supervised procedures to master lumbar epidural technique with an adequate success rate.[7,8] Kopacz and colleagues[9] suggest that 45 spinal and 60 epidural procedures must be done to achieve a 90% success rate. These figures are similar to mastery of frequently used technical procedures in other specialties (eg, flexible fiberoptic sigmoidoscopy by family practice residents); however, these are aggregate statistics and likely underestimate the needs of some students.

It seems it would take considerably more experiences to attain success in peripheral nerve techniques, particularly those of the lower extremity. Rosenblatt et al[4] showed that more than 10 interscalene blocks must be accomplished before the student attains even 50% autonomy. Konrad and coworkers[7] have shown that at least 70 axillary block experiences are required before a success rate of 85% can be achieved. Thus, when compared to available data, it is very unlikely that student nurse anesthetists are performing enough peripheral nerve blocks to develop a requisite proficiency.

Establishing general numerical minimums does not assess students' technical or clinical competence. Perhaps unique measurable criteria need to be established for various techniques. Students must also develop nontechnical proficiency, such as patient selection and perioperative management of regionally anesthetized patients, including the physiology and pharmacology associated with regional anesthesia. Experience must be gained with the management of intraoperative sedation as well as identification of and management of complications. The ability to analyze and apply outcomes data is also important to anesthesia practice.

Student Nurse Anesthetist Training

Success by graduate nurse anesthetists on the National Board on Certification and Recertification of Nurse Anesthetists' Certification Examination suggests only that the graduates' theoretical (ie, cognitive) knowledge is adequate for entry level to practice. As with all written examinations, it cannot evaluate regional anesthesia clinical skills.

In most regards, the history of regional anesthesia training of student nurse anesthetists parallels that of anesthesiology residents. That the RRC is concerned about the adequacy of resident training in regional anesthesia should be a harbinger of concern for the Council on Accreditation of Nurse Anesthesia Educational Programs (COA) as well. Although statistics are not available for nurse anesthesia educational programs (NAEPs), it should be fair to assume that considerable discrepancies exist among programs in regard to the quantity and quality of training in regional anesthesia. We can only speculate that access to clinical material and interprogram variability is similarly problematic. This may be particularly so in programs collocated with anesthesiology residencies where access to clinical cases is highly competitive.

Although formal course work focused on regional anesthesia has a long tradition in didactic curricula, inclusion of regional anesthesia in NAEP clinical curricula has been measured. In 1990, the COA outlined the requirement for administration and/or maintenance of 30 regional anesthesia cases. Actual administration was "strongly encouraged."[10] In 1994, the COA informed NAEPs that "Administration of regional anesthetics . . . will be required by the year 2000."[11] In 1999, the COA began requiring administration of a minimum of 25 regional anesthetics, including 5 spinal blocks, 5 epidural blocks, and 5 peripheral blocks (type not specified).[12] A footnote advised that the number of spinals and epidurals was to increase to 15 each by 2003. In 2004, the total number of regional anesthesia cases required remained the same, but the specific stipulations by technique were removed.[13]

Most recent data (2008) indicate that graduates (N = 2,057) report an average of 109 ($\pm$ 61) actual administrations of regional anesthesia techniques. These include 45 (± 28) spinal blocks, 43 (± 34) epidural blocks, and 21 (± 23) peripheral blocks during training. Management of regional anesthesia techniques fares better in that graduates report an average of 130 (± 68) cases. Although not specifically recorded, epidural experience appears to be gained primarily during obstetrical rotations in which graduates report an average of 44 (± 43) epidural analgesia for labor cases.[14] As with all statistics, caution must be used when drawing conclusions or implying correlations from data. This is especially true in that some of the studies mentioned previously state only "regional anesthesia" and did not classify by type of technique or patient population. Care must be taken when comparing statistics because anesthesiology residencies are 48 months duration, not including fellowships, and are almost exclusively clinically based, while NAEPs average 28 months duration and include a substantial amount of didactic education as well as clinical experiences.

The 2006 AANA Practice Profile Survey states that the following percentage of full-time CRNAs (N = 13,217) report performing the following anesthesia techniques as part of their current practice: intravenous regional, 71%; spinal, 67.5%; epidural, 55.1%; brachial plexus, 23.1%; pain management, 17.6%; and ophthalmologic block, 4.9%.[15]

Scope of Practice

In addition to spinal and epidural techniques, there are more than 40 different combined and peripheral nerve block techniques. Thus, it is understandable that a student is not likely to become proficient in specific procedures during the basic training cycle. This lack of proficiency is further aggravated by the technical variations introduced by different anesthesiologist and CRNA clinical instructors.

So, in which techniques should a graduate SNA be proficient? Hadzić[16] offered an attractive approach. He divided the current 40-plus techniques into 3 categories, ranked by degree of difficulty, time required to master, and potential for complications (Table 15.1). The student is introduced first to the essential (basic) techniques, then to the more complex (intermediate) techniques, and lastly, to the advanced techniques. Clearly, access to clinical material and the ability of the student are critical to this approach.

It may be reasonable to expect students to achieve a high level of proficiency with common blocks (eg, spinal, epidural) in average patients during basic training; however, achieving the save level of proficiency in patients with significant surgical comorbidities and anatomical anomalies may be beyond the scope of basic clinical training. It is unlikely that students will have the opportunity to become proficient in the intermediate and more advanced techniques during their basic training. Competition for clinical cases may severely limit SNAs' opportunities for all but the most basic spinal and epidural techniques.

Even if cases are available, students should not attempt more advanced techniques until they have demonstrated proficiency with the basic techniques. To have a student try and fail at a more complex technique may deter use of regional anesthesia in the future.

Table 15.1. Regional Anesthesia Techniques Ranked by Degree of Difficulty, Time Required to Master, and Potential for Complications

Basic Techniques	Intermediate Techniques	Advanced Techniques
Superficial cervical plexus block	Deep cervical plexus block	Continuous interscalene brachial plexus block[b]
Axillary brachial plexus block[a]	Interscalene block[b]	Continuous infraclavicular brachial plexus block[b]
Intravenous regional anesthesia (Bier block)[a]	Supraclavicular block[b]	Thoracic paravertebral block: single-injection, continuous
Wrist block	Infraclavicular block[b]	
Digital nerve block	Sciatic nerve block: posterior approach	Thoracolumbar paravertebral block
Intercostobrachial nerve block	Genitofemoral nerve block	Combined lumbar plexus/ sciatic blocks
Saphenous nerve block[b]	Popliteal block: all approaches	Lumbar plexus block
Ankle block[b]	Suprascapular nerve block	Continuous femoral nerve block[b]
Spinal anesthesia[a]	Intercostal nerve block	
Lumbar epidural anesthesia[a]	Thoracic epidural anesthesia: single injection or continuous	Sciatic nerve block: anterior approach
Combined spinal-epidural anesthesia[a]	Lumbar plexus block[b]	Anterior sciatic nerve block: para femoral technique
Femoral nerve block[b]	Combined lumbar plexus/sciatic block	Obturator block
	Continuous femoral nerve block[b]	Continuous sciatic block: posterior approach
	Sciatic nerve block: anterior approach and parafemoral technique	Continuous popliteal nerve block: intertendinous and lateral approaches
	Obturator nerve block	
	Continuous sciatic nerve block[b]	
	Continuous popliteal block: all approaches	
	Cervical epidural anesthesia	
	Cervical paravertebral block	
	Maxillary nerve block	
	Mandibular nerve block	
	Retrobulbar and peribulbar nerve block	

(Adapted from Hadzić A, Vloka JD.[16])

[a] Indicates the author's opinion of techniques in which student nurse anesthetists should demonstrate competency before graduation.

[b] Indicates the author's opinion of techniques to which student nurse anesthetists should receive significant exposure before graduation.

Taxonomy: Learning Domains

The problem of rote learning by students has been recognized for more than 4 centuries.[17] Educators universally agree that the educational process must not only provide knowledge about things, it also must provide the capability and competence of the student to actually *do* things. The development of educational theories provided an approach to creating educational objectives based on the behaviorist perspective of identifying what the student is able to do as a result of the educational activity.[18,19]

Bloom's taxonomy,[20] or variations thereof, continues to be the most widely used framework of its kind in education and training. This is largely because of its simplicity, clarity, and effectiveness for explaining and applying learning objectives and teaching methods, and for measuring learning outcomes. Bloom's work, known as *Bloom's Taxonomy of Learning Domains* or *Bloom's Taxonomy of Educational Objectives* was introduced in 1956 in an attempt to assist in the design and assessment of learning activities.[20] His original work introduced and discussed 2 unique domains, the *cognitive domain* and the *affective domain*. Numerous authors, adding more relevance to the field of academic education, have expanded his seminal work by introducing a third domain, the psychomotor domain.

Definition of Taxonomy

Taxonomy provides a coherent structure for planning, designing, assessing, and evaluating training and learning effectiveness. Models serve as a kind of checklist by which we can ensure that teaching is planned in such a manner as to deliver the necessary learner development. They provide a template by which the validity and coverage of training can be assessed.

More often than not, training is limited to nonparticipative, unfeeling attempts to transfer knowledge (eg, those endless boring lectures), recognizing that such teaching is focused on fact transfer and rote recall of information (the lowest level of learning). Bloom felt that learning should focus on mastery of subjects and the promotion of higher forms of thinking, rather than simply transferring facts. He attempted to establish a system of developing educational learning objectives that could be properly measured to ensure mastery of a subject. Thus, elements of the domains within his taxonomy are structured from the very simple (eg, memorizing facts) to the more complex (eg, analyzing or evaluating information). The complete Bloom's taxonomy comprises a structure of 3 overlapping domains. Depending on the publication referenced, the details of these domains may vary, particularly the third domain.

Given that Bloom was a behaviorist, it is not surprising that his taxonomy is a structured hierarchy that assumes a cumulative nature of learning—that student advancement to the next level of learning is dependent on previous success in the lower level. However, taken from a cognitivist's view, the outcome of an education experience should ultimately focus on the modification of the student's ability to do certain things. In this context, Bloom's Taxonomy of Educational

Objectives could more appropriately be titled Taxonomy of Cognitive Abilities of the Graduate.

Those new to clinical education need not be threatened by the academic jargon or the apparent complexity of taxonomies. Academics write for other academics. Thus, at first look, their terminology and processes may appear complex. They truly are relatively simple and logical models.

Taxonomy can be defined as a structure to help the teacher to plan for each developmental stage of a student's growth. Domain can be defined as a category. Although domains often appear in shorthand forms such as KSA (knowledge-skills-attitude), or do-think-feel, Bloom's original terminology included:

- *Cognitive domain:* Intellectual capability (ie, knowledge, or ability to think). This relates to the intellectual or rational dimension of a student's experience.
- *Affective domain:* Feelings, emotions, and behavior (ie, attitude, or ability to feel). This relates to the emotional or feeling dimension of a student's experience.
- *Psychomotor domain:* Learning of manual and physical skills (ie, the ability to move, act, or manipulate the body to perform a physical movement: the ability to do). This relates to the bodily movement associated with preconscious cognitive functioning.

From the perspective of the health sciences, the 3 domains may be seen as:

- *Cognitive domain (knowing):* Relates to the knowledge of and ability to work with information and ideas. Relates to the acquisition of knowledge, intellectual skills, and abilities (eg, diagnosis of disease, and developing strategies for treatment options).
- *Affective domain (feeling):* Relates to the ability to organize, articulate, and live and work by a coherent value system germane to the capabilities achieved through education. Relates to the ability to deal with feelings, emotions, mindsets, and values. This includes the nurturing of desirable attitudes for personal and professional development (eg, allaying the concerns and fears of patients and their families as they experience surgery, displaying mutual trust and respect in working with members of the healthcare team, and upholding high ethical standards in practice).
- *Psychomotor Domain (doing):* Relates to acquisition of skills that require varying levels of well-coordinated physical activity and precise manipulative procedures (eg, selection of anesthesia equipment, and performing a specific regional anesthetic technique).

Effective learning, particularly when training, is expected to result in measurable behaviors, and should touch on all levels of each of the domains when relevant to the student. In this instance, the student is expected to demonstrate knowledge and intellect (cognitive domain), attitude and beliefs (affective domain), and the ability to effect physical and bodily skills, to act (psychomotor domain).

The domains are traditionally represented in matrix form, as a checklist or template for designing learning programs or lesson plans. Within the domains, categories (or levels) are organized in order of complexity. An essential premise of Bloom's taxonomy is that each level must be mastered before progressing to the next and that a student must demonstrate mastery of the simpler form before progressing to more complex levels. Thus, the categories within a domain are considered increasingly complex levels of learning development (Table 15.2). In this regard, the psychomotor domain may perhaps be the most versatile to maneuver within when planning and providing clinical training.

Table 15.2. Domains of Bloom's Taxonomy

Level	Cognitive domain	Affective domain	Psychomotor domain[22]
	Knowledge	Attitude	Skills
1	Recall data	Receive (awareness)	Imitation (copy) (see then do)
2	Understand	Respond (react)	Manipulation (follow instructions) (hands-on practice)
3	Apply (use)	Value (understand and act)	Develop precision (practice, practice, practice)
4	Analyze (structure/ elements)	Organize personal value system	Articulation (combine, integrate related skills) Integration Learner knows *why.* Learner knows *when.*
5	Synthesize (create/build)	Internalize value system (adopt behavior)	Naturalization (automate, become expert) (Learner can perform the skill while concurrently performing other tasks.)
6	Evaluate (assess, judge in relational terms)		

Objectives and learning activities for an introductory course may be appropriately concentrated in the lower levels, and objectives and learning activities for a course in the later semesters normally will be concentrated in the upper levels. This does not imply, however, that teachers should only convey information to learners and expect only memorization from them in the lower levels. Analysis and evaluation of information is essential in the practice of anesthesia. It is imperative that higher-order thinking skills are encouraged and taught even from the beginning.

The Psychomotor Domain

Because the scope of this chapter is limited to a discussion of the acquisition of psychomotor skills, seeking more in-depth understanding of the cognitive and affective domains from other sources is encouraged.

Bloom's initial work focused on the cognitive domain.[20] His later work focused on the affective domain.[21] Most recently, numerous authors, most notably Dave,[22]

Table 15.3. Comparison of Psychomotor Domains

Dave	Simpson	Harrow
Imitation (copy)	Perception (awareness)	Reflex movement
Manipulation	Set	Basic fundamental movements
Develop precision	Guided response	Perceptual abilities
Articulation	Mechanism	Physical abilities
Naturalization	Complex overt response	Skilled movements
None	Adaptation	Nondiscursive
None	Origination	None

Simpson,[23] and Harrow[24] have expanded Bloom's model to include a third domain, the psychomotor domain or skills (Table 15.3). Dave's adaptation is the simplest and easiest to apply in a corporate environment. Because they offer different advantages and emotional perspectives, Harrow's and Simpson's models of the psychomotor domain are particularly useful for adults learning entirely new and challenging physical skills (eg, those requiring additional attention to awareness and sensory perception and mental and emotional preparation). This is especially true when students must step out of their comfort zones as they address sensory, perception (and by implication, attitudinal), and preparation issues (eg, a threatening task such as that first epidural anesthetic).

When taken collectively, taxonomy concepts are useful in the planning and design of the university-level educational process, including lesson plans and materials, and the evaluation of learning. As nurse anesthesia educators, we should find taxonomies useful as a framework for ensuring that we are using the most appropriate type of learning required of our mission; however, we must remember that learning design and evaluation for a given learning event need not cover all aspects of a given taxonomy. Emphasis should be placed on only those aspects that are appropriate to that event.

When planning a learning activity, the teacher must decide which domain the desired learning best fits. When it was first introduced, the psychomotor domain addressed primarily physical movements. This domain has evolved to include other professional and social skills such as interpersonal communications (eg, provider-to-provider, provider-to-patient, provider-to-family, telephone skills, and public speaking), and manual tasks (eg, airway management, regional anesthesia techniques, and computer keyboard skills) that are important in the field of anesthesiology.

Psychomotor skills may require speed, tools, or equipment; are not evaluated by written means; and must be performed and observed to determine the student's mastery of the skill. An example of a learning activity in the psychomotor domain is performing an epidural anesthetic technique. A nonexample is identifying the various indications for performing an epidural.

Clinical Teaching and Learning

Clinical instruction is one of the most enriching activities a teacher can do. Opportunities for directly demonstrating procedures, observing and guiding learner technical skills, and providing immediate substantive feedback to learners are without comparison in other teaching formats. Although complex, clinical teaching is a powerful personal and interpersonal experience, and fundamental principles define the roles that learners and teachers assume.

Learning in the clinical anesthesia environment requires dynamic interpersonal communication between 2 people: a learner and a teacher. Considerable commitment and effort is required of both learner and teacher.

The Role of the Teacher

The role of the teacher includes the knowledge, attitudes, and skills that he or she brings to the learning relationship. Too often, teachers in the health sciences feel they must be a font of knowledge and skills that they will impart on learners. We know from our own experiences (both as learners and as teachers) that this is an impossible feat. Certainly, knowledge of the material and ability to perform a task are necessary; however, they are not sufficient to guarantee successful learning. As clinical teachers, we assume multiple roles in our interactions with learners. Adapted from Ulian's[25] work, most behaviors and characteristics of (perceived) excellent clinical teachers fall into 4 roles.

1. In the role of anesthetist, the teacher is the expert and primary source of knowledge. There is substantial difference between the anesthetist's and learner's experience and knowledge of the profession. As a member of the profession and socializing agent, the anesthetist helps uphold professional standards and is ultimately responsible for evaluating the learner's competency.
2. In the role of teacher, the teacher is aware of the needs and aspirations of the learner. The teacher listens and encourages learners but is also aware that he or she will not be able to provide the learners with everything they need.
3. In the role of supervisor, the teacher demonstrates skills and procedures, provides the learner opportunities for guided practice, observes and evaluates learner performance, and provides feedback.
4. In the role of person, the teacher must nurture an atmosphere of trust in which learners are safe and comfortable offering their ideas, thoughts, and feelings. This does not necessarily require that the teacher like the learners, only that he or she accepts their needs. As a person, the teacher may provide substantial personal support outside the clinical environment and may serve as a role model.

The Role of the Learner

The role of the learner includes the experiences and knowledge that the learner brings to the learning relationship. It is important that teachers be aware of the different types of learners to individualize their approach. Learners bring numerous needs, problems, and anxieties to the learning relationship. Teachers must realize they cannot be all things to all learners. Anesthesia learners may be categorized as follows: [26]

- *Compliant learners* are the typical good students. They work hard, are task oriented, show little emotional turmoil, and are primarily oriented toward truly understanding the material. They are generally compliant with the teacher's directions.
- Anesthesia students are often *anxious dependent learners*. They are very dependent on the teacher for knowledge and support. They may be difficult to engage in discussion and prefer the lecture format with copious handouts and notes. They are overly concerned about grades and are anxious about being evaluated. Their feelings of incompetence and anxiety often inhibit learning.
- *Independent students* are generally older than their peers and may have completed previous graduate work. They often appear confident and unthreatened by the teacher, attempting to form peer relationships with them. They approach material calmly, objectively, and often in creative ways.
- Because of their pessimism and low self-esteem, *sniper students* have trouble forming productive relationships with authority figures. They are often elusive when confronted with issues and may become hostile when corrected or given negative feedback.
- *Silent Students* are most noticeable by what they do not do. They often feel vulnerable and helpless. Interestingly, they typically do not exhibit the anxiety of the anxious dependent learner.

Conditions for Effective Learning

Teachers must be mindful of the conditions or external influences that affect the learning process. The study of nurse anesthesia requires maturity and discipline. Student nurse anesthetists are adult learners. Their clinical education should follow the doctrines of adult education. Unfortunately, such is not always the case because nurse anesthesia educators are frequently not aware of these tenets. The following 4 principles of adult learners are particularly noteworthy.

1. Adult learners are normally *eager to apply what they learn* as soon as possible. Thus, many find the front-loaded curriculum format frustrating. Teachers should strive to make all material presented clinically relevant.
2. Adult learners *enjoy learning principles and concepts*. They benefit from solving problems rather than simply learning facts. Unfortunately, because of the sheer density and breadth of medical information, there are numerous facts that simply must be memorized. Nurse anesthesia learners have a substantial

clinical experience base before entering their course of study. It is wise to use this clinical experience to emphasize application, rather than simple retention, as a base of discussion and to enhance their clinical reasoning and problem-solving skills. Such discussions often take the "what if" format.

3. Adult learners *enjoy active participation in the learning process.* Incorporating them into the development of appropriate learning objectives is important. Although it can be argued that learners do not know what they need to know, the knowledgeable teacher can guide and negotiate with learners as to what learning should take place, given the resources available. This generally leads to enhanced motivation and participation.

4. Adult learners *need to know about their progress.* Formative feedback (ie, feed-back intended for the sake of improving performance) will help them evaluate their own progress. The clinical environment provides numerous opportuni-ties for the teacher to evaluate competence (eg, summative evaluation). Teachers' comments, particularly negative ones, play a critical role in helping a student learn and perform a skill appropriately, make better decisions, and change professional behavior. Timely, well-intentioned, and appropriate feed-back is critical to instilling learner confidence in the learner-teacher relation-ship and enhancing progress toward the learning objective.

Principles of Clinical Teaching

Learner training must be provided at an appropriate level. This should begin in nonthreatening situations such as laboratory settings. Once basic skills are acquired, the learner may be placed in more advanced clinical settings, such as supervised performance on actual patients.

Clinical teaching in anesthesia generally takes place in the immediate preopera-tive preparation area, the surgical or obstetric suite, or the immediate postoperative recovery area. These interactions provide the cornerstone for teaching and learning the knowledge, skills, and attitudes of anesthesia. Unique to this experience is the fact that the patient is present and an active participant. There are 4 fundamental objectives of these interactions:

1. *Teaching should be based on patient-related data and information.* During clinical interactions, teaching focuses on the patient's history, the physical examination, diagnostic study findings, and often, procedures. Procedures, in particular, provide a unique opportunity to teach psychomotor skills and provide the occasion to demonstrate appropriate anesthetist-patient interaction skills. During procedures, the patient's words and reactions must always be incorpo-rated into the activity and the learning process.

   Typically, patient data is reviewed with learners in the patient's absence before an actual encounter. The intent is to discuss relevant findings to prepare learners for the time spent with the patient. Aberrations in findings and the teacher's insights and previous experiences can be freely discussed. Time must be allowed for questions from the patient and family. Closure to the visit should focus on the patient's immediate concerns and on ensuring that no confusion or ambiguity persists on the part of the provider or patient. It must be clear to all that the patient is of central importance throughout the encounter.

2. *Clinical teaching must respect the patient's dignity and comfort.* This feature is paramount. When properly conducted, clinical learning encounters are positive experiences for both learners and patients. The patient, teacher, and learner must be comfortable during the interaction. Demonstrating concern and respect for the patient is reassuring and serves to minimize distress and anxiety regarding the medical situation and about the procedure.

   It is very important to introduce yourself and your role, and then introduce any learners. The teacher should clearly state his or her purpose and request permission of the patient (eg, "I'm here to discuss your anesthesia care, but first I'd like to ask you a few questions about your medical history." or "Is it okay if I take a look at your epidural catheter?"). This is particularly important when the encounter will involve physically touching the patient for whatever reason. In some cases, it is helpful for the teacher to revisit the patient alone in order to clarify any misunderstandings.

   Care must be taken to clearly, and in layperson's terms, describe any technical procedure(s) you plan to perform. All communications, including technical discussions, should make the patient feel included. As part of the problem-solving process, the patient should be encouraged to participate in the discussion with the teacher and learners. Conclusions and recommendations should be communicated clearly. Again, it may be helpful for the teacher to reiterate and summarize the key points of the discussion, particularly when an invasive procedure (eg, regional anesthesia) is planned. A parting optimistic statement to the patient (eg, "We'll take good care of you.") will serve to relieve anxieties.

3. *Psychomotor skills are best taught in the clinical environment.* Clinical interactions allow the teacher to demonstrate (and learners to directly observe and practice) the technical elements of procedures as well as psychosocial aspects such as concern and caring. This is not taught by lecture but rather by example. In the clinical environment, the learning of psychomotor clinical skills is often exemplified by the saying, "See one, do one, teach one." Interestingly, educational research actually supports this methodology.

   Clinical interactions are fundamental to teaching and learning psychomotor skills in anesthesia. The decreasing time and volume of clinical experiences in NAEPs should be of concern. In addition to diagnostic and therapeutic procedures, physical examination and problem solving skills are best learned in this environment. Once the fundamentals of technical skills are mastered, emphasis should be focused on problem solving. When the patient is made aware that your discussion of "what ifs" is a learning encounter, he or she will be reassured and may actively engage in the discussion.

As previously discussed, central to the basis of most taxonomies of learning psychomotor skills is a clearly organized series of steps, building on one another until the skill is properly learned and executed. The overall skill is broken into discrete components and presented and learned sequentially until the entire skill is mastered. It is generally best for the teacher to initially present (actually perform) the overall skill set in its entirety, discuss and demonstrate its components, and then have the learner attempt the skill with close supervision. The initial demonstration provides the boundaries of what is acceptable and a sense of desired outcome.

For this to be effective, the teachers must remember that they are the experts and can likely perform the demonstrated skill in their sleep. Indeed, this is a hallmark of mastery; however, when teaching new skills (eg, regional anesthesia techniques) the learners, more often than not, "don't know what they don't know." The effective teacher closely monitors learners' level of comprehension and ability and matches teaching to that level. For example, a student nurse anesthetist may need to first be made aware that an epidural is an appropriate technique for a given patient situation. This is followed by a review of the proper equipment and pharmaceuticals and then an overview and demonstration of the technical aspects. By now the learners begin to appreciate what they do not know and anticipate learning more. These steps parallel those of taxonomies previously described.

4. *Clinical teaching is a unique opportunity to provide learners with feedback.* Teacher evaluation of learners is perhaps most effective when done during clinical interactions. Both formative and summative feedback is of value. In educational parlance, feedback refers to the process of sharing information with learners about their current performance with the intent that they may improve it with future experiences. Such feedback may be negative or positive. Negative feedback is given in the hope of changing unacceptable behavior, while positive feedback is given to strengthen appropriate behavior.

Criticisms are intended to make the learner feel bad; they are not negative feedback. Compliments are meant to make the learner feel good; they are not positive feedback. Neither is helpful in improving performance. Feedback, rather, should be informative, consisting of observations and judgments intended to help the learner improve.

Rather than evaluative, feedback should be descriptive. For example, while observing a learner attempt an epidural placement, a teacher's comment, "Geez, you really are clumsy!" would be evaluative and of little support. A more descriptive and less pejorative feedback statement would be: "Perhaps next time you should try holding the Tuohy needle like this . . ." Such descriptive feedback is unambiguous and provides suggestions for improvement.

Feedback should be as specific to the task as possible. For example, a learner has properly performed a preoperative evaluation. A teacher's compliment such as "Nice job" does not reinforce the learner's specific favorable behavior. A more helpful statement would be: "I am particularly pleased with your interview technique and your ability to focus on that patient's concerns with spinal anesthesia. I think she now better understands what happened with her previous experience and what to expect today."

Timing of feedback is also critical. It should be provided as soon after the experience as practical. A summative evaluation after a week or month of clinical experiences does not provide learners the opportunity to adjust their behavior in response to the feedback. Indeed, they may not even remember the events being evaluated.

Learning Alternatives

The time-honored process of teaching regional anesthesia directly on preoperative patients is less than ideal. Fundamental to anesthesia training is an adequate and appropriate patient caseload and acuity mix. Learning regional anesthesia, particularly peripheral nerve blocks, is greatly enhanced when separate, properly equipped anesthetizing locations are used before entering the surgical theater. Adequate staffing to allow the learner time to prepare and perform the technique is critical as well. When a learner will be mentored by multiple teachers, ideally the teaching staff should have previously come to an agreement on the "one best way." This minimizes unnecessary stress on learners because they do not have to learn each instructor's technique in addition to the fundamentals of the skill being learned. Numerous methods are available to teach regional anesthesia and are described below.

Audiovisual

Interactive educational programs on CD-ROM and DVD have proliferated in recent years. Many have been adapted to personal handheld devices, allowing the anesthetist to review information immediately before performing a technique.[27] Realistic graphics enhance many of these offerings.

3D Animation

Some instructors are incorporating the use of virtual-reality models for teaching peripheral nerve and plexus blocks. One such model incorporates clear schematic drawings, relevant video clips, and live demonstrations. Others have used short 3-dimensional virtual-reality animations to demonstrate the steps in performing a peripheral nerve block. Animation allows the superficial anatomy to appear transparent while showing landmarks and geometry of needle placement.

Cadaver and Animal Models

Cadaver preparations allow an in-depth review of relevant anatomy and geometry associated with blocks. Blocks on anesthetized animals provide real-time experience with enhanced feel of tissue planes. The latter is particularly useful when learning perineural catheter techniques.

A group of anesthesia practitioners has described a unique embalming method that more closely mimics tissue conditions of living patients (ie, color, soft consistency, and movability) while allowing flap dissection to demonstrate anatomical planes. They also describe simulation of pulsatile landmarks by implanting latex tubing along peripheral arterial routes in the extremity of cadavers.[28,29]

Supplemental Equipment

Use of the peripheral nerve stimulation has long allowed visual confirmation of needle placement. More recently, ultrasound-guided needle placement has gained considerable popularity.[30]

Videotape

Videotaping a learner performing a technique provides the opportunity for timely critique by both teacher and learner and opportune feedback.[31] Unfortunately, this does not evaluate the learners' cognitive skills.

Simulation

When possible, demonstration and practice on life-size plastic simulation models allow the learner the opportunity to see and get a feel for the technique before actually attempting it on a live patient. Simulation often includes "green grocer models," using commonly available produce (eg, oranges, bananas, bread) that mimic human tissue layers.[32]

Virtual Model

One innovative company, Energid Technologies (Cambridge, Massachusetts), has described its efforts to develop a localized virtual patient model for regional anesthesia simulation training.[33] Their model reportedly captures the reflexive responses during nerve block stimulation by combining advanced technologies in tissue deformation, motor nerve stimulation model, and haptic feedback rendering. Currently, fiscal considerations limit the availability of such devices.

Personal Experience

Personal experience with the anesthesia and surgery process can be informative. One interesting report discusses residents' responses following the experience of receiving regional techniques themselves as compensated volunteers.[34] The researchers reported that they learned to be more sensitive to patient concerns and to communicate better with their patients about the anesthetic plan. They also came to appreciate the value of sedation and the discomfort associated with local anesthetic infiltration, paresthesias, and nerve stimulators.

Regional Block Rotation

The paucity of exposure to peripheral nerve block techniques has given rise to unique methods for teaching. Because consistency is helpful, it would be ideal if learners were allowed a defined rotation during which they were assigned only to patients who had a high likelihood of receiving regional techniques. This may provide the learner an opportunity to perform several blocks per day under direct mentorship. This repetition of techniques in a short period of time, particularly peripheral nerve blocks, is designed to increase the learner's awareness of the role of regional anesthesia applications. It also boosts the learners' confidence in selecting these techniques as part of their anesthesia care plan and enhances their technical skills. Clearly this is an ideal situation that currently exists in few NAEPs. From personal experience, this is not common in many anesthesiology residencies either.

Using such a system, Duke University Health System (Durham, North Carolina) anesthesia residents increased their experience from a median of 66 spinal blocks (59-74) to 107 spinal blocks (92-123) per student, and a median of 133 epidural blocks (127-142) to 233 epidural blocks (221-241) per student.[35] Their exposure to peripheral nerve blocks increased even more dramatically from a median of 80 (58-105) to 350 (237-408). One must keep in mind, however, that these numbers were gained over a 4-year residency period and numerous perioperative area assignments.

Although this approach was encouraging for 1 teaching program, a national survey in the same year showed less favorable results.[36] Of all responding anesthesiology residencies, 58% offered a specific peripheral nerve block rotation, and 61% of those rotations were 1 month long. Formal didactic instruction was provided during 69% of these rotations. Interestingly, multimedia, manikins, and cadaver dissection were used infrequently (13%-25%), suggesting these were strictly clinical experiences. Surprisingly, on average, residents performed only 2 supraclavicular and 10 axillary brachial plexus techniques. Perhaps this was 48% of the time these blocks were performed in the operating room and not a specific regional anesthetizing area (eg, block room).

A disadvantage to this approach is that, once the patient is blocked, learners turn over the intraoperative management to another anesthesia provider and thus may not appreciate that there is more to regional anesthesia than needle placement. They do not follow their patients into the operating room and do not manage their patients intraoperatively. Therefore, they do not learn to anticipate, recognize, and manage the failed or partial block or the complications and adverse effects associated with their blocks.

Although most adverse events during a regional anesthetic are benign (but not unimportant), such as the patient moving during surgery or otherwise harmless physiologic alterations, they do require a degree of experience and finesse to manage. In other situations, complications (eg, bradycardia, hypotension, seizure, or airway difficulties) may be devastating.[37] The interpersonal relationship between the provider and patient, which is very important to the overall success of blocks in the awake patient, may be diminished by this approach as well.

Regional Anesthesia Fellowship Training

Fellowship programs offer anesthesiology residents the greatest opportunity to become highly skilled in regional anesthesia. In 2005, approximately 12 active fellowship programs existed in the United States and Canada.[38] To minimize the differences in the quality and quantity of regional anesthesia experience in these fellowships, program administrators have recently published consensus-based guidelines for regional anesthesia fellowships in North America.[39]

In my opinion, the AANA should closely watch the development of regional anesthesiology fellowship training and, in those instances, where possible, partner with them to provide regional anesthesia experiences for SNAs. A fundamental tenet of being a professional is the ability to pass on (teach) information to others. Regional anesthesia fellows should be encouraged to mentor other learners as part of their educational process.

Continuing Education Opportunities

Continuing education meetings, such as regional anesthesia hands-on workshops, serve a valuable purpose by providing didactic information and limited demonstrations of evolving techniques. They also provide the opportunity for learners to communicate directly with experts in the field and with learner colleagues. Workshops also enhance learning at both the entry level and for learners desiring to update their skills.

As the technology becomes available, we can expect to find more computer-based high-fidelity learning opportunities. Virtual reality applications will enhance the anatomical and technical manipulations associated with various techniques. As the cost of electronic imaging technology decreases, which we experienced with noninvasive blood pressure monitoring technology and pulse oximetry technology, we will undoubtedly see an increase in its clinical use.

Hands-on Workshops

The AANA Regional Anesthesia Workshops (spinal/epidural and upper/lower extremity) have consistently been sold out since their inception in 1993 and 1995, respectively. Participants in these workshops are CRNAs who did not have the opportunity to learn regional anesthesia in their generic programs, those who had didactic but limited clinical experience, and those in both situations who have not practiced regional anesthesia consistently since graduation and who wish to update their knowledge and skills.

Future Directions

Advances in student training in regional anesthesia have been slow but steady. The increasing demand by both surgeons and patients and rapid development of newer pharmacologic preparations, continuous catheter techniques, and ultrasound-based techniques require that all anesthesia providers become more adept in regional anesthesia. It is best to develop a solid base of knowledge and competency during the formative training years and a desire to continue learning after graduation.

The Instructional Process

Regardless of the domain, there are fundamental steps in the overall instructional process. Table 15.4 is an example of a lesson plan adapting Dave's psychomotor domain to teach the physical skills associated with placing a spinal anesthetic.

Table 15.4. Lesson Plan Example

Learning objective: To demonstrate basic skills placing an epidural anesthetic			
Steps	**Instructor**	**Learner**	**Type of instruction**
1. Imitation	Provide content knowledge.	Learner listens to and observes instructor.	Explanation Demonstration
	Demonstrate the entire skill, including all steps, without interruption.	Learner imitates instructor.	Guided practice
	Provide learner opportunity to imitate the skill.		
2. Manipulation	Reduce skill into essential steps and actions; explain each step and action.	Learner repetitively attempts specific steps.	Guided practice Feedback
	Provide learner opportunity to imitate each step.	Learner attempts entire skill.	
	Provide learner opportunity to imitate entire skill.		
3. Precision	Provide learner time to practice independently.	Learner practices until able to perform with no mistakes.	Independent practice
		Learner increases speed of performing skill.	
4. Articulation	Provide learner time to practice independently.	Learner fine tunes ability to perform skill.	Independent practice
5. Naturalization	Evaluate learner's entire performance.	Learner performs skill with only minimal supervision.	Evaluation

(Adapted with permission from Romiszowski A.)[40]

Proposed Regional Anesthesia-Specific Psychomotor Domain Taxonomy

Technical procedures such as regional anesthesia should be analyzed to determine the skills necessary to perform them appropriately and safely. Included in this chapter is a regional anesthesia-specific adaptation of the psychomotor domain for the reader's consideration. It is modeled in part after a presentation by Ferris and Aziz.[41] The example used is for epidural anesthesia, but it can be easily adapted for any technique.

This hierarchy builds on the fundamental recognition of the equipment and materials required of the skills of regional anesthesia. It continues through several levels of the skills in handling and using the materials to achieve desirable outcomes, followed by the ability to create and execute a plan that will achieve a desirable result. It ends with a means to evaluate the results and plan for improvements in outcomes.

1. *Recognition of the equipment and materials used in the epidural anesthesia technique:* The fundamental practical skill competence in regional anesthesia is the ability to recognize the materials and tools of the trade. This is essential for both an effective technique and personal and patient safety. For example, the learner must know and understand the various components of an epidural technique such as the unique design of the tip, the association of the hub notch to the tip orifice, the significance of the markings on the shaft of the needle, the various markings on the epidural catheter, and the purpose and function of the Luer hub. This level of competence involves learning how to recognize the equipment and materials associated with the technique to be performed.

2. *Proper care and handling of equipment and materials used in regional anesthesia techniques:* Our tools must be handled appropriately. In addition to sterility, personal safety (eg, needle sticks) and patient safety (eg, correct drugs) must be paramount. Learners must be properly instructed and observed using acceptable techniques throughout procedures so that these risks can be identified and preempted. This level of competence involves learning how to care for and safely handle equipment and materials.

3. *Basic operation of equipment and materials used in regional anesthesia techniques:* Basic to the epidural technique is the learner's ability to properly hold and put to use the necessary equipment. This includes preparing solutions, draping materials, the epidural needle, various syringes, the epidural catheter and Luer adapter, and taping materials. These tasks, when accomplished in a sequence, should result in the completion of a universally acceptable technique. This is not the time for clinical instructors to offer their "pearls of wisdom" but rather to offer a most basic unitary technique. This level of competence involves learning how to operate equipment and materials while incorporating elements of safety associated with their use.

4. *Competent operation of equipment and materials used in regional anesthesia techniques:* At this level, the learner is becoming confident and competent with the equipment and materials of epidural anesthesia. This level builds upon the previous level in that the learner is now able to perform the complete sequence of tasks associated with the epidural technique in an acceptable manner. For example, the learner can appropriately set up the epidural kit, prepare the patient, perform the loss-of-resistance technique, place the epidural catheter, and prepare and tape the catheter. This level of competence involves the ability to consistently and safely perform the technique.

5. *Expert operation of equipment and materials:* This level is identified by the learner's ability to repetitively use equipment and materials in rapid, efficient,

effective, and safe manner. The learner is now able to perform the tasks with the correct outcome in the broader context of the techniques application rather than simply on the narrow context of placing the needle or catheter. An example of this level of competence is a learner's ability to appropriately perform epidural techniques in a safe and fluid manner.

6. *Planning the work process:* At this level, the learner is able to analyze system requirements to prioritize work to be done. The process of work planning requires an intimate understanding of surgical or obstetrical schedule requirements, patient information, and anesthesia provider availability and capability. This may require the ability to discern the order of operations to effectively and efficiently produce the desired outcomes. An example of this level of competence is a learner's ability to prioritize and then appropriately perform epidural techniques concurrently in a series of multiple patients in a safe and fluid manner.

7. *Evaluation of patient outcomes and implementation of improvements:* At this level, the learner is able to review the overall quality of the epidural technique and process. He or she is able to identify deficiencies and actions that could be taken to either correct or prevent the faults through appropriate planning. This level of competence represents the highest level of achievement and is highlighted by the ability to critically review previous actions.

Summary

Ideally, student nurse anesthetists would be independently proficient in basic regional anesthesia techniques upon graduation. This ideal is not currently being accomplished. More highly skilled clinical instructors and increased access to clinical patient opportunities are needed. True mastery would perhaps best be accomplished by the establishment of postgraduate fellowship programs modeled after, or perhaps integrated with, those of anesthesiologists. Until that time, nurse anesthesia educators must develop methodologies for teaching regional anesthesia that emphasize not only technical skills but also patient management and evaluation of learner competency.

Educational taxonomies may be used to develop improved methods to train and assess anesthetists in regional anesthesia techniques. They provide guidance for the design, delivery, and evaluation of learning experiences as well as a simple, quick, and easy checklist when planning and executing learning episodes. They encourage a variety of teaching and learning methods. In checklist format, they help minimize the risks of overlooking some vital aspects of the learning experience. The teacher should consider these as tools in their toolbox. As such, tools are most useful when the user controls them, not vice-versa.

Despite criticism, Bloom's (and others') taxonomy of educational objectives remains influential in the development of educational programs. The taxonomies in the first 2 domains (cognitive and affective) have been used extensively in primary and secondary education, where educators generally have an extensive theoretical background in education. Clinical educators in the health sciences have historically had little formal training in the concepts that underlie the educational process.

Although it is the latest addition to taxonomies, the psychomotor domain seems to have been developed for the primary and secondary educational levels, in which learners have a substantial need to develop the elements of psychomotor skills. It also has meaningful application for higher education, where competence in the physical motor skills associated with the performance of the professional practice (eg, regional anesthesia) are to be mastered.

How a taxonomy is applied will differ depending on the educational level of the learners. Professional education, such as nurse anesthesia, is generally consumed by young adults with a strong academic background and a high degree of previous sophisticated clinical experience. Thus, their educational experience focuses on the need to develop knowledge, attitudes, and skills pertaining to the specific practices of anesthesiology.

The intent of this discussion has been to guide clinical instructors in their quest to establish a rational process of educational activities leading to planned outcomes. I hope that clinical instructors will be better able to develop graduate anesthetists who have a coherent set of practical skills that lead to competence in regional anesthesia.

A reasoned design in developing clinical practicums should enable more efficient use of equipment and instructor resources as the kind and amount of experience provided will be targeted to gain the maximum effect. A further benefit of planning clinical practicums around logical objectives should be the ability to design formal assessment of the learners' practical skills and overall patient care.

Regional anesthesia has become a popular method of providing anesthesia and analgesia for numerous surgical and obstetrical procedures. The ultimate success in performing regional anesthesia techniques lies in clinicians' innate ability to use appropriate psychomotor skills. The current focus solely on recording the number of regional techniques performed during a generic program is inadequate because it does not address the following questions:

- How is competency defined?
- How many repetitions of a specific nerve block are enough to establish competency?
- How do learners become skilled in overall patient care? Performance of techniques is not enough. Care of the patient throughout the regional anesthetic experience requires the practitioner to learn pharmacology, complications, and regional anesthesia-related outcomes.

References

1. Bridenbaugh LD. Are anesthesia resident programs failing regional anesthesia? *Reg Anesth.* 1982;7:26-28.

2. Kopacz DJ, Bridenbaugh LD. Are anesthesia residency programs failing regional anesthesia? the past, present, and future. *Reg Anesth.* 1993:18(2):84-87.

3. Kopacz DJ, Neal JM. Regional anesthesia and pain medicine: residency training—the year 2000. *Reg Anesth Pain Med.* 2002:27(1):9-14.

4. Rosenblatt MA, Fishkind D. Proficiency in interscalene anesthesia-how many blocks are necessary? *J Clin Anesth.* 2003;15(4):285-288.

5. Smith MP, Sprung J, Zura A, Mascha E, Tetzlaff JE. A survey of exposure to regional anesthesia techniques in American anesthesia residency training programs. *Reg Anesth Pain Med.* 1999;24(1):11-16.

6. Hadzić A, Vloka JO, Kuroda MM, Koorn R, Birnbach DJ. The practice of peripheral nerve blocks in the United States: a national survey. *Reg Anesth Pain Med.* 1998;23(3):241-246.

7. Konrad C, Schuepfer G, Wietlisbach M, Gerber H. Learning manual skills in anesthesiology: is there a recommended number of cases for anesthetic procedures? *Anesth Analg.* 1998;86(3):635-639.

8. Schuepfer G, Konrad C, Schmeck J, Poortmans G, Staffelbach B, Jöhr M. Generating a learning curve for pediatric caudal epidural blocks: an empirical evaluation of technical skills in novice and experienced anesthetists. *Reg Anesth Pain Med.* 2000;25(4):385-388.

9. Kopacz DJ, Neal JM, Pollock JE. The regional anesthesia "learning curve": what is the minimum number of epidural and spinal blocks to reach consistency? *Reg Anesth.* 1996;21(3):182-190.

10. Standards and Guidelines for Accreditation of Nurse Anesthesia Educational Programs. Park Ridge, IL: Council on Accreditation of Nurse Anesthesia Education Programs; 1990.

11. Standards and Guidelines for Accreditation of Nurse Anesthesia Educational Programs. Park Ridge, IL: Council on Accreditation of Nurse Anesthesia Education Programs; 1994.

12. Standards and Guidelines for Accreditation of Nurse Anesthesia Educational Programs. Park Ridge, IL: Council on Accreditation of Nurse Anesthesia Education Programs; 1999.

13. Standards and Guidelines for Accreditation off Nurse Anesthesia Educational Programs. Park Ridge, IL: Council on Accreditation of Nurse Anesthesia Education Programs; 2004.

14. National Board on Certification and Recertification of Nurse Anesthetists. Annual Report: Summary of NCE / SEE Performance and Transcript Data. Park Ridge, IL: American Association of Nurse Anesthetists; 2008.

15. *Practice Profile Survey.* Park Ridge, IL: American Association of Nurse Anesthetists; 2006.

16. Hadzić A, Vloka JD. *Peripheral Nerve Block, Principles and Practice.* New York, NY: McGraw Hill Professional; 2004:1-5.

17. Butterfield S. *Educational Objectives and National Assessment.* Bristol, PA: Open University Press; 1995:46.

18. Airasian PW. The impact of the taxonomy on testing and evaluation. In: Anderson LW, Sosniak LA, eds. *Bloom's Taxonomy of Educational Objectives: A Forty-year Retrospective.* Chicago, IL: The National Society for the Study of Education; 1994:82-102.

19. Rohwer WDJ, Sloane K. Psychological perspectives. In: Anderson LW, Sosniak LA, eds. *Bloom's Taxonomy of Educational Objectives: A Forty-year Retrospective.* Chicago, IL: The National Society for the Study of Education; 1994:41-63.

20. Bloom BS. *Taxonomy of Educational Objectives, Handbook 1: The Cognitive Domain.* New York, NY: David McKay Co; 1956.

21. Krathwohl DR, Bloom BS, and Masia BB. *Taxonomy of Educational Objectives: Book 2: Affective Domain.* New York, NY: David McKay Co; 1999.

22. Dave RH. *Psychomotor Domain.* Berlin, Germany: International Conference of Educational Testing; 1967.

23. Simpson E. *The Classification of Educational Objectives, The Psychomotor Domain.* Vol. 3. Washington, DC: Gryphon House; 1972.

24. Harrow A. *A Taxonomy of the Psychomotor Domain: A Guide for Developing Behavioral Objectives.* New York, NY: David McKay Co; 1972.

25. Ullian JA. National Society for Performance and Instruction. Medical student and resident perceptions of clinical teaching. *Healthcare Chapter News.* 1986;1(4):4-5.

26. Mann RD, Arnold S, Binder J, et al. *The College Classroom: Conflict, Change and Learning.* New York, NY: John Wiley: 1970.

27. Delbac A, Eisenach JC, Albert N, et al. Peripheral Nerve Blocks on DVD: *Upper and Lower Limb Package.* Version 2.0. [DVD] New York, NY: Lippincott Williams & Wilkins; 2005.

28. Schwarz G, Feigl G, Kleinert R, et al. Pneumatic pulse simulation for teaching peripheral plexus blocks in cadavers. *Anesth Analg.* 2002;95(6):1822-1823.

29. Feigl G, Anderhuber F, Schwarz G, Dorn C, Fasel J, Likar R. Training methods for regional anaesthesia: evaluation and comparison. [in German]. *Anaesthetist.* 2007;56(5):437-443.

30. Grau T, Bartusseck E, Conradi R, et al. Ultrasound imaging improves learning curves in obstetric epidural anesthesia: a preliminary study. *Can J Anaesth.* 2003;50(10):1047-1050.

31. Birnbach DJ, Santos AC, Bourlier RA, et al. The effectiveness of video technology as an adjunct to teach and evaluate epidural anesthesia performance skills. *Anesthesiology.* 2002;96(1):5-9.

32. Leighton BL. A greengrocer's model of the epidural space. *Anesthesiology.* 1989;70(2):368-369.

33. Hu J, Lim YJ, Tardella N, Chang C, Warren L. Localized virtual patient model for regional anesthesia simulation training system. *Stud Health Technol Inform.* 2007;125:185-90.

34. McDonald SB, Thompson GE. "See one, do one, teach one, have one": a novel variation on regional anesthesia training. *Reg Anesth Pain Med.* 2002;27(5):456-459.

35. Martin G, Lineberger CK, MacLeod DB, et al. A new teaching model for resident training in regional anesthesia. *Anesth Analg.* 2002;95(5):1423-1427.

36. Chelly JE, Greger J, Gebhard R, Hagberg CA, Al-Samsam T, Khan A. Training of residents in peripheral nerve blocks during anesthesiology residency. *J Clin Anesth.* 2002;14(8):584-588.

37. Liguori GA, Kahn RL, Gordon J, et al. The use of metoprolol and glycopyrrolate to prevent hypotensive/bradycardic events during shoulder arthroscopy in the sitting position under interscalene block. *Anesth Analg.* 1998;87(6):1320-1325.

38. Neal JM, Kopacz DJ, Liguori GA, Beckman JD, Hargett MJ. The training and careers of regional anesthesia fellows—1983-2002. *Reg Anesth Pain Med.* 2005;30(3):226-232.

39. Hargett MT, Liguori GA, Beckman TO, Neal JM. Education Committee in the Department of Anesthesiology at Hospital for Special Surgery. Guidelines for regional anesthesia fellowship training. *Reg Anesth Pain Med.* 2005;30(3):218-225.

40. Romiszowski A. The development of physical skills: instruction in the psychomotor domain. In: Reigeluth CM. *Instructional Design Theories and Models: A New Paradigm of Instructional Theory.* Vol II. Mahwah, New Jersey: Lawrence Erlbaum Associates; 1999.

41. Ferris TLJ, Aziz SM. A psychomotor skills extension to Bloom's taxonomy of education objectives for engineering education. Presented at: Exploring Innovation in Education and Research; March 1-5, 2005; Tainan, Taiwan.

Chapter 16

Mentoring: The Teacher as a Mentor

Bernadette Henrichs, CRNA, PhD, CCRN

The flowers of all tomorrows are in the seeds of today.

–Native American Proverb

Key Points

- Mentoring involves taking an active role in helping the inexperienced student nurse anesthetist to develop into a Certified Registered Nurse Anesthetist both professionally and personally.

- A mentor serves as a protector, supporter, teacher, counselor, advisor, leader, role model, nurturer, listener, sponsor, promoter, and friend to the student.

- Ideally, the mentor and the student should *not* be assigned randomly, but the literature has supported the success of the matching of mentors and students by a third party. Personality types and styles of learning should be considered when a mentor is paired with a student.

- Mentoring differs from precepting in length and depth of involvement. Precepting normally lasts for a specified, short period of time, but mentoring often involves the building of a close bond that can last a lifetime.

- Mentoring involves work, dedication, time, discipline, honesty, creativity, and a positive attitude.

- Mentoring includes setting goals. These should include both specific and broad goals and include short-term and long-term tasks.

- Mentoring involves 4 phases: initiation, cultivation, separation, and redefinition.

- Mentoring can lead to job recruitment and retention.

- Mentoring can lead to the student's desire to serve as a mentor in the future.

- Mentoring can be a rewarding experience for both the mentor and the student.

271

Introduction

Change can be exciting . . . stressful . . . uncertain. Consider the intensive care nurse who has been accepted into a nurse anesthesia program. Emotions range from exuberance and eagerness to fear and self-doubt. The transition from intensive care nurse to nurse anesthetist is extremely stressful. The student will be taught new information about anesthesia in the academic setting and will learn psychomotor tasks he or she has never performed in the operating room. The student needs guidance and support to help face the challenges and overcome the struggles ahead. Who can help this person get through this exciting, yet difficult, experience? The student must be able to turn to someone for support, someone who understands what the student is experiencing and can provide assistance and counsel not only through the clinical and academic struggles but also through the emotional hurdles. *The student needs a mentor.*

Definition

The meaning of the word "mentor" dates back to ancient Greek mythology. In Homer's epic poem, *The Odyssey,* King Odysseus was forced to leave his home to participate in the siege of Troy. During his 10-year absence, the king asked his good friend Mentor to educate his son. Mentor "nurtured, protected, taught, and guided" the King's son throughout those 10 years.[1] Thus, the concept of "mentoring" was established.

Mentoring is defined as "a process by which persons of rank, achievement, and prestige instruct, counsel, guide, and facilitate the development of others identified as protégés."[1] Mentoring involves the association of an experienced member and an inexperienced member of a specific organization. In anesthesia, the experienced professional, the Certified Registered Nurse Anesthetist (CRNA) or the anesthesiologist, takes an active role in helping the protégé, the inexperienced student nurse anesthetist, to develop professionally and personally. "The mentor plots the course; the protégé makes the journey."[2]

Mentoring vs Precepting

Mentoring differs from precepting. Precepting is an orientation technique and occurs over a specified period of time. For instance, the student may be assigned a preceptor during the first few weeks of clinical training in the operating room or within a specialized rotation. The preceptor assists the student in learning the role of a nurse anesthetist but, because of its limited time frame, an emotional connection is not likely to develop between the preceptor and student.[3] The goal of precepting is to orient the person to the roles and responsibilities of a new job; whereas, the goal of mentoring is to build a relationship with the student through personal, one-on-one nurturing.

Mentoring is a longer and much more involved process.[1] It generally lasts from the time the student starts school until he or she starts working as a CRNA. If the mentor and the student build a close bond, a mutual, supportive, open, and trusting relationship can extend into a friendship that can last a lifetime.

Mentors should be clinical experts in their field. Clinical expertise, according to Fagerlund and Kusy,[4] "has been the primary strength of nurse anesthetists and the focus of nurse anesthesia educational programs." Nurse anesthetists who are willing to teach will "probably find they are able to have more influence on the changes taking place within healthcare than are the individuals who have not developed these skills."[4]

Mentors "exude qualities of wisdom, teaching, reliability, and caring within a strong personal and emotional relationship."[5] Mentoring often involves "fiery emotions" where the "sharing of intense personal feelings and values forms the foundation for deep interpersonal relationships."[5]

Are we really mentoring our student nurse anesthetists? According to Hand and Thompson,[6] nurse anesthesia faculty members are confused about what is involved in mentoring. They state that "the use of the terms 'mentor' and 'mentoring' have now been rendered banal and essentially meaningless."[6] Some instructors feel that there should be a definite division between student and instructor. They believe instructors should not build close relationships with students, and that the student should be somewhat afraid of the instructor. Is this fear model an effective method of teaching? Many disagree. A more effective teaching and learning environment often exists "when the person develops a relationship"[7] with the student. A mentor should be looked upon by the student as an advisor and counselor.[7]

Hand and Thompson[6] state that many faculty members feel that "teaching, providing clinical instruction, supervising student experiences, serving as role models, serving as preceptors, and acting as sponsors are synonymous with mentoring"; however, mentoring is described as a deeper relationship. Anesthesia faculty members questioned whether it was possible for anesthesia faculty to expend the time and energy to mentor the students in addition to serving as preceptors. Although mentoring has advantages over precepting, the authors felt that being a good academic instructor or clinical preceptor was more valuable and important for the development of student nurse anesthetists. When serving as mentors, they felt that it may be more beneficial "to focus our energies on the continued growth and development of our clinical faculty."[6] Still, they stated that "mentoring is a tremendously beneficial process and should be encouraged whenever there is a mutual agreement between the involved parties."[6]

Roles and Responsibilities of a Mentor

What are the responsibilities of a mentor? A true mentor plays several roles in the student's life. The mentor should provide information, instruction, advice, guidance, and encouragement to help the student develop the intellectual and technical skills needed to engage in safe clinical practice. A mentor should not only teach the student to perform clinical tasks, such as inserting an endotracheal tube, but also provide social support. The mentor should help the student develop professionally. A mentor will "model, inform, confirm or disconfirm, prescribe, or question."[3] A mentor will also "protect, promote and support . . . act as a counselor, providing advice, guidance, oral support and nurturing."[3]

Mentoring "demands hard work, discipline, rigour, creativity, honesty and integrity."[8] It requires effort by both individuals. The personalities and learning styles of those involved must be taken into account.[8] The mentor should strive constantly to determine the most effective manner by which the student learns and then adjust the teaching style to fulfill the established goals.

An effective mentor has strong leadership qualities. A leader is "visible, committed, and knowledgeable,"[2] and is "calm, confident, and predictable."[2] The leaders of the anesthesia community should step forward to mentor the inexperienced. The mentor may not only serve as a teacher but also as a "coach, positive role model, developer of talent, opener of doors, protector, sponsor, and successful leader."[2] Because of such leadership characteristics, the nurse anesthetist leader has the capability to make the mentoring process a success.

A strong leader will guide others into their professional roles and "*intentionally* influence another individual or a group in order to accomplish a goal."[5] A charismatic leader will motivate, excite, and move individuals to reach their goals; thus, a person with strong leadership abilities should not waste such talent and should mentor others. The mentor should "give the protégé the authority to set goals, dream, grow, and surpass the achievements of the teacher."[5]

If the relationship between the instructor and the student is successful, the rewards will be priceless. The functions of a good mentor are described by Busen and Engebretson (Table 16.1).[1] If these functions are achieved throughout students' educational experience, they will be molded successfully into their professional roles in a manner that will affect their future careers positively. Mentoring can have such a lasting influence that the student may decide to serve as a mentor later on. The process can then continue with each new group of students, making the path to becoming a CRNA less stressful and more successful.

Phases of the Mentoring Process

The mentoring relationship can be divided into 4 phases: initiation, cultivation, separation, and redefinition. In the initiation phase, a relationship between the mentor and the student is established.[3] This relationship will determine the success of the mentoring process. If the personalities of the mentor and the student clash, the process may not be successful; however, in this situation, the student is more likely to have a successful experience if there is more than 1 instructor involved in the training. If the student doesn't get along well with the mentor with whom he or she has been matched, changing the mentor assignment should be considered, if possible. If the personalities of the mentor and the student "click" and they are paired together, the process has a much higher chance of being successful and lasting indefinitely.

The second phase of mentoring, the cultivation phase, involves building a relationship and establishing and accomplishing goals. The student and mentor must sit down together and write specific goals for the student's time in nurse

> **Table 16.1. Functions of a Good Mentor**
>
> Demonstrate role expertise.
>
> Promote role socialization.
>
> Provide a vision by being a role model.
>
> Provide reflection that enables the student to determine how and why decisions are made.
>
> Help the student understand how such decisions influence positive outcomes.
>
> Share values and customs.
>
> Provide support through listening, befriending, and expressing positive expectations.
>
> Help to make the experience special.
>
> Challenge the student by constructing hypotheses and engaging in spirited discussions.
>
> Set high standards and demand performance.
>
> Empower the student to reach autonomy through competency, self-confidence, and responsibility.
>
> Open doors and facilitate important contacts.

Adapted with permission from Busen and Engebretson.[1]

anesthesia school. The functions involved in the development of this relationship and the student's career should be mutually beneficial.

The third phase of mentoring, the separation phase, involves the mentor gradually allowing the student to become more independent in the tasks being learned. The guidance and teaching that were previously necessary are no longer needed. The relationship between the student and mentor will change dramatically because of the growth and development of the student in knowledge of nurse anesthesia.

In the final phase of mentoring, the redefinition phase, the student becomes a graduate of the nurse anesthesia program. The mentoring process will either end, or it will evolve into a long-term relationship. With some individuals, the friendship continues and grows deeper and closer throughout a lifetime.

Advantages of Mentoring

Mentoring can be beneficial for a number of reasons (Table 16.2). When an instructor works side-by-side with a student and teaches new tasks, the learning process is enhanced. The mentor can give feedback and positive reinforcement, and the student may become more self-confident and optimistic about his or her performance.[3] Mentoring should "bridge the gap between school and the early years" of practice; however, when the relationship with the student endures, these strong ties can help later when the protégé needs advice and counseling.[9]

Students who have mentors have a distinct advantage over those who do not have mentors.[6] Advantages of a successful mentoring program for the student

Table 16.2. Advantages of Mentoring

Decreases stress of the student.

Offers advice, support and empathy to the student.

Enhances the learning process.

Provides guidance and helps the student learn new tasks.

Increases professionalism and prevents "eating our young."

Promotes self-confidence and optimism of the student.

Promotes role socialization and professional networking.

Builds friendships between the mentor and the student.

Enhances recruitment of students after graduation.

Provides personal satisfaction to mentor.

Provides job enrichment and professional growth of mentor.

Increases the chance of being successful in one's profession.

include decreased stress, advice, empathy, and an outlet to express feelings. Positive relationships between the mentor and the student may also increase professionalism and prevent the concept of "eating our young,"[9] the common practice of experienced practitioners making things difficult for student nurse anesthetists. Why this practice occurs is uncertain, but it may prevent successful mentoring.

The mentor also benefits from the relationship with the student. Advantages include the personal satisfaction of having played a role in another person's growth, job enrichment and professional growth for the mentor, and new friendships.

Mentoring has advantages for the institutions that employ the students after graduation. Research shows that nurses who were mentored have more job satisfaction and tend to stay in their jobs longer than nurses who were not mentored.[10] Mentoring helps a student to become acclimated to the work environment of the institution and become familiar with the socialization process of its employees. Mentoring can mold the student into a successful leader in the field. Once the student completes training and looks for employment, improved job satisfaction and the intent to stay at the training institution can be satisfying outcomes of the mentoring experience.[9]

Disadvantages of Mentoring

Although mentoring can guide the student to career success, disadvantages to mentoring do exist (Table 16.3). Fortunately, the disadvantages are few and the advantages far outweigh them. Mentoring is not an easy task. The mentor must be willing to invest time, patience, and knowledge. One of the greatest disadvantages is the time commitment required. The mentor must be available to help the student. "Preparation . . . is essential."[11] Investing extra time means going above and beyond the call of duty. Financial compensation for the extra time invested usually is not given. Not only is the mentor serving in this role during normal educational days, but the role may be extended to nights, weekends, or holidays

> **Table 16.3. Disadvantages of Mentoring**
>
> Difficulty of mentoring
> Time commitment involved
> Possibility of mentor—student mismatch
> Lack of financial compensation
> Knowledge, skill, and responsibility involved
> Lack of availability of mentor
> Schedule conflicts

as well. In fact, mentoring is a 24-hour commitment. The student may need the assistance of the mentor at an unpredictable time. A truly dedicated mentor will be reasonably available and ready to give the student the support needed, no matter the time of day. This is especially true for emotional support. The mentor may also give extra time to help the student with additional tutoring. An effective mentor must be "ready to give generously and unselfishly of the extensive time, experience, knowledge, and personal ability that is desperately needed for seeking out and nurturing our successors."[12]

The success of a student may be hindered without mentoring. Published reports in the literature state that individuals in the business world who do not have mentors have lower positions within organizations, and those with mentors rise to higher status within similar organizations.[13]

Effective Mentoring

According to Faut-Callahan,[5] mentors should not be assigned if they are to be effective. Assigning 2 people to work together and expecting that relationship to build into an intense commitment is unrealistic. Ideally, the mentor and the student should be able to choose each other; however, this may be a difficult task. The literature has supported the success of matching mentors and students by a third party.[14] Personality types and styles of learning should be considered when a mentor is paired with a student. This consideration can only improve the outcome of the experience and increase its chances of success.

Because the mentor is a teacher and role model for the student, mentoring is similar to parenting. It is an investment in "the future of the nursing profession, just as parenting is an investment in the future of the human race."[15] It involves mutual respect between the mentor and the student. There must be an unstated trust between the individuals for the process to be successful. Communication between the mentor and student must be open and uninhibited. Successful mentoring requires the mentor to listen more than talk when working with the student. It is important for the mentor to consider the student's moral beliefs and values and to share his or her own values and beliefs.[16]

The student should feel comfortable asking questions, and should never feel that a question is stupid. The mentor should be knowledgeable in answering the questions; thus, the mentor should be a well-respected expert in the field, "the best of the best" as an instructor in anesthesia. When the mentor does not know an answer, he or she should admit it. This gives the mentor and student the opportunity to work together to find the answer to the question. Thus, mentoring can become a learning experience for both the student and the instructor.

Ineffective Mentoring

Ineffective mentoring can occur when the student and the mentor do not have a "positive synergy" or "chemistry."[1] A personality match must exist or the relationship will not be successful. If a positive relationship does not develop, the learning process will be inhibited.

When a mentoring relationship becomes negative, frustration and dissatisfaction may lead to lower performance by the student, both academically and clinically. A potential solution to the mismatch is to pair the student with a different mentor if possible; however, valuable time has been lost in the development of the mentor–student relationship.

Another reason for ineffective mentoring may be that the student does not respect the instructor and does not view the mentor as a good practitioner. The student may doubt the mentor's leadership abilities as a CRNA. If the student views the mentor as a negative role model, the process will not be a success. A mentor who is not admired will not be able to guide and instruct the student. The student may doubt every word that the mentor says.

If a mentor carries out the role in a domineering, controlling fashion, ineffective mentoring may occur.[17] If the mentor acts superior to the student and does not teach in a respectful manner, the student may feel inferior, and learning will be prevented. Being too controlling and not allowing independence may lead to resentment and lack of self-confidence in the student. Being too critical or out of touch with the student's feelings will lead to a negative experience; however, being too passive with teaching and guidance may also pose problems. If the direction and support are not given, the student may not be able to learn the tasks necessary to become a successful CRNA. The mentor must achieve a balance of providing guidance and allowing independence. This balance is crucial to the development of the student into a confident, competent nurse anesthetist with outstanding clinical skills.

Promoting Success Through Mentoring

Nurse anesthetists must mentor students entering the field of anesthesia to promote students' success. Mentors can help the student learn the role professionally, master the clinical tasks, be knowledgeable, and make wise decisions in the delivery of anesthesia. They can respond to the student's call for help, share strategies for handling difficulties, help the student to stay positive, and encourage success. "Anesthetists who fail to mentor their junior colleagues jeopardize the future of nurse anesthesia and do a disservice to their patients, their communities, and their profession."[2]

Being a mentor can result in a tremendous feeling of emotional satisfaction and professionalism. Not only does the student grow and develop throughout the educational experience, but so does the mentor. Learning never stops, despite the vast amount of information and experience gained with time. The mentor can help the student make the path to a nurse anesthesia career "a bed of roses, not obstacles."[18] The experience can be motivating and invigorating for both individuals. The relationship between the mentor and student "represents the bond between the past and the future."[8] It can open the door for future possibilities in one's professional career. Not only does the process assist in role modeling; it may also assist the student nurse anesthetist to reach professional excellence in nurse anesthesia.[1]

Examples of Mentoring Programs

Because of the potential benefits of mentoring, schools of nurse anesthesia have set up a variety of programs. The Nurse Anesthesia Program at the Goldfarb School of Nursing at Barnes-Jewish College, St Louis, Missouri, tries to pair the new students with the same CRNA for several days in a row when they start clinical training. By doing this, the new student gains some familiarity with the clinical instructor and will be less stressed by the newness of the experience. New students are also paired with students from the previous class. The more advanced students are instructed to call the newer students at the start of the program to offer support and guidance. They help to answer any questions the new students may have, including those related to housing and transportation. Throughout the program, the senior students serve as resources for questions the newer students may have, including queries about their academic courses, their clinical rotations, the rules and regulations of the program, and social activities.

A mentorship program has been used successfully at the Hospital of St Raphael School of Nurse Anesthesia, New Haven, Connecticut, since 2004 (J. Thompson, written communication, January 29, 2008). Each student is paired with a CRNA by the director of the program. The intent is to match the student to a CRNA with similar interests or personalities. They may have common situations such as being enrolled in a nurse anesthesia program while raising a family, having similar intensive care unit experience, or having relocated to attend the nurse anesthesia program. Having similar personal issues, they may be able to support each other more effectively because of a better understanding of each other's situations.

If the match between the student and the CRNA is not a good fit, the student is then encouraged early in the program to choose another CRNA from the list of volunteer mentors. The student and the CRNA must get along well with each other so that they feel comfortable sharing their thoughts and concerns.

During the first few weeks of clinical experience in the operating room, when the education and training can become very stressful, the student is encouraged to ask the mentor for guidance. Informal meetings, phone calls, and emails between the mentor and the student are encouraged. Students are also encouraged to be honest when they talk to their mentors about their clinical experience, so it is vital that discussions remain confidential to build trust. The mentor is encouraged to provide guidance, understanding, and support to the student throughout the nurse anesthesia program. Many lasting friendships have been formed from this early association, and former students often volunteer to serve as mentors once they become CRNAs.

In 2005, the Nurse Anesthesia Program at the University of Pittsburgh School of Nursing won the Crystal Apple Award from the American Association of Nurse Anesthetists Education Committee for its mentoring program. The program was developed to provide a confidential, structured plan for student nurse anesthetists to reach out to CRNAs who serve as role models. As part of the program, interested CRNAs attended a workshop on mentoring. The CRNAs attended lectures on the definition of mentoring and learned about key mentoring concerns, student learning styles, normative modeling, and the elements of effective clinical evaluation. The CRNAs were taught to help the students develop their clinical skills, offer knowledge and information, provide feedback and advice, offer networking opportunities, and provide emotional support.

A mentoring coordinator initially met with the first-year student nurse anesthetists to describe the program. Students were subsequently paired with CRNAs based on key traits and interests that were identified using questionnaires of mentors and students. Mentors signed contracts stipulating that they meet with their students at least once a month throughout the 28-month program. The mentoring coordinator conducted ongoing monitoring of the mentors and the students via phone calls and emails. Responses from the students at the end of the program were highly favorable. Positive feedback from the mentors also demonstrated the success of the mentoring program.

The program has been ongoing since 2005 and is sustained by support from the Department of Anesthesia at the University of Pittsburgh. Both CRNA and student nurse anesthetist satisfaction scores have been consistently high. Interestingly, survey data of the students suggest that, although they value their assigned mentors, they prefer to identify and interact with mentors of their own choosing. This is consistent with the mentoring literature and likely reflects the reality of the difficulty of finding good matches given individual and generational diversity (J.M. O'Donnell, written communication, March 28, 2008).

Summary

Mentoring can be a rewarding experience, not only for the student nurse anesthetist, but also for the CRNA serving as a mentor. Friendships between them can develop into lifetime relationships. Mentoring can also result in a successful, positive outcome for the profession of nurse anesthesia as a whole. Students who have favorable experiences with mentors are more likely to serve as mentors for future student nurse anesthetists. The support given to a future student will help keep the mentoring tradition alive and ensure continuity. Thus, the future of our profession depends on the success of having CRNAs serve as mentors for our student nurse anesthetists.

References

1. Busen NH, Engebretson J. Mentoring in advanced practice nursing: the use of metaphor in concept exploration. *Internet J Adv Pract Nurs.* 1999;2(2):1-10. http://www.ispub.com/ostia/index.php?xmlFilePath=journals/ijanp/vol2n2/mentoring.xml. Accessed December 20, 2007.

2. Pollock GS. We are all leaders. *AANA J.* 1996;64(3):225-227.

3. Walker WO, Kelly PC, Hume R. Mentoring for the new millennium. http://med-ed-online.org/f0000038.htm. Accessed December 20, 2007.

4. Fagerlund K, Kusy M. Teaching, learning, and leading. *AANA J.* 1999;67(1):45-47.

5. Faut-Callahan M. Mentoring: a call to professional responsibility. *AANA J.* 2001;69(4):248-251.

6. Hand R, Thompson E. Are we really mentoring our students? *AANA J.* 2003;71(2):105-108.

7. Kerfoot KM. Leadership, civility, and the "No Jerks" rule. *Nurs Econ.* 2007;25(4):233-237.

8. Centeno AM. How to enjoy your mentee's success and learn from it. *Med Educ.* 2002;36(12):1214-1215.

9. Stachura LM, Hoff J. Toward achievement of mentoring for nurses. *Nurs Adm Q.* 1990;15(1):56-62.

10. Prevesto P. The effect of "mentored" relationships on satisfaction and intent to stay of company-grade US Army Reserve nurses. *Milit Med.* 2001;166(1):21-26.

11. Burns C, Beauchesne M, Ryan-Krause P, Sawin K. Mastering the preceptor role: challenges of clinical teaching. *J Pediatr Health Care.* 2006;20(3):172-183.

12. Frohlich ED. A renewed call to mentor. *Hypertension.* 2000;36:309-311.

13. Zey M: *The Mentor Connection.* Homewood, IL: Irwin Publishing; 1984:77-88.

14. Connor MP, Bynoe AG, Redfern N, Pokora J, Clark J. Developing senior doctors as mentors: a form of continuing professional development: report of an initiative to develop a network of senior doctors as mentors: 1994-1999. *Med Educ.* 2000;34(9):747-753.

15. Brown BJ. Comments from the editor. *Nurs Admin Q.* 1990;14(1):vii-viii.

16. Hagenow N, McCrea MA. A mentoring relationship: two viewpoints. *Nurs Manage.* 1994;25(12):42-43.

17. Ehrich L, Tennent L, Hansford B. A review of mentoring in education: some lessons for nursing. *Contemp Nurse.* 2002;12(3):253-264.

18. Kelly JW. Messages from the anesthesia pioneers. *AANA Foundation Newsletter.* 2003;2:2.

Chapter 17

Student Evaluation in the Clinical Area

Lynne M. Van Wormer, CRNA, MSN

Key Points

- Evaluating student clinical practice complies with the requirements of the Council on Accreditation of Nurse Anesthesia Educational Programs, protects the public, meets institutional standards, and satisfies student expectations.

- There are different types of evaluations, each serving a specific purpose, such as daily assessment or self-evaluation.

- An evaluation should be clear, specific, and appropriate to the level of proficiency expected.

- Reflective learning is a key feature of assisting the clinical student to progress.

- The instrument used to evaluate clinical performance should be competency based.

- Good documentation of a student's poor performance is critical to assist both the student and the program in formulating a specific plan of remediation. If remediation fails, good documentation serves as a tool in substantiating dismissal from the program.

Introduction

Evaluation of clinical performance is an integral part of a nurse anesthesia educational program. This chapter lists objectives for developing clinical evaluations and for evaluating clinical performance. Types and elements of clinical evaluations and the components of an instrument for evaluating clinical performance are discussed. Barriers to evaluation in the clinical setting are enumerated. A case study at the end of the chapter demonstrates the evaluation process.

Objectives of Evaluation

The evaluation of student clinical practice serves several objectives. These include protecting the public, satisfying student expectations, meeting institution requirements, and complying with the standards of the Council on Accreditation of Nurse Anesthesia Educational Programs (COA). Additionally, student clinical evaluation can serve as a guide for employer evaluation of the newly hired Certified Registered Nurse Anesthetist (CRNA), as well as alumni evaluation of the program and the education they received. Finally, the American Association of Nurse Anesthetists (AANA), the professional organization of CRNAs, has the objective "to develop and promote educational standards in the field of nurse anesthesia."[1] This implies clinical competence as well as didactic knowledge.

Public accountability has become a major factor in both clinical practice and clinical education. Today's healthcare consumer has access to all kinds of information regarding quality of care. One such resource is the Institute of Medicine (IOM). The IOM released a report on April 8, 2003, titled *Health Professions Education: A Bridge to Quality*. This document calls for nursing practice education "that prepares individuals with interdisciplinary, information systems, quality improvement and patient safety skills and expertise."[2] Other areas of emphasis in the IOM's report that can be linked to clinical evaluation of performance include practicing evidence-based medicine and delivering patient-centered care. In addition to publications by the IOM, the public has access to documents from state health departments and articles in journals, magazines and newspapers, as well as the Internet. The easy availability of information has led to a more educated consumer who demands accountability from all aspects of the healthcare system, including the educational components.

Students' expectations regarding evaluation of clinical practice usually center on specific tasks and outcomes. This is especially true in the early part of their clinical experience. Frequently, students' expectations of experiences they should have and tasks they wish to master are unrealistic based on their didactic knowledge and previous skill achievements. At that stage, they perform best when demonstrating technical skills comprising specific objectives. They want to know exactly what is expected of them and how each task will be graded. As they progress through the program, students' expectations evolve to include a desire to be assessed on the correlation of clinical performance with didactic knowledge. Interwoven throughout students' expectations is a desire to know how well their performance has prepared them for the certification examination and the real world.

Institutions set forth performance benchmarks for programs and students. A minimum acceptable grade is part of an institution's policies. This information is typically published in general information documents, the student handbook, and the institution's website. Programs are usually required to post students' grades to the registrar's office at regular intervals, usually by semesters.

The COA ensures the academic quality of educational offerings of nurse anesthesia programs. This is done by the promulgation of standards that educational programs must meet to be accredited. The following COA standards address the need for clinical evaluation of students.

Standard III (Program of Study) lists several criteria that require evaluation of clinical performance. They are C5, C7, C16, C17, C18, C19, and C20.[3(pp4-7)] The aspects of evaluation delineated in this section encompass professional socialization, certification, competency, safety, call experience, perianesthesia continuum, critical thinking, communication skills, and professional responsibility.

Standard IV (Program Effectiveness) looks at criteria that examine the quality of student enhancement of the educational process. Specifically, criteria D4a and D4b require formative evaluation, summative evaluation, and student self-evaluation[3(p9)] (discussed in the next section).

Standard V (Accountability) mandates that programs be responsible to their communities of interest. Criterion E7 requires cumulative records of educational activities, whereas E13 addresses clinical supervision ratios as they relate to patient safety and student knowledge and ability.[3(pp10-11)] The COA considers a program's community of interest to be the same stakeholders that were identified as being concerned with student clinical evaluation. Additionally, documentation of educational activities is a program indicator of compliance with COA standards.

Nurse anesthesia educational programs survey employers of recent graduates to determine if the graduates have received appropriate didactic and clinical knowledge and experience to prepare them to be safe, competent practitioners. Although this is not clinical evaluation of individual students per se, it is an indicator of the clinical experience.

Alumni of nurse anesthesia educational programs are also surveyed approximately 1 year after completion of their program. Once again, this assists the program leaders in evaluating the appropriateness and scope of the clinical experience they provide to students. It can also indicate clinical experiences needing more emphasis or exposure.

Types of Clinical Evaluations

Different types of evaluations may be used when assessing the clinical performance of learners. Each type serves a specific purpose. The types are formative, summative, terminal, task-specific, 360°, and self-evaluation.

Formative Evaluations

Formative evaluations are used to provide an ongoing, daily assessment of performance. The evaluation is used to motivate learners, diagnose their strengths and weaknesses, provide feedback, and help them develop self-awareness. Reflective learning should be included as part of the formative evaluation. In my opinion, a formative evaluation should consist of both a written and verbal component. Many preceptors delay giving the student a written evaluation at the end of a clinical day. Reasons given for this practice include the fact that it is late and both the student and preceptor are tired. The preceptor or student may have a commitment that precludes taking the time for an immediately written evaluation.

A simple method for introducing the student to reflective learning in the clinical area while giving verbal feedback is the use of a brief postclinical conference at the end of a clinical day. The preceptor can ask the student a few leading questions, such as: "What do you think that you did well today? What could you have done better?"

The preceptor can then give specific, pertinent, objective-based feedback. The written formative evaluation should follow the same criteria used during the verbal exchange. There should be no surprises. Appendix 17.1 (at the end of this chapter) is an example of an objective-based daily clinical evaluation used at my institution. This form is used throughout the entire clinical experience. It indicates student level and defines expectations for each level. Also included is a section for specific comments about achievements and areas needing improvement. The components of the stated objectives found in Appendix 17.1 are identified in detail in Appendix 17.2, which contains a definition of competency levels and a guide for clinical faculty.

Summative Evaluations

Summative evaluations serve a different purpose than formative ones. Summative evaluations are used to pass or fail a learner. They can also be used to allow a student to progress to different objectives. Each clinical semester should have a summative evaluation specific for that point in the program. The objectives for a first clinical semester should not be the same as those for the final clinical semester. Appendix 17.3 provides an example of a summative evaluation for a student's first clinical semester. Notice that many of the objectives reflect the need for close supervision during the initial clinical practicum.

Terminal Evaluations

Terminal evaluations are given at the completion of a nurse anesthesia educational program. These evaluations serve 2 purposes: to ensure suitability for work and to predict future success. Appendix 17.4 contains the summative evaluation of the last clinical semester in my institution's educational program. This also serves as the student's terminal evaluation.

Task-Specific Evaluations

Task-specific evaluations are useful during simulation exercises. These are used to measure mastery of certain psychomotor skills, such as intubation or insertion of a central line. When developing task-specific evaluations, the instructor usually needs to break down a complex skill into smaller steps. Steps usually must occur in a specified order. Objectives should include a degree of acceptable performance on each step and on the total skill.

360° Evaluations

A 360° evaluation is more oriented to peers or customers and is not useful when learning new skills. The 360° performance evaluation is based on feedback from every individual who comes in contact with the student being evaluated.[4] In the case of a student nurse anesthetist in the clinical area, feedback should come from, at minimum, the clinical instructor, the anesthesiologist, the surgeon, residents, nurses, and scrub technicians. Although many of these individuals would be willing to give input verbally as to a student's performance, it is my experience that few will commit to doing so in writing. This type of evaluation is not mandated by the COA, and not all programs use it.

Self-Evaluations

A very important part of the clinical evaluation process is the student's self-evaluation. Such evaluation is mandated by the COA. Most students have a realistic assessment of their progress. At my institution, students are expected to complete a self-evaluation at the end of each clinical semester. They are encouraged to be specific and to delineate achievements. The objectives delineated on the self-evaluation form completed by the student are identical to the objectives listed on the summative evaluation form for that clinical semester.

Elements of Clinical Evaluations

Clinical evaluations should be based on objectives appropriate to the level of proficiency expected and observed. Specific behaviors in relation to clinical performance, which encompass the affective, cognitive, and psychomotor domains, should be assessed.

The *affective domain* is concerned with objectives pertaining to appreciations, attitude, emotions, and values.[5] An example of an objective meeting this criterion is identification of biopsychosocial problems that might affect the anesthetic management of the patient.

The *cognitive domain* includes objectives related to knowledge or information.[5] Objectives that evaluate a student's ability to synthesize a patient's history and laboratory results and to develop a plan of care would fall into this category.

The *psychomotor domain* is the easiest to evaluate in the clinical area. It comprises objectives assessing basic motor skill and physical movement.[5] The student's ability to insert an intravenous catheter would be a skill defined as within the psychomotor domain.

Values such as work ethic should also be included. Assessing values can easily become subjective unless explicitly defined. Including definitions in clinical syllabi makes it clear to the student which values will be evaluated. A clinical evaluation should be factual, descriptive, clear, concise, and constructive, as well as timely. The evaluation needs to be behaviorally directed and based on change-able items. For example, if a student is having difficulty performing intubations, a written observation may state that today, while attempting laryngoscopy, the student did not sweep the blade to move the tongue out of the way. Such a critique clearly and concisely delineates, in a timely manner, the fact that the student is not using proper technique to accomplish a specific task.

The Instrument

The instrument used to evaluate clinical performance needs to be competency based. The skill set needed for safe anesthesia practice should form the matrix of the summative and terminal evaluations.

Working backward from those criteria, the instructor should develop perform-ance objectives to test a student's clinical proficiency based on didactic knowl-edge, clinical experience, and length in the program.

The instrument must be reliable and valid. *Reliability* means the repeatability of the measurement.[6] Will each student who successfully performs a task receive the same grade? Additionally, if one student performs the same task in the same manner, will he or she receive the same grade? A *valid* instrument is accurate; it has a strength of conclusion, inference, or proposition.[6] An example of validity would be testing the accuracy of the information in the anesthesia record (the observed outcome, or conclusion) after the important information was reviewed in conference.

In addition, the instrument should have a grading scale that is simple, consis-tent, and easy to interpret. The scale should be consistent with university or program criteria. If it varies from the university's or program's scale, that fact should be published in the clinical syllabus. It should be clearly defined how many evaluations below standard are allowed and what the consequences of receiving multiple poor evaluations will be. For examples of grading scales that are applicable to clinical evaluations, please refer to Appendices 17.1 through 17.3.

Barriers to Effective Evaluations

Several barriers to effective evaluations exist. Sometimes CRNAs do not fill out evaluations. This is especially true if the student has not performed well. Reasons given for not documenting poor performance include not wanting to be the "bad guy," ("Everyone else says what a great job Mary is doing"; "It's the first time I've observed of poor performance").

Another barrier exists when a CRNA tells the student what a great job he or she has done and then writes an observation of poor functioning. Such a situa-tion may require the program faculty to educate the CRNA as to how this sends mixed messages to the student and is not conducive to improving performance. A third barrier is the CRNA who always gives only positive feedback. This is usually done because the CRNA does not want the student to be put on proba-tion or terminated.

A phenomenon that can also occur with a student who has performed poorly on a few occasions is what I classify as "ganging up" on the student. In this situation, in addition to giving evaluations based on previous performance, a group of anesthesia practitioners discuss the student and decide as a group how the student executes clinical tasks. The evaluation is then based on a preconceived expectation of poor performance as opposed to actual observation of the task at hand. If evaluations are consistently being filled out incorrectly or the clinical faculty puts little effort into making meaningful observations, program faculty members need to examine the situation. At faculty business meetings, an in-service on current clinical objectives and expectations can go a long way toward improving documentation of clinical performance. Giving specific examples of appropriate documentation will often result in better compliance by clinical faculty. If a program has multiple clinical sites, a process for giving summative evaluations to students off campus should be in place. Two options are via computer or telephone.

Case Study: Addressing Evaluations of Unacceptable Performance

Unacceptable clinical performance, when documented, must be acted on in a timely and stepwise fashion. The following case study demonstrates this.

Susie has been in clinical practicum for 6 months. The first clinical semester was 4 months long. Although not outstanding, Susie passed her first clinical semester with a grade of B. In this program, a passing grade in all anesthesia courses is a B or better. Some of the clinical faculty have verbally expressed concern about Susie's ability to manage an airway. The program clinical coordinator takes Susie to the simulation laboratory and has her demonstrate mask management and intubation. Again, Susie's performance is acceptable but not great. It is now 2 months into the second clinical semester, and Susie receives 2 daily evaluations that cite a lack of knowledge of proper drug dosages and her continued difficulty with establishing an airway.

Program faculty members meet with Susie to counsel her about her poor evaluations. They ask about any personal issues, then place her on written warning and probation. They give her a remediation plan that clearly defines areas of deficiencies and a plan of correction with measurable objectives and a timeline for reevaluation. In addition, they offer Susie counseling services. She refuses. The faculty sends the documentation to the college progress committee. Susie does not improve. Daily evaluations continue to identify her lack of didactic knowledge and inability to establish an airway. During this time, program faculty offers Susie one-on-one time in the simulation area and oral discussions of commonly used anesthetic drugs.

It is now the end of the second clinical semester, and Susie receives a C on her summative clinical evaluation. Susie is dismissed from the program due to failure of an anesthesia course. This is consistent with the program's written policy. Written documentation is present to justify the program's action.

Summary

Evaluation of clinical performance is an integral part of a nurse anesthesia education program. Objectives for developing clinical evaluations and for evaluating clinical performance include ensuring patient safety, satisfying student expectations, meeting institution requirements, and complying with COA standards. Types of clinical evaluations include formative, summative, terminal, task-specific, 360°, and self-evaluation. The components of an instrument for evaluating clinical performance should include being clear, specific, and appropriate to the level of proficiency expected; being competency based; and providing written documentation. When evaluations are not performed effectively, program faculty should work to correct the situation with an in-service or other means.

Appendix 17.1. Daily Clinical Student Evaluation

Albany Medical College Center for Nurse Anesthesiology—Nurse Anesthesiology Program

Date: _____

Student name:

_____

	Student level (*please circle*)				
	Clinical year 1		Clinical year 2		Senior residency
	Winter I	Spring/Summer I	Fall II	Winter II	Summer II/Fall III
	Jan 1-May 31	June 1-Aug 31	Sept 1-Dec 31	Jan 1-April 30	May 1-Graduation
	Course 502L	503L	504L	604L	607L

Level 1: Learning
Is gaining didactic knowledge.
Is observing and gaining psychomotor skills.
Requires close supervision/instruction.

Level 2: Readiness
Has didactic knowledge and psychomotor skill.
Correlates theory and skill with assistance.
Requires help setting priorities.
Is close to moderate supervision/instruction.

Level 3: Development
Applies didactic knowledge and psychomotor skills.
Correlates theory and skill.
Is organized and plans for problems.
Requires moderate overall assistance.

Level 4: Competent
Applies principles accurately at all times.
Provides correct rationale for patient management.
Applies appropriate problem solving to complex situations.
Requires minimal assistance.

Objectives	1	2	3	4	Comment on strengths and areas needing improvement
Preanesthetic assessment: Interviews and examines patient in relation to anesthetic management.					
Creates anesthetic care plan and shows ability to revise plan.					
Organizes resources, selects proper equipment, anesthetic agents, and accessories.					
Ensures proper positioning and safety of patient.					
Induction: Demonstrates skill in anesthetic administration and airway management.					
Maintenance: Demonstrates skill in the maintenance of anesthesia care based on patient needs.					
Fluid management: Demonstrates skill in assessing and managing intraoperative fluid therapy.					
Emergence: Demonstrates skill in caring for the patient emerging from an anesthetic.					
Accurately monitors and records patient status.					
Postanesthesia: Evaluates the postanesthetic condition in relation to the anesthetic given.					
Personal attributes: Demonstrates professionalism, communication and rapport with patient and healthcare team. Demonstrates cultural competency.					

Faculty name (print):   Clinical site: _____

_____

Faculty signature:

_____

(Reproduced with permission from The Albany Medical College Center for Nurse Anesthesiology, Albany, New York.)

Appendix 17.2. Clinical Faculty Guide to Assist in Development of Student's Daily Clinical Evaluation

Albany Medical College Center for Nurse Anesthesiology

Competence levels:
1 = Close supervision/instruction
2/3 = Moderate supervision/instruction
4 = Minimal direction

	Clinical year 1		Clinical year 2		Senior residency
Course	**502L**	**503L**	**504L**	**604L**	**607L**
Section I: Preoperative evaluation and assessment					
1. Performing and recording an accurate preanesthesia history and physical	1	2/3	4	4	4
2. Making a determination if pathology exists, which may have implications to anesthesia and/or surgery	1	2/3	4	4	4
3. Reviewing all laboratory, x-ray, and electrocardiographic information and identifying abnormal findings that have implications to anesthesia and the incorporation of the information into the formulation of the anesthesia care plan	1	2/3	4	4	4
4. Identification of biopsychosocial and pharmacological problems that might affect the anesthetic management of the patient	1	2/3	4	4	4
5. Recording appropriate preanesthetic progress notes, to include counseling of patient and/or families	1	2/3	4	4	4
6. Selecting the appropriate preoperative medication, to include recommending or writing the order	1	2/3	4	4	4
7. The formulation of a proposed anesthesia nursing care plan	1	2/3	4	4	4
8. Communicating, collaborating, and/or consulting with other healthcare team members in making decisions	1	2/3	4	4	4
Section II: Interoperative evaluation					
1. Organization, selection, and appropriate testing of resources, ie, agents, equipment, accessories	1	2/3	4	4	4
2. Checking, identifying, and reporting defective equipment so it may be serviced	1	2/3	4	4	4
3. Receiving, identifying, and preparing the patient for anesthesia and surgery	1	2/3	4	4	4
4. Checking the patient's chart for accuracy and completeness	1	2/3	4	4	4
5. Application of monitoring equipment	1	2/3	4	4	4
6. Starting intravenous infusions (start with appropriate needle and/or catheter) and administering physiological fluids	1	2/3	4	4	4
7. Inserting a central venous pressure line(s) and attachment to the appropriate monitor	1	2/3	2/3	4	4
8. Interpreting venous pressure measurements	1	2/3	4	4	4
9. Performing an arterial puncture and/or arterial catheter insertion	1	2/3	4	4	4
10. Interpreting blood-gas analysis results and taking corrective measures when indicated	1	2/3	4	4	4
11. Providing for the safety of both the patient and operating room team to include proper positioning of the patient, proper grounding of the electrical equipment and evacuation of anesthesia gases from the room, and appropriate infection control measures	1	2/3	4	4	4
12. Implementing the anesthesia nursing care plan, making necessary adjustments as indicated by the patient's biopsychosocial condition, and type of surgical procedure	1	2/3	4	4	4
13. Recording appropriate information accurately, completely, and legibly on the anesthesia record	1	2/3	4	4	4
14. Recognizing an obstructed airway	1	2/3	4	4	4
15. Taking appropriate measures to correct an obstructed airway	1	2/3	4	4	4
16. Performing tracheal intubations	1	2/3	4	4	4
17. Assisting and/or controlling ventilation	1	2/3	4	4	4
18. Management of fluid intake and output (eg, blood loss, urinary)	1	2/3	4	4	4
19. Decision-making ability in solving problems as they arise during anesthesia management	1	2/3	2/3	4	4
20. Administering blood components when indicated	1	2/3	4	4	4
21. Utilizes appropriate criteria for an endotracheal extubation	1	2/3	4	4	4
22. Demonstrates decision-making skills in patient emergence	1	2/3	4	4	4

23. Performing regional anesthesia techniques	1	2/3	4	4	4
24. Ability to incorporate theoretical framework in clinical practice throughout perioperative course	1	2/3	4	4	4
25. Communicating, collaborating, and/or consulting with other healthcare team members in making decisions	1	2/3	4	4	4
Section III: Postoperative evaluation					
1. Appropriate monitoring in transporting the patient from the operating room to the PACU	1	2/3	4	4	4
2. Reporting patient's pertinent preoperative and intraoperative data to the recovery room personnel	1	2/3	4	4	4
3. Completing all records in the appropriate format	1	2/3	4	4	4
4. Cleaning and maintaining anesthesia equipment/supplies	1	2/3	4	4	4
5. The follow-up postoperative evaluation of the patient	1	2/3	4	4	4
6. Communicating, collaborating, and/or consulting with other healthcare team members in making decisions	1	2/3	4	4	4

PACU indicates postanesthesia care unit.
(Reproduced with permission from Albany Medical College Center for Nurse Anesthesiology, Albany, New York.)

Appendix 17.3. Summative Evaluation of Clinical Practice, First Clinical Semester

Albany Medical College Center for Nurse Anesthesiology
Winter Semester I (January 1 – May 31)

Student's name:_____

Score Key:
0 = Not acceptable. Poor correlation of didactic knowledge and clinical performance.
1 = Close supervision/instruction needed. With coaching, the student can correlate didactic knowledge with clinical performance.
2/3 = Moderate supervision/instruction needed. The student is developing proficiency correlating didactic knowledge with clinical performance.
4 = The student demonstrates outstanding performance in technical skills and correlation of didactic and practicum knowledge.
N/A= Not applicable at this time; not observed.

ALL SCORES OF 2 OR BELOW MUST BE COMMENTED UPON IN
EVALUATION/COMMENTS

At the end of Practicum Laboratory 502L, the graduate student will be able to:

Score
_____ 1. Prepare a written anesthetic care plan with assistance from anesthesia provider to include:
a. Discussion of history and physical, current medications, pathophysiology, and anesthetic implication/rationale.
b. Types of anesthetics and considerations, including premedication, if indicated; maintenance and emergence with assistance.
c. Advanced monitoring and additional equipment.
d. Fluid replacement.
_____ 2. Identify and locate all types of anesthetic equipment and related anesthetic supplies within the operating room area.
_____ 3. Set up and test all anesthesia machines currently in use to ensure proper functioning.
_____ 4. Perform preoperative anesthesia assessment for assigned patients:
a. Review patient's medical record and document pertinent information, including cultural biases, on preanesthetic sheet.
b. Recognize abnormal laboratory values (list, note, record).
c. Obtain medical history from patient (or family).
d. Recommend appropriate premedication after consultation with anesthesia provider.
_____ 5. Record all pertinent data on the anesthetic and related records.

6. Demonstrate manual dexterity in the performance of (but not limited to) the following tasks:
   a. Properly position the patient on the operating room table.
   b. Follow infection control guidelines related to anesthesia practice.
   c. Prepare an intubation set according to established guidelines.
   d. Draw up and correctly label and compute dosage of all necessary drugs.
   e. Properly place and interpret all noninvasive standard monitoring equipment.
   f. Perform venipuncture for catheter insertion or drawing blood specimen.
   g. Manage an airway with assistance:
      1) Establish and maintain airway.
      2) Maintain adequate mask fit.
      3) Recognize an obstructed airway.
      4) Insert an oral and/or nasal airway.
      5) Perform uncomplicated oral endotracheal intubations with assistance.
   h. Manage regional anesthesia with assistance.
7. Recognize cardiac dysrhythmias and other common complications, such as hypotension, and discuss appropriate care and corrective measures.
8. Demonstrate knowledge of appropriate sequencing and technique for emergence.
9. Provide an accurate and complete report to post anesthesia care unit personnel.
10. Interpersonal relationships:
    a. Demonstrates reliability, punctuality, maturity, professionalism, cultural sensitivity, and effective communication skills.
    b. Accepts instruction and constructive critique.
    c. Functions effectively among anesthesia and surgical team members.
11. Adheres to policies pertaining to drug accountability.
12. Completes postoperative assessment on assigned patient.

Total Score: _____

(Total score is a composite of subscores. Any critical deficiency in a subcategory will result in a total score less than the composite.)

Evaluation/comments (Include clinical strengths and areas needing improvement.):

_____   _____
Clinical director's signature   Graduate student's signature

_____
Date

(Reproduced with permission from The Albany Medical College Center for Nurse Anesthesiology, Albany, New York.)

Appendix 17.4. Summative Evaluation of Clinical Practice, Final Clinical Semester

Albany Medical College Center for Nurse Anesthesiology
Fall Semester II (May 1 - Graduation)

Student's name: _____

Score Key:
0 = Not acceptable. Poor correlation of didactic knowledge and clinical performance.
1 = Close supervision/instruction needed. With coaching the student can correlate didactic knowledge with clinical performance.
2/3 = Moderate supervision/instruction needed. The student is developing proficiency correlating didactic knowledge with clinical performance.
4 = The student demonstrates outstanding performance in technical skills and correlation of didactic and practicum knowledge.
N/A = Not applicable at this time; not observed.

ALL SCORES OF 2 OR BELOW MUST BE COMMENTED UPON IN EVALUATION/COMMENTS

At the end of Practicum Laboratory 607L the graduate student will be able to:

_____ 13. Perform a preanesthetic interview and assessment.
_____ 14. Develop an individualized anesthesia care plan.
_____ 15. Administer anesthesia based on sound physiological and pharmacological principles to all types of patients for all surgical procedures.
_____ 16. Demonstrate manual dexterity in the performance of (but not limited to) the following tasks:
    a. Utilize a broad variety of monitoring equipment safely and effectively, including but not limited to electrocardiogram, precordial stethoscope, direct arterial pressure, central venous pressure, blockade monitor, O_2 analyzers.
    b. Position or supervise positioning of patients to ensure optimal physiological function and patient safety.
    c. Utilize mechanical ventilators effectively.
    d. Administer regional anesthesia.
    e. Manage regional anesthesia.
_____ 17. Utilize accepted physiological principles in the management of fluid therapy and electrolyte balance.
_____ 18. Evaluate blood loss and make sound clinical judgments for accurate replacement.
_____ 19. Recognize and manage perioperative complications.
_____ 20. Provide an accurate and complete report to PACU personnel:
    a. Complete postoperative assessment on assigned patients.
    b. Recognize postoperative complications; institute appropriate treatment.
    c. Complete postoperative assessment on assigned patients.
_____ 21. Function as a team member in cardiopulmonary resuscitation.
_____ 22. Demonstrate organizational skills and adaptability.
_____ 23. Interpersonal relationships:
    a. Demonstrates reliability, punctuality, maturity, professionalism, cultural sensitivity, and effective communication skills.
    a. Accepts instruction and constructive critique.
    c. Functions effectively among anesthesia and surgical team members.
_____ 24. Adheres to policies pertaining to drug accountability.
_____ 25. Completes postoperative assessments on assigned patients.

Total Score: _____

(Total score is a composite of subscores. Any critical deficiency in a subcategory will result in a final score less than the composite.)

Evaluation/comments (Include clinical strengths and areas needing improvement.):

_____   _____
Clinical director's signature   Graduate student's signature

_____
Date

References

1. American Association of Nurse Anesthetists. Bylaws and Standing Rules of the American Association of Nurse Anesthetists. Park Ridge, IL: American Association of Nurse Anesthetists; 2008.

2. Institute of Medicine. Health professions education: a bridge to quality. Institute of Medicine website. April 8, 2003. http://www.iom.edu/CMS/3809/4634/5914.aspx. Accessed March 25, 2009.

3. Standards for Accreditation of Nurse Anesthesia Educational Programs. Park Ridge, IL: Council on Accreditation of Nurse Anesthesia Educational Programs; 2008:4-11.

4. Sparks R. 360° performance evaluation. Missouri Business website. http://www.missouribusiness.net/cq/2002/360_performance_eval.asp. Accessed March 25, 2009.

5. O'Bannon B. Classifying objectives. University of Tennessee Knoxville Educational Technology Collaborative website. http://edtech.tennessee.edu/~bobannon/classifications.html. Accessed April 23, 2008.

6. Colosi L. Reliability and validity: what's the difference? Social Research Methods website. http://www.socialresearchmethods.net/tutorial/Colosi/lcolosi2.htm. Accessed March 25, 2009.

Chapter 18

From Novice to Expert: How Registered Nurses Become CRNAs

Elizabeth Monti Seibert, CRNA, PhD

Key Points

- The novice-to-expert model provides instructors with one way of assessing a student nurse anesthetist's clinical growth and development.

- Five levels of nursing practice—novice, advanced beginner, competent, proficient, and expert—are distinguished in the novice-to-expert model.

- Changes in behavior, not the passage of time, indicate movement from one stage to another and maturation into the role of nurse anesthetist.

- Although student nurse anesthetists enter nurse anesthesia programs with critical care skills, novice students need new rules to guide their behavior because they lack experience in the anesthetic environment.

- Advanced beginners recognize some important aspects of anesthetic situations, are beginning to feel somewhat comfortable in the clinical area, and demonstrate marginally acceptable performance.

- Competent students demonstrate greater confidence because of improved situational awareness and technical and organizational skills that enable them to prioritize and respond more quickly in complex situations.

- Proficient students have achieved an identity as nurse anesthetists and are able to perform appropriately in myriad challenging anesthetic situations. The proficient student is exemplified by the recently graduated student nurse anesthetist.

- The expert level of practice is unlikely to be attained by student nurse anesthetists because it requires a tremendous amount of experience in a variety of situations and development of an intuitive ability to accurately identify the most important aspects of a problem without needing to consider a range of alternatives.

Introduction

The transition from registered nurse (RN) to Certified Registered Nurse Anesthetist (CRNA) is a transformational journey. Although the journey is exciting and invigorating, it can be perilous. Student nurse anesthetists (SNAs) are eager to take the journey, but the culture, customs, and language of the new country are unfamiliar and disconcerting. Like many travelers, SNAs need experienced guides to make the trip more enjoyable and less dangerous. In the clinical practicum, CRNA preceptors assume the role of guide and mentor for SNAs by pointing out important sights, introducing them to new experiences, and alerting them to hazards along the way.

Unfortunately, CRNAs have not had the benefit of a guide to help them learn how to provide clinical instruction. Other than their own experiences as learners or suggestions made by seasoned clinical instructors, few maps are available to guide the novice CRNA preceptor. Therefore, identifying patterns of learning and behavior that SNAs exhibit at various stages of their training may be helpful for clinical instructors. Because nurse anesthesia programs rely on preceptor evaluations of student clinical performance, the reliability of evaluation also may be improved if behaviors that students commonly exhibit as they evolve into competent entry-level practitioners can be quantified. The purpose of this chapter is to briefly review one theory of how beginners learn to become competent healthcare providers and to identify characteristics of SNAs at various stages in the clinical practicum.

Like all adult learners, student nurse anesthetists enter a new learning situation with a well-established identity as capable, competent adults, and in the case of SNAs, as successful critical care nurses. The process of becoming a CRNA challenges students' existing knowledge and skills as well as their image of themselves as expert nurses and leaders within their units. To achieve success and graduate from a nurse anesthesia program, students must construct new personal and professional identities as CRNAs.[1]

Surprisingly little information is available about how RNs become CRNAs. Although undergraduate grade point average and science grade point average are acknowledged as factors contributing to successful academic outcomes, studies have not identified other factors that lead to achievement of clinical competence as a nurse anesthetist. Surveys of nurse anesthesia educators and practitioners describe a core set of knowledge and skills that CRNAs need,[2] but other than the National Certification Examination, valid methods for demonstrating competence in these skills are not available. Experienced CRNAs learn to incorporate new knowledge into practice by first learning basic principles, then by trying out the new information in practice situations, and finally, by accumulating enough experience in various situations to place the knowledge in context.[3] Student nurse anesthetists may learn in a similar manner, but specific learning processes of SNAs have not been described. Nurse anesthesia clinical instructors must look to the general educational and nursing education literature for suggestions about how students acquire new knowledge and skills.

The practice of nurse anesthesia, like many other health professions, involves both science and art. Course work in anatomy, physiology, chemistry, pharmacology, and other sciences augmented with instruction in technological aspects of anesthesia management provides the scientific basis of the profession. However, the mere acquisition of knowledge is not sufficient to ensure competent practice. The true art of the profession lies in the ability to organize knowledge so that it may be applied to specific patients in specific situations. This is the crux of the issue: What differentiates expert practitioners from novices or those who are merely competent?

Novice-to-Expert Framework

Benner's[4] landmark study of practicing nurses described how clinicians learn and accrue knowledge through experience in a variety of situations. Using a qualitative approach, Benner sought to capture the knowledge embedded in nursing practice and identify differences between theoretical and practical knowledge. Basing her work on the Dreyfus Model of Skill Acquisition, Benner and her colleagues distinguished 5 levels of nursing practice—novice, advanced beginner, competent, proficient, and expert—and described common features of each level as well as implications for teaching and learning.[4,5]

Benner recognized that, although nursing has a theoretical base, skilled practice does not rely on knowledge alone.[6] The distinction between theoretical and practical knowledge is described as the difference between "knowing that" and "knowing how." "Knowing that" refers to an individual's knowledge base and the ability to recall facts and rules, but "knowing how" refers to the incorporation of knowledge and experience into innate knowledge so a practitioner can make decisions intuitively.[7] The difference between "knowing how" and "knowing that" can be explained by a simple scenario: A CRNA may have a "gut feeling" that something is wrong with a patient and then respond reflexively to intervene. A student observing the CRNA's performance will ask for the CRNA's reasons and rationale, only to be frustrated when the CRNA cannot provide a ready answer or states that he or she "just knows." Students want solutions or to "know that" while expert CRNAs "know how" from the experience of repeatedly applying knowledge and judgment in patient care situations.[4]

Although Benner's model is only one perspective on how individuals achieve expertise, the novice-to-expert model has relevance for CRNA clinical instructors for several reasons. First, much of nurse anesthesia education occurs in patient care situations, not in the classroom. Practitioners develop expertise through repeatedly encountering real-life situations. Theoretical knowledge provides a foundation, but it must be interpreted in the context of the clinical situation. Clinical instructors have the situational awareness that SNAs lack and thus can guide SNAs' development. Second, the model identifies learning needs in the various stages, providing a guideline for structuring learning activities to meet the needs of students in each stage. Third, the model lends itself to the development of evaluation tools. Because nurse anesthesia programs are expected to graduate competent entry-level practitioners, the model can help educators determine acceptable performance characteristics that SNAs should achieve at different stages of training.[4,5] Finally, the model may help CRNAs recognize their own level of clinical prowess, appreciate the mastery they have attained, and identify areas for further growth.

The remainder of this chapter describes characteristics of each stage of the model, followed by examples of behaviors SNAs might exhibit at that level. I have incorporated suggestions for clinical instruction throughout each section. Readers should understand that these descriptions are not the result of research, but are based on my observations of student nurse anesthetists in clinical settings, from discussions with clinical and didactic faculty, and from listening to students describe the joys and frustrations of their clinical journeys.

The Novice Student

The novice-to-expert model assumes that, although beginners have certain basic abilities, they lack experience in the new role and situations where they must act.[4,8] Learning must begin somewhere.[6] To provide some context, novices are given rules and cues in the form of theoretical knowledge to guide their actions. Although rules provide structure, they also limit the novice because rules cannot cover all possible situations or actions. Rules may limit flexibility because of their prescriptive nature and because students must remember the rule and how to apply it. Thus, novice SNAs must take classroom knowledge and previous nursing experience and begin to apply it to new situations.

Nearly all SNAs are unfamiliar with the operating room environment because most nursing programs do not include operating room experience in their curricula. The first step in helping novice SNAs feel comfortable in their new roles is an adequate orientation to the physical structure of the operating room and anesthesia department, the roles of key personnel, and pertinent policies and procedures. The orientation should also include information about where students may take a break, store or buy their lunch, find textbooks, and locate online reference materials, if available. Any areas that are off-limits for students should also be identified. The clinical site coordinator may conduct the orientation, or students may be teamed up with another student to ease the transition.

Most students entering the operating room for the first time are eager, enthusiastic, motivated, and anxious. Although they are impatient to immerse themselves in clinical experiences, students are also afraid of making mistakes, hurting patients, and being embarrassed by their lack of knowledge and skills. The whole process of anesthesia administration is mysterious, because most SNAs have not seen a complete general anesthetic from induction through emergence. The fact that there are many ways to achieve the same goal in anesthesia is frustrating for novice SNAs, who crave the structure offered by definitive guidelines, rules, and procedures that are more common in nursing practice.

Knowledge and skills acquired in critical care nursing are thought to best prepare SNAs for nurse anesthesia practice. Accreditation standards for nurse anesthesia educational programs require that applicants have at least 1 year of acute care experience defined as: "Work experience during which an RN has developed as an independent decision maker capable of using and interpreting advanced monitoring techniques based on knowledge of physiological and pharmacological principles."[9] Quantifying applicants' skills in these areas has been difficult for most nurse anesthesia programs.

Clinical instructors may assume that all beginning SNAs have a similar background or that SNAs have intensive care unit experience similar to the preceptor's own. However, differences in acute care unit acuity and autonomy, years of experience, and basic nursing preparation mean that novice SNAs vary greatly in their ability to use and interpret basic monitors, titrate vasoactive and sedative drugs, and apply knowledge to practice. In addition, the amount of didactic instruction and hands-on training that novice students receive before entering clinical education is not standardized among nurse anesthesia programs. Preceptors are then faced with identifying the strengths and weaknesses of the basic knowledge and skills novice SNAs possess.

The novice stage is characterized by uncertainty and frustration. Students are unsure what to do and when to do it because they lack context for their actions. Although novice SNAs may have dealt with events such as hypotension, hypoxia, and sepsis as critical care nurses, the context in which these situations occur in the operating room is poles apart from their previous experience and requires different actions. Clinical instructors must identify salient features of anesthesia for novice SNAs so they can learn what events are expected and what are not. For instance, beginners learn about the induction, maintenance, and emergence phases of anesthesia in the classroom. Novices may observe these events in a patient, but they may be unable to recognize characteristics of each stage because they have not been immersed in the experience before. Preceptors can help place the events in context by pointing out cardinal signs of each stage and discussing how these may be differentiated from other similar events.

A great source of student frustration is the result of unclear guidelines and practices among instructors. For example, beginning students are often frustrated when trying to organize their equipment and set up medications when CRNAs in a department do not agree on a common setup. When each CRNA prepares equipment and drugs differently, students feel compelled to learn individual preferences rather than a routine. Because most CRNAs are creatures of habit, they expect students to set up their way and are annoyed when students do not. Nothing disconcerts a novice more than starting the day with a disgruntled instructor; novices feel they can do nothing right and performance rapidly deteriorates. As a result, learning anesthesia is overshadowed by pleasing the preceptor.

Student anxiety is decreased when instructors set clear expectations. Anxiety is common among new students, and miscommunication can occur if preceptors assume that novice students understand what they are saying. Beginning students are frequently overwhelmed by the complexity and rapidity of events in the operating room and are unable to concentrate on what is important, particularly during induction and emergence. Therefore, preceptors should discuss their expectations of the student roles and responsibilities *before* patients are seen or arrive in the operating room. For example, if the instructor says: "I want you to focus on airway management," the student may assume that he or she will also give the drugs and watch the monitors while managing the airway. Because novices need rules, preceptors should be explicit about who will do what: "Once the monitors are on, you can start preoxygenating the patient. After you've preoxygenated for 3 minutes or the end-tidal oxygen is greater than 90%, I'll give the induction drugs. After the patient is asleep, check the lash reflex and then try to ventilate. I want you to use your precordial stethoscope so you can tell if you're ventilating or if the airway is obstructed." A less prescriptive technique is to ask students to describe what they intend to do and ascertain their understanding of their role.

An old adage states that a child must crawl before walking. Similarly, novice SNAs must acquire a core set of knowledge, skills, and attitudes before advancing to more difficult tasks. Knowledge, skills, and attitudes correspond to Bloom's cognitive, psychomotor, and affective domains of learning.[10] In each domain, learning progresses from simple to complex. Understanding these basic concepts can help preceptors identify and design learning experiences that help students acquire new skills and progress to more difficult concepts.

Preceptors should direct novice students toward learning the basic psychomotor skills of the profession. Generally, instructors will have no problem achieving this goal because novice students perceive these tasks as what a nurse anesthetist does.[1] Basic skills that novices must learn include preparing of the anesthesia machine, drugs, and equipment; performing a preoperative history and physical assessment (including listening to heart sounds and lung sounds and evaluating the airway); establishing venous access; applying and using basic monitors; establishing and maintaining the airway using a bag and mask; performing endotracheal intubation; and completing the anesthesia record. Frequently, the novice SNAs are so focused on intubation that the preceptor must remind students to attach the circuit and ventilate the patient, check the breath sounds, and turn on volatile agents. Students may find that preparing a detailed list of the steps involved in the induction process helps organize their thinking.

Novice SNAs need guidance in organizing tasks to develop routines that provide structure and ultimately become habits. Basic monitoring with the senses (look, listen, feel) should be encouraged because novices often are more intent on watching the monitors or automated anesthesia record system instead of the patient. Instructors can give guidance on developing scanning techniques for surveying the patient, surgical field, and monitors. Preceptors should require that novices use a consistent method for setting up equipment and drugs. Just as pilots use preprinted checkout forms, students should be encouraged to develop and use checklists or notes to guide them through the set-up process. CRNAs should share any "pearls" or mnemonics they have found useful such as MSMAID (ie, machine, suction, monitors, airway, IV, drugs).

The anesthesia care plan is another area in which beginners often struggle. Novices' care plans frequently take a cookbook approach, miss important patient or surgical issues, and show lack of individualization. When looking for information on which to base a care plan, students often consult well-known textbooks that offer generic plans for various surgical procedures. They frequently give little attention to different techniques of airway management, use of alternative drugs for induction or maintenance, or techniques other than general anesthesia. Because students often spend considerable time developing care plans, preceptors should take time to read and comment on written care plans. While understanding that, at this point, students are trying to learn the basics, preceptors can help SNAs develop good care plans by asking them to prioritize the patient's problems and potential surgical issues, identify the anesthetic implications of each, propose interventions when needed, and provide a rationale for the intervention. Instructors will find that some students fail to recognize the importance of the care plan to learning and dismiss it as busy work. With these students, preceptors can emphasize the role of repetition in buttressing knowledge, and they can reinforce expectations for written care plans.

In summary, novice SNAs begin to identify with their new role through repeated performance and accomplishment of recognizable tasks that they feel represent nurse anesthesia practice. As students gain confidence in their ability to execute basic psychomotor skills, they are able to more fully participate in more demanding aspects of patient care such as planning and implementing an individualized anesthetic for each patient, making interventions in response to changes in physiologic parameters, and recognizing the stages of anesthesia. Most beginners progress from the novice to advanced beginner stage within a few months of entering clinical practice. How quickly an individual SNA advances depends on the student's determination, the amount of time spent in clinical practice, the number and type of cases that the student is exposed to, and the willingness of instructors to allow students to gain necessary experiences.

The Advanced Beginner

The advanced beginner is the student who has acquired enough experience to recognize important aspects of situations and who is beginning to feel somewhat comfortable in the clinical area.[4] Aspects are identifiable global attributes of a patient or situation that require previous experience to recognize.[4] According to Benner, advanced beginners "demonstrate marginally acceptable performance."[4] Although the advanced beginner is still focused on tasks, the student does not feel as overwhelmed by the environment, begins to place situations in context from participating in similar events, can identify situational cues as a result, and is able to make some interventions based on previous experiences.

In contrast to novice SNAs, advanced beginners have achieved certain milestones. They are able to perform routine preparation of the anesthesia machine, basic airway equipment, and drugs in about 30 minutes at the start of the day. Planning and preparation for successive cases begin to occur during the preceding case. Their psychomotor skills with venous access, airway management, and manipulation of the anesthesia machine are improving. Because less effort and energy are required to complete these technical tasks, students can concentrate on improving techniques, making interventions, and applying knowledge to practice.

Advanced beginner SNAs continue to struggle with mask ventilation and will not always recognize airway obstruction or failure to ventilate. Although their intubation skills are improving, students often perceive "production pressure" and think laryngoscopy and intubation must be performed quickly. Because their skills are not yet well developed, rushing through intubation may lead to lip lacerations and chipped teeth. At this stage, students' attention should be directed toward good body mechanics and correct airway management techniques.

Many novice and advanced beginner SNAs exhibit poor body mechanics while masking the patient or intubating, a practice that increases student fatigue and can lead to failure. One technique that can make mask ventilation less tiring for students is to lean back slightly while ventilating, using body weight as leverage rather than forearm or hand strength. Posture should be corrected if a student tends to bend over when ventilating or intubating. Simple techniques such as making sure the table is at the student's waist level and the patient's head is at the top of the bed may improve success with laryngoscopy. Very short students may need a platform if the table is too high for them.

Preceptors can assist advanced beginner SNAs with improving basic airway management techniques. During mask ventilation, instructors should help students recognize and correct airway obstruction. Although the precordial stethoscope appears out of favor as a monitoring device with many CRNAs, its use can help students identify and correct airway obstruction. When intubation is planned, using nondepolarizing neuromuscular blocking agents to slow the pace of induction will give students a few minutes to practice mask ventilation while the paralytic is taking effect. The additional time may also allow students to relax a little before tackling intubation. Although every CRNA has his or her own favorite tricks of the trade, the need for good basic intubation practices such as sniffing position, sweeping the tongue, staying off the lips and teeth, and identifying pertinent anatomy should be reinforced at this point.

Advanced beginners can identify certain salient points of anesthesia, and they are starting to place them in context. Preceptors can guide SNAs by providing cues or guidelines about what to look for or expect in a given situation. One such guideline might be that systolic pressure less than 20% to 25% of baseline is hypotension and should be treated by administering fluids, placing the patient in the head down position, decreasing volatile agents, or administering vasopressors. However, this guideline does not distinguish subtle nuances of treating hypotension. Nuances are fine distinctions between situations that affect the decision or intervention made. For example, a CRNA discusses the need for preoxygenation of all patients before induction and describes methods to accomplish this. The student grasps the concept and decides that using 4 deep breaths is an effective way to achieve preoxygenation; however, the student fails to consider patient conditions, such as morbid obesity, that might require a different technique. The guideline was good, but the student lacks sufficient experience to interpret the rule in light of differences in patient pathophysiology. Instructors can help students identify distinctions of common anesthesia events and share their rationales for making decisions and instituting interventions.

Because the judgment necessary to recognize nuances comes from experience, advanced beginners are dependent on the instructor's knowledge. Although they want to assert their capability and judgment, advanced beginners are unsure and question their ability to make meaningful contributions to a case. At this point, SNAs doubt their interpretation of events and are hesitant to voice their opinions because they are afraid that others will think them inept or unknowledgeable. For example, when a patient becomes hypotensive in the period between induction and incision, a student may cycle the blood pressure cuff several times to verify the correctness of his or her assessment. Next, the student may timidly suggest an intervention or ask permission to initiate a treatment: "Is it okay if I give 5 mg of ephedrine?" An SNA who is very unsure may appear frozen and unable to act. This type of situation is a good opportunity for the instructor to discuss alternative treatments or what the CRNA might do in a similar scenario.

Advanced beginners are still anxious, especially when confronted with new or challenging clinical situations. Although anxiety may improve vigilance, anxiety may also limit learning and impede decision making. Many novices and advanced beginners express the fear that they will be solely responsible for the patient's entire care. A closely aligned fear is that the instructor will leave the student's side, abandoning the student (and patient) to a variety of imagined perils. Students may think that the preceptor's primary role is as an instructor, when that role is actually secondary to providing patient care. Advanced beginner SNAs should be reassured that they will be allowed to participate in cases to the extent possible, depending on their level of preparedness, the patient's acuity, and the complexity of the surgical procedure. Although advanced beginners generally require constant supervision, students should know how, when, and who to call for help if the CRNA must leave the room. To determine a student's capability for greater independence, an instructor can review possible scenarios that might occur during the CRNA's absence and ask how the student would manage each event.

Advanced beginners are still task-oriented and procedure-oriented. They are trying hard to make sense of situations by developing routines. Even small deviations from routine may derail a student. Advanced beginner SNAs often report that their day is "ruined" (and their performance disintegrates) after they miss an intubation or IV start, or forget a portion of the drug or airway setup. Because students are focused on personal ability to execute a task rather than on patient care, inability to perform a skill is perceived as a personal failure. The advanced beginners quickly begin to doubt their ability, leading to a vicious cycle of performance anxiety, self-flagellation, and further failure. Kindness and tact are imperative when CRNA instructors assess the performance of advanced beginners because an SNA's enthusiasm and spirit can easily be crushed by harsh criticism.

Prioritization is another area in which the advanced beginner SNA needs support. Because guidelines are often generic, they do not help the student decide what to do first or when to do it. The student may know that a volatile agent must be turned on after endotracheal tube (ETT) placement is verified but may wait to do so until the ETT is secured, the ventilator is turned on, gas flows are adjusted, and esophageal stethoscope and airway or bite block are placed. Similarly, a student may focus on a task such as completing the anesthesia record and not notice alarms or changes in vital signs. Preceptors can redirect the student's attention by asking: "What's that noise?" or "What do you think that means?" while pointing out the alarm or vital sign change.

Advanced beginner SNAs feel little accountability for patient care. Lack of ownership may stem from previous critical care experience in which nurses lacked autonomy and decisions were physician-driven or protocol-driven. Advanced beginners focus on performing tasks and developing routines and doubt their knowledge and abilities. Therefore, advanced beginners often feel that responsibility for decision making rests with those who have superior knowledge and experience. In addition, students entering the profession may underestimate the amount of responsibility that nurse anesthetists assume for patient care. Clinical instructors may observe this lack of ownership when students assume that they can leave at 3:00 PM even though the case will finish at 3:30 PM. This perception can be reinforced when instructors take over a case or are too prescriptive. To gain a sense of ownership and confidence, advanced beginners must start making interventions based on their assessments and then observe firsthand the results of their decisions. In other words, students must be allowed to make good and bad decisions.

If advanced beginners are to develop competence, they must be allowed opportunities to work through new and challenging situations.[5] Student nurse anesthetists must learn to deal with the ambiguity of decision making and take responsibility for the results of their decisions. Every CRNA can recall particular experiences that helped him or her grow as a practitioner and that honed judgment and skills. Benner calls these events *paradigm cases* because they make a major impact on the learner.[4] CRNAs often share their paradigm cases with students by telling stories of various experiences and what they learned as a result. Advanced beginner SNAs must begin to compile their own know-how based on different patient care issues that exemplify certain concepts and provide concrete guides for future actions. Because paradigm cases also reveal developing competencies, students should be encouraged to share their experiences with their peers or other anesthesia providers.

Preceptors should not assume that advanced beginner SNAs have good rationale for their actions. Students at this level have limited knowledge, misunderstand concepts, or apply theoretical knowledge inappropriately. Instructors should attempt to elicit the depth of the student's knowledge. For example, when asked to describe succinylcholine, a student may appropriately respond that it is a depolarizing neuromuscular blocking agent but may be unable to explain the process of depolarization. The instructor can clarify or explain misunderstood or unknown concepts or direct the student to review the topic and return to the instructor with an answer. Nurse anesthetists who have been practicing for a while may hesitate to ask questions because they have forgotten the information or because they fear that the student knows more than the preceptor. Instructors can overcome this anxiety by admitting that time has dimmed their theoretical knowledge and by asking the student to refresh the instructor's memory. Another technique instructors can use is to develop several stock questions (and answers) to ask students. Alternatively, preceptors may wish to become local experts on a certain topic or type of case. As students become aware that an instructor is knowledgeable on a subject, they will come to expect questions about this topic from the CRNA or will consult the CRNA for expertise.

Through continued practice and exposure to different patient conditions, surgical procedures, and anesthesia providers, the advanced beginner SNA gradually develops competence. This is an incremental process that might be characterized as "2 steps forward, 1 step back." With repeated practice and over time, the student takes more steps forward and fewer steps back. In my opinion, students graduate to the competent level when they are able to manage a general anesthetic with minimal assistance for a healthy patient (American Society of Anesthesiologists physical status I or II) undergoing a simple surgical procedure (eg, a hysterectomy, laparoscopic cholecystectomy, laminectomy, or similar procedure). Although variations in nurse anesthesia educational programs prohibit generalizations about when an SNA will achieve this milestone, a student should probably advance to the competent stage after participating in 150 to 200 anesthetics or 6 months of full-time clinical experience.

The Competent Student

The competent student demonstrates improved technical and organizational skills and increasing knowledge and awareness of clinical situations.[5] Although he or she still has much to learn, the competent SNA demonstrates sufficient familiarity with a variety of basic anesthesia situations for which he or she can make appropriate decisions and function with less preceptor intervention. When faced with circumstances similar to previously encountered events, competent SNAs are able to identify significant aspects of a situation, eliminate those that are insignificant, and most importantly, anticipate events that may occur. As a result, competent students can limit the range of possible choices that can be made and focus on what needs to be done.[5]

Improved organizational ability enables competent SNAs to deal with complex situations more easily. Less time and effort are wasted on unnecessary tasks, and students are not as easily overwhelmed when things do not go perfectly. Because they are better organized, competent SNAs function more calmly and efficiently. As an example, preoperative evaluation is more thorough, focused, and accomplished in less time. Patients are speedily transported to the operating room and induction is accomplished smoothly and proficiently. Competent students take great pride in their ability to multitask and often describe a day as going well when they skillfully manage numerous demands.[5]

The competent SNA's organizational skills now extend to anticipatory planning.[5] The competent student plans ahead for the day rather than just the first case, anticipating what is needed and preparing equipment and supplies in advance. Not only can the student complete tasks in a timely manner, he or she also can plan for events that might occur with a patient or surgical procedure. Care plans are improved as a student anticipates what might happen when a patient's coexisting disease and the surgical procedure intersect. The morbidly obese patient, for example, is recognized as potentially having a difficult airway. Therefore, the student considers appropriate airway management techniques, has the necessary equipment available, positions the patient appropriately for intubation, and plans alternatives to the primary plan. Adverse intraoperative events that accompany specific procedures are expected, and the student will have a second IV, fluid warmer, central line, and vasoactive drugs prepared when large volume shifts or hemodynamic changes are expected.

Prioritization is also improved in competent students. Although advanced beginners might know what needs to be done, their actions are haphazard because students do first what they know best how to do.[5] Competent SNAs are able to identify what is most important and do that first. The ability to prioritize implies that students are able to make better judgments about critical aspects of situations and to use their time efficiently. As described in an earlier example, novice or advanced beginners focus on a task such as completing the anesthesia record while ignoring alarms or vital sign changes. Competent students can receive sensory input from numerous sources, identify changes needing intervention, and implement a response. Unlike proficient students who function seamlessly, competent students must still analyze the possibilities of each situation and think through the options. Advanced beginners' grasp of situations was limited by tunnel vision; competent SNAs see the big picture.

Compared with advanced beginners, competent students' psychomotor skills are vastly improved, and their movements are smoother and more fluid. Competent students complete endotracheal intubations easily on the first attempt most of the time, even when the airway is somewhat difficult. Although able to accomplish intubation quickly, competent students realize the value of taking time to visualize structures, using the right hand to manipulate the larynx, and directing those present to assist them. Manual dexterity has improved to the point that students do not need to think about each step as it is performed. Therefore, competent students are able to assess their own skills and consider alternative steps if what they are doing is not working.

Competent SNAs are much more comfortable with their skills and abilities and, as a result, may settle into routine methods of delivering an anesthetic. Although this beginning mastery is to be appreciated, there is some danger that students will become complacent and that their growth will slow. Stagnation can be prevented by continuing to expose students to more challenging patients and procedures. Students usually need little encouragement to try using different drugs and techniques, but instructors can stimulate experimentation by suggesting alternatives. Another way to broaden the student horizons is to ask students to teach the instructor something new. Getting out of one's comfort zone can be a growth experience for both students and instructors.

Competent SNAs assume greater personal and ethical responsibility for patient care. Accountability is evident when a student carefully checks the patient's medical records for necessary diagnostic studies or requests additional studies, discusses a proposed anesthetic plan with the instructor and provides rationale for decisions, and accepts responsibility for making mistakes without being defensive. Students at this level are aware that their actions can sometimes cause harm to patients, and they feel devastated after making an error that might compromise a patient. The competent student is becoming a patient advocate, interceding with the surgeon or other team members when decisions might jeopardize patient safety. Advocacy may be seen when a student suggests the use of extra padding to protect a patient during positioning, asks a surgeon to stop manipulations that cause a vagal response, or questions whether a certain technique is appropriate based on the patient's coexisting diseases.

Procedural rules or guidelines are no longer necessary or relied on because some decisions are becoming internalized. Having gained sufficient experience with a variety of patients and surgical procedures, competent students have begun to develop their own rules for dealing with perioperative events.[5] Competent SNAs have a basic plan for delivering an anesthetic and intervening when anticipated events occur. They have encountered enough situations to acknowledge the significance of various physiological changes and recognize deviations from normal. For example, the student recognizes the potential for hypotension in the period between induction and incision and automatically adjusts volatile agents and increases fluids when blood pressure begins to decrease rather than waiting for repeated measurements to confirm hypotension. Students trust that their observations and judgment are accurate and do not need continual affirmation from instructors that their decisions are correct. Competent students are better able to make a case for what they want to do.[5]

Although competent students have a basic action plan in place, they are also able to individualize the plan in regard to existing patient pathophysiology.[5] They recognize the implications of disease states and adjust the anesthetic plan to avoid placing the patient at risk. Thus, competent students understand that a systolic blood pressure of 85 mm Hg may be acceptable in a young, healthy patient but not in a patient with hypertension and coronary artery disease. When different or unusual situations occur, competent students can reason through potential interventions and request help if unsure what to do. Competent SNAs also recognize areas in which their knowledge is limited and spend considerable time reviewing previously learned material or looking up new information.

Students at this level begin to doubt the knowledge and wisdom of their instructors and other members of the healthcare team.[5] Students previously perceived the knowledge of other clinicians as superior, but they may now become critical of CRNAs and anesthesiologists whose judgments or rationale they perceive as faulty or unreliable, particularly if they have observed poor outcomes as a result of these decisions. Although this demonstrates an ability to discern the effectiveness of different courses of action, students may challenge the instructor's knowledge and authority during this stage. For example, a student may refuse to carry out a direct order or may do something he or she was instructed not to do. Of course, this behavior generally infuriates the instructor and may place the patient at risk while exposing the student's overconfidence and ability to accept instruction. The situation also reflects the limits of the student's theoretical and experiential knowledge. When the time is right, the clinical instructor should discuss this situation with the student and attempt to elicit the rationale for his or her behavior.

Competence as an SNA should not be confused with competence in a new graduate of a nurse anesthesia program. The competent SNA moves toward proficiency as he or she continues to gain further experience with demanding cases, encounters some infrequently occurring anesthetic situations, and manages more patients who deviate from the norm. Again, this transformation occurs incrementally. Students may demonstrate proficiency in some areas and, at the same time, exhibit competent or advanced beginner abilities in other areas. A student may be quite proficient with psychomotor or patient assessment skills and competent in managing most major general surgery cases but may appear at the advanced beginner stage when confronted with cardiac procedures, major trauma, or transplant cases. According to Benner et al: "Change, not passage of time, is the defining characteristic of experience."[5] Therefore, proficiency is not necessarily related to the number of months that a student has been in clinical practice but to changes in behavior that indicate maturation of knowledge, skills, and behavior as a nurse anesthetist.

The Proficient Student

As competent entry-level practitioners, students who are soon to graduate exemplify the proficient level of the novice-to-expert model. Students at this point are able to see situations as a whole because they are able to synthesize previous experiences and understand the meaning of an event without systematically analyzing each aspect.[4,5] Proficient SNAs understand normal responses to anesthesia and surgery and recognize when events deviate from what is expected. Although deeply involved and connected to the patient when managing an anesthetic, proficient SNAs have the ability to mentally step back and see the big picture in light of the patient's physiologic responses to intraoperative events. Proficient students are able to zero in on the most important aspects in a rapidly changing environment and make decisions without needing to consider myriad options.

Proficient students recognize the relevance of subtle nuances that might have been overlooked by the competent student. Proficient students are able to place these nuances in context, recognize their implications, eliminate certain options, and generate an appropriate plan of action. For example, when a proficient student administers anesthesia to a patient who has coronary artery disease and who is undergoing a carotid endarterectomy, he or she quickly identifies potential causes of hypotension, acknowledges ramifications for the patient, and initiates interventions to correct the problem. Having participated in enough similar cases and having confidence in his or her judgment, the student does not need to weigh and eliminate all possible causes of hypotension. The proficient performer is beginning to show signs of intuitive decision making that epitomize expert practice.

The technical skills of proficient SNAs are excellent. Students are adept at performing basic tasks such as IV insertion and airway management with endotracheal tubes and laryngeal mask airways, although they may still need experience with regional blocks or alternative airway management devices. Unfortunately, students sometimes confuse mastery of these skills combined with admirable organizational and time management ability as indicative of expertise. Students may feel overly responsible or become overly confident, resulting in the potential for humbling errors.

Proficient students seek improved patient outcomes in their practice.[5] No longer content with merely performing tasks quickly and efficiently, they seek to prevent common problems and minimize adverse events. For proficient students, emerging a patient no longer means recognizing when to remove the ETT. Instead, they plan the emergence so that the patient wakes up without coughing on the ETT; is free from nausea, vomiting, and excessive pain or sedation; and is able to be discharged from the recovery room in a short time.

Giving information to patients is an area where proficient students differ from those who are competent.[5] For instance, the competent student might recite a laundry list of all possible anesthetic complications when obtaining informed consent. The proficient student will adjust discussion of possible adverse anesthetic events based on his or her reading of the patient's and family's ability to understand and readiness to learn. The student does not withhold important information or try to deceive the patient but tailors the information to what the patient needs and wants to know.[5]

A heightened sense of responsibility is characteristic of proficient SNAs, who often think they must do everything themselves and do not take advantage of help offered by other clinicians. While outwardly acknowledging the need to function as part of the operating room and anesthesia teams, students mistake the ability to manage all parts of an anesthetic without assistance as proficiency. In reality, this behavior demonstrates insecurity because more seasoned clinicians readily seek help, share tasks, and request consultation when needed. Failing to share responsibility for a patient may also contribute an unnecessary burden when adverse events occur. When students feel unrealistically responsible for a patient, they may blame themselves for events that were unforeseeable, unpredictable, and unpreventable.

Proficient students may become complacent in expanding their knowledge base or feel that information learned in the classroom is not practical or useful.[4] Some students may think that they know it all because their knowledge is more current than their instructor's or may think that they have seen it all if their case numbers are high. Such students may begin demonstrating unprofessional behaviors such as wandering in late to the clinical site, failing to call the instructor for induction or emergence, or refusing to consider the instructor's suggestions. Fortunately, most soon-to-graduate students do not fall into this category, but those who do can be challenging for the instructor.

Although they have not yet passed the National Certification Examination, proficient students have achieved an identity as nurse anesthetists. Their ability to perform appropriately in myriad challenging anesthetic situations has been confirmed by instructors, surgeons, and other operating room personnel. Although still a little anxious in new situations, proficient students feel that they are able to meet clinical challenges because they have confidence in their own abilities. Because they are no longer deeply engaged in learning new skills and knowledge, proficient students are able to expand their view of the nurse anesthetist's role as a patient care advocate and member of the healthcare system. Students now begin to evaluate how different anesthesia practice models affect CRNA practice, to identify and discuss professional issues, and to consider involvement in state and local professional associations.

The Expert Practitioner

The expert is easy to recognize, but identifying attributes of the expert practitioner is more difficult. Experts have gained a tremendous amount of experience in a variety of situations and have developed an intuitive ability to accurately determine the most important aspects of a problem without needing to consider a range of alternatives. According to Benner, experts do what normally works in a situation.[4] This is not to say that an expert does not consider other possibilities, diagnoses, or interventions, but that the expert does not need to methodically evaluate each option to make a judgment. Experts have difficulty verbalizing how they make decisions or respond to specific events, often replying, "It depends," when asked what course of action they would take in a particular situation. This answer suggests that experts consider a broad range of choices based on ingrained theoretical and experiential knowledge.

Experts anticipate potential events that may occur with a given patient or situation and plan for them. Experts are prepared to deal with various possibilities and are flexible enough to rapidly switch courses of action. Experts recognize subtle changes in a patient's condition and act before a crisis occurs. Within their work settings, experts are those individuals consulted by their peers for their superior knowledge and ability—they are the "go-to" persons.

Experts can make wrong decisions or evaluations of a situation. In these cases, experts revert to more analytic problem solving.[4] However, even expert practitioners revert to the novice role when confronted with a new drug, technique, or unfamiliar situation. Untoward events such as malignant hyperthermia, cardiac arrest, and anaphylaxis happen infrequently in anesthesia. Therefore, even experienced CRNAs may need rules or algorithms to guide their practice when these unique events occur. Simulation centers with whole body simulators allow practitioners to experience these rare occurrences and develop a degree of comfort in dealing with them.

In my estimation, SNAs cannot achieve the expert level of practice. At a minimum, graduates of nurse anesthesia programs are expected to demonstrate the knowledge and skills deemed by the profession to represent entry-level competence; however, the majority of graduates have not had sufficient experience in a wide range of situations to develop the intuitive decision-making skills that characterize expert practice. Indeed, not all CRNAs reach the expert stage, but expertise is something all CRNAs can strive to achieve.

Summary

The novice-to-expert model provides one way of examining and assessing a student nurse anesthetist's clinical growth and development. The normal "growth pattern" for SNAs demonstrates slow but steady progression with occasional hesitations along the way. As with normal human growth and development, students advance at different rates. Some students grow rapidly; others take longer to achieve the same growth milestones. All have periodic growth spurts when things suddenly come together ("ah-ha" moments). A few students will not progress much beyond the advanced beginner stage, a condition I have dubbed "failure to thrive." These individuals may even perform competently in situations where cases are simple, patients are healthy, and adequate support or supervision is available. However, the student who is not growing and progressing does not adapt when confronted with more difficult cases or patients, unusual or emergent situations, or rapidly changing circumstances. The novice-to-expert model can help educators distinguish students who are meeting the expected growth trajectory from those who are not.

A limitation of the novice-to-expert model is that it fails to take into account the important role that clinical instructors play in modeling behavior. Students construct an image of the ideal qualities of a CRNA based on the admirable and not so admirable qualities of their clinical and didactic instructors.[1] Generally, students hold their instructors in high esteem and view them as mentors. Positive instructor traits might be making a difference in patient care, acting as a patient advocate, and possessing clinical acumen and excellent technical skills. However, none of these traits is important if an instructor makes a student feel humiliated, threatened, or unwelcome. Clinical preceptors must recognize the impact their actions have on students, and that instructors can facilitate or hinder learning according to the value that the instructors place on certain knowledge or skills.[11] Students gain confidence in their skills and ability to function in a range of situations through repeated practice and confirmation by others that they are making progress.[1] Preceptors can facilitate a working relationship with students through having a friendly and open demeanor, discussing their rationale for decision making, and sharing clinical pearls.

References

1. Stockhausen LJ. Learning to become a nurse: students' reflections on their clinical experiences. *Aust J Adv Nurs.* 2005;22(3):8-14.

2. McShane F, Fagerlund KA. A report on the Council on Certification of Nurse Anesthetists 2001 Professional Practice Analysis. *AANA J.* 2004;72(1):31-52.

3. Wren KR. Learning from a nurse anesthetist perspective: a qualitative study. *AANA J.* 2001;69(4):273-277.

4. Benner PA. *From Novice to Expert: Excellence and Power in Clinical Nursing Practice.* Commemorative ed. Upper Saddle River, NJ: Prentice-Hall, Inc; 2001.

5. Benner PA, Tanner CA, Chesla CA. *Expertise in Nursing Practice: Caring, Clinical Judgment and Ethics.* New York, NY: Springer Publishing Company, Inc; 1996.

6. O'Connor AB. *Clinical Instruction and Evaluation: A Teaching Resource.* Sudbury, MA: Jones and Bartlett Publishers; 2001.

7. Dreyfus HL, Dreyfus SE. *Mind Over Machine.* New York, NY: The Free Press; 1986.

8. Dreyfus HL, Dreyfus SE. The relationship of theory and practice in the acquisition of skill. In: Benner PA, Tanner CA, Chesla CA, eds. *Expertise in Nursing Practice: Caring Clinical Judgment and Ethics.* New York, NY: Springer Publishing Company, Inc; 1996.

9. Standards for Accreditation of Nurse Anesthesia Educational Programs. Park Ridge, IL: Council on Accreditation of Nurse Anesthesia Educational Programs; 2006.

10. Clark DR. Learning Domains or Bloom's Taxonomy. http://www.nwlink.com/~donclark/hrd/bloom.html. Accessed September 15, 2008.

11. Teunissen PW, Scheele F, Scherpbier AJ, et al. How residents learn: qualitative evidence for the pivotal role of clinical activities. *Med Educ.* 2007;41(8):763-770.

Section III

Didactic Education

Chapter 19

Teaching Processes, Methods, and Lesson Planning

Lawrence H. Truver, CRNA, MSNA

Key Points

- Andragogy is a theory for adult learning that specifies that learners are self-directed and encourages learning by experience and example using problem-solving skills.

- Bloom's taxonomy is a classification that divides educational objectives into 3 domains: cognitive (basic knowledge), psychomotor (technical skills), and affective (behavior and attitudes).

- Important components of a lesson plan are a title page with references and course information, an introductory statement, learning objectives, and a properly sequenced outline of lecture content.

- Objectives for a lesson plan should specify what knowledge, task, or behavior the instructor expects of the learner.

Introduction

The focus of this chapter is the preparation and execution of an effective lesson plan for the didactic curriculum. In addition to clinical experience, a review of current materials allows an instructor to incorporate the latest information and research findings into the literature. After briefly considering some of the theoretical background of teaching and learning, the chapter will emphasize planning and presenting a formal lecture. This will include an examination of the components of a lesson plan, along with suggestions for teaching resources and instructional aids. An important consideration is that an instructor's choice of teaching methods can make a major difference in the amount of knowledge retained (Table 19.1).

Theoretical Foundations

Theories that address teaching and learning have filled volumes in the disciplines of education and psychology. This discussion will be limited to a few pioneers who developed the fundamental principles of teaching intellectual skills to adult learners.

Gagne and coauthors[1] described different types of learning that require various forms of instruction. Their 5 major categories of learning are verbal information, intellectual skills, cognitive strategies, motor skills, and attitudes. Gagne et al theorized that various internal and external conditions are necessary for each type of learning. Their philosophy includes a hierarchy for learning, organized according to complexity. They described processes involved with effective learning such as stimulus recognition, response generation, procedure following, use of terminology, discriminations, concept formation, rule application, and problem solving. By incorporating these instructional strategies, a teacher can help students to gain maximum benefit from the presentation.

Knowles[2] developed a theory specifically for adult learning called andragogy. His premise is that learners are self-directed and should take responsibility for critical thinking. Knowles labeled various assumptions for instructional design geared toward the adult learner. He believed that adults need to know why they should learn something and that the topic should be of value to them. In addition, andragogy encourages learning by experience and example using problem-solving skills. Suggested strategies for teaching mature students, such as student nurse anesthetists, should include case studies, role playing, and simulation.

Table 19.1. Learning/Teaching Method and Retention of Information	
Learning/teaching method	Information retained (%)
Reading assignments	10
Listening to lecture	20
Visual aids	30
Lecture with visual aids	50
Discussion of material	70
Information applied to real-life experiences	80
Material taught to someone else	95

Criterion-referenced instruction is, in great part, attributed to Mager.[3] He described methods for designing and presenting instructional programs based on mastery learning and performance-oriented instruction. The critical aspects of Mager's theory include identification of what needs to be learned (goal/task analysis), specification of outcomes (performance objectives), determination of how objectives will be evaluated (establish the criterion), evaluation of the extent to which objectives have been met (criterion-referenced testing), and development of objective-based learning modules. Mager suggested that a multimedia format allows learners to set their own pace for mastering outcomes. Although this last feature is difficult to maintain in a tightly structured and sequenced anesthesia curriculum, his emphasis on teaching according to measurable objectives is well suited for the scientific nature of the material taught in anesthesia school.

Rogers and Freiburg[4] may have set the stage for others with their theories of experiential learning. Basic to their concepts is the acknowledgment of 2 types of learning. Cognitive or meaningless learning involves things such as memorizing vocabulary or multiplication tables. Experiential learning, or substantial learning, refers to applied and meaningful material. For our students, there is actually a place for both of these levels of instruction. The student must memorize drug doses and minimum alveolar concentrations as entry-level knowledge required in the operating room; however, the instructor will be able to facilitate experimental learning of material that will ultimately affect the conduct of anesthesia. Rogers and Freiberg[4] emphasized the importance of learning to learn and being open to change. This is especially important in a discipline that evolves with each new drug that is marketed or each surgical technique that is introduced.

Application and Integration: The Teaching Process

Although each instructor will need to develop his or her own style of teaching, the principles described can be incorporated to develop a process of instruction. For graduate students in a nurse anesthesia program, some of the groundwork has already been laid. The students are registered nurses who have participated in careers as healthcare professionals. As such, most anesthesia students maintain a high degree of self-motivation because they typically have made major financial and personal sacrifices to return to school. The instructor's role is to build on students' past experiences and provide guidance toward an advanced degree. Also, with the high level of autonomous function held by a nurse anesthetist, it is easy to stress the importance of the material presented. Consider the example that the instructor has been asked to present a lecture on the pharmacology of intravenous induction agents. With emphasis on the potential impact on patient safety, the learners gain a sense of the clinical relevance of the material. After the instructor establishes the motivation to learn and gains the students' attention, another important step in the teaching process is to develop objectives for the learner. This topic will be addressed in the following sections.

As described by several theorists, the role of the instructor is different when dealing with adult learners compared with younger students. Rather than merely presenting a lecture, the teacher must facilitate discussions and provide resources for self-learning. This assists in making the subject meaningful and in recruiting the students to actively participate in the teaching process. By emphasizing the ultimate goal of providing safe anesthesia, the instructor is able to optimize the conditions for learning and the degree of student involvement that are consistent with philosophies of adult education. An advantage that a Certified Registered Nurse Anesthetist has compared with a basic science instructor, for example, is that he or she is able to call on personal clinical experience to develop the importance of a topic. Students are receptive to stories from the trenches that contribute something beyond what they read in a textbook. Telling the students how a task was performed last week or how to administer an anesthetic goes a long way toward establishing a meaningful learning environment.

Another important component of the teaching process involves the evaluation of learning. Although this is often left to examination questions, it should also include class discussion and around-the-room questioning to ensure that students are grasping the key points. If the program has an anesthesia simulator, it can be used to enact an anesthetic. The students can be evaluated by how they administer anesthesia to a simulated patient.[5] Evaluation can be facilitated by developing appropriate objectives and proper construction of a lesson plan. As just described, the adult student should participate in self-evaluation, and the instructor should encourage feedback about the presentation. This should include formal evaluations of the instructor, along with informal questioning to determine students' retention of the material. Often, a course director will have a specific tool for assessing an instructor's effectiveness, and this information ideally will be discussed at the end of the semester.

Principles of Educational Objectives

Essentially, objectives can be referred to interchangeably in terms of learning, instruction, behavior, and/or performance. A common thread to the instructional theories that have been reviewed is the importance of preparing measurable learning objectives. One of the most popular resources for the development of objectives is Bloom's *Taxonomy of Educational Objectives*.

Bloom's Taxonomy

Bloom's taxonomy is a classification of the different objectives and skills that are established for students.[6] The model was proposed in 1956 by a panel including Benjamin Bloom, a well-known educator. The taxonomy, developed by Bloom and others, bears his name because it was first in the alphabetic list of authors. This hierarchical taxonomy divides educational objectives into 3 domains, with learning at higher levels being dependent on prerequisite knowledge and skills from lower levels. According to Bloom's taxonomy, these domains include the following: cognitive (basic knowledge), psychomotor (technical skills), and affective (behavior and attitudes).

Within the cognitive domain, emphasis is on basic knowledge and the development of intellectual skills. This includes the recall or recognition of specific facts and concepts that serve in the development of one's knowledge base. There are 6 major categories, which are listed in order in Table 19.2, starting from the simplest behavior to the most complex. The categories can be thought of as degrees of difficulty that must be mastered in sequence. The instructor should begin with simple goals such as gaining and comprehending information. Intermediate goals could include application and analysis of the lecture content. Finally, the advanced learner will be expected to accomplish tasks such as synthesis and evaluation.

The psychomotor domain includes the development of technical skills that require practice to establish competency. Categories ranging from basic to advanced skills also are listed in Table 19.2. In this domain, the student will begin with tasks of perception and preparation. At the next level, the learner should be expected to give guided responses and defined mechanisms. In the final stages, the instructor should facilitate the student's ability to adapt and originate new techniques.

The affective domain involves the manner in which students behave, including their feelings, values, motivations, and attitudes. The 5 major categories are described in the final section of Table 19.2, from the simplest behavior to the most complex. In this domain, the level of objectives expands from the basics of receiving and responding, to more complex goals such as assigning values, organization, and internalization. An important aspect of writing objectives is consideration of the expected standards or level of performance of the student, including the advanced expectations within several domains of learning.

The Taxonomy Table

Over the years, Bloom's taxonomy has been reviewed and revised multiple times. One noteworthy adaptation was suggested by Anderson and coauthors.[7] They recognized an important drawback with regard to the 1-dimensional nature of the original hierarchy as demonstrated by the following:

Knowledge → Comprehension → Application → Analysis → Synthesis → Evaluation

Their revised taxonomy for learning, teaching, and assessing includes 2 dimensions in a tabular format as shown in Table 19.3. According to this new model, objectives can be written or critiqued using the taxonomy table.

As displayed in Table 19.3, the dimensions are types of knowledge and levels of cognitive processes. The 4 general types of knowledge include factual, conceptual, procedural, and metacognitive. Factual knowledge involves discrete bits of information such as terminology, details, and elements. Conceptual knowledge is a more complex and organized form that includes classifications, generalizations, theories, and structures. The procedural category of knowledge considers how to do something by employing algorithms, techniques, and methods. The metacognitive realm encompasses strategic knowledge, conditional knowledge, and self-knowledge.

The categories of the cognitive process range from those commonly found in objectives such as *remember, understand,* and *apply,* to the less frequently encountered levels of *analyze, evaluate,* and *create. Remembering* involves retrieval of

Table 19.2. Categories Associated With the 3 Domains of Learning

Domain category	Learning goal
Cognitive domain (knowledge)	
Knowledge	Recall data or information.
Comprehension	Understand the meaning and interpretation of instructions and problems.
Application	Use a concept in a new situation or unprompted use of an abstraction.
Analysis	Separate material or concepts into component parts to understand organization.
Synthesis	Assemble parts to emphasize the creation of a new meaning or structure.
Evaluation	Make judgments about the value of ideas or materials.
Psychomotor domain (skills)	
Perception	Use senses to guide motor activity from stimulation to translation.
Set (mind-sets)	Make dispositions that determine one's response to different situations.
Guided response	Incorporate activities such as imitation, trial and error, and practice.
Mechanism	Perform tasks with some confidence and proficiency.
Complex overt response	Accomplish skillful completion of difficult tasks.
Adaptation	Develop and modify skills to fit special requirements.
Origination	Create new skills to address a particular situation or specific problem.
Affective domain (attitude)	
Receiving phenomena	Demonstrate awareness, cooperation, and selected attention.
Responding to phenomena	Exhibit active participation and motivation.
Valuing	Attach worth to a particular object, phenomenon, or behavior.
Organization	Compare, relate, and synthesize value systems.
Internalizing	Behave in a manner consistent, predictable, and characteristic of the learner.

information from long-term memory. *Understanding* is defined as constructing the meaning of various forms of communication. *Applying* means carrying out a procedure for a given set of circumstances. *Analyzing* is the ability to determine relationships, as well as overall structure and purpose. *Evaluating* includes making criterion-based and standard-based judgments. Finally, *creating* is putting elements together to make an original product.

To construct or evaluate an objective using the taxonomy table (Table 19.3), the verb is considered with regard to the desired cognitive process and the noun is in context of the type of knowledge to be achieved. Consider the following example: "The student will be able to *recall* the intubation *dose* for succinylcholine." The verb *recall* implies the cognitive process of remembering, and a drug *dose* is a type of factual knowledge. Therefore, this objective would be categorized into cell A-1 (factual-remember) according to the taxonomy table. Over the course of instruction, a desirable goal for writing objectives is to address as many cells on the table as possible. According to Pickard,[8] the revised Bloom's taxonomy can be used as a tool to clarify and communicate to teachers, students, parents, and school patrons the intended outcomes resulting from instruction.

Table 19.3. The Taxonomy Table

		Cognitive processes					
		1. Remember Recognizing Recalling	2. Understand Interpreting Exemplifying Classifying Summarizing Inferring Comparing Explaining	3. Apply Executing Implementing	4. Analyze Differentiating Organizing Attributing	5. Evaluate Checking Critiquing	6. Create Generating Planning Producing
K n o w l e d g e	A. Factual	A1	A2	A3	A4	A5	A6
	B. Conceptual	B1	B2	B3	B4	B5	B6
	C. Procedural	C1	C2	C3	C4	C5	C6
	D. Metacognitive	D1	D2	D3	D4	D5	D6

(Adapted from Anderson[7] with permission by Allyn & Bacon/Pearson Education.)

The New Taxonomy

More recently, Marzano and Kendall[9] described a new taxonomy that has several revisions to the work of Anderson et al, but it maintains the 2-dimensional nature of the taxonomy table. Although these new schemes are certainly useful, their departure from the classic domains could be problematic to some educators. An alternative strategy will be suggested in the next section that maintains the original domains of learning but also considers 3 levels of learning.

Writing the Objectives

By targeting material toward the appropriate level or domain of learning, an instructor can help the student nurse anesthetist develop critical thinking skills. This is especially important because this final level of understanding is required to deliver safe anesthesia care. For example, after accomplishing the cognitive task of memorizing numerous induction doses, a student nurse anesthetist must be able to critically evaluate which patients require a dose adjustment. With well-constructed and sequenced objectives that address the various stages of learning, the instructor and students are able to measure progress toward their ultimate goals.

When establishing learning objectives, the instructor analyzes instructional needs to determine the appropriate goals for the students. This begins with a description of the overall learning goal for a topic. The instructor then defines the smaller tasks or specific learning objectives. There are several key components of behavioral objectives. For one, the desired behavior should be specific and measurable. To measure an objective, the instructor must be able to confirm that the desired outcome was obtained. With regard to lecture material, this often includes the ability to write an appropriate examination question to determine the student's level of comprehension. When presenting the learner objectives, one should also state the conditions of learning, including suggested resources and methods for obtaining information.

When constructing objectives for a lesson plan, the instructor may benefit from a few guidelines regarding terminology. The instructor should avoid vague expressions such as "to understand" or "learn about." Instead, he or she should specify what knowledge, task, or behavior is expected of the learner. A set of objectives can be introduced with a statement such as the following: "At the conclusion of this lesson, the student nurse anesthetist will be able to . . . ."

For suggested terminology, Table 19.4 provides examples of action verbs that the instructor can use when writing measurable objectives for different levels of performance within common domains of learning. It incorporates the grid arrangement from the previously described taxonomy table (Table 19.3) to allow for targeted construction of objectives. It also can provide a tool for evaluating the scope of objectives for a lecture or course.

For use in writing an objective, the cells of the table can be thought of in terms of a battleship-type game, in which the instructor targets the different domains and levels of performance. For example, a lecture or laboratory exercise on subarachnoid blocks could include the following objectives and methods of evaluation:

Objective:	Identify the ligaments encountered with the midline approach. (Cell A1, basic level–cognitive domain)
Evaluation:	Multiple-choice question: Identify the most superficial ligament contacted by the spinal needle. Cadaver laboratory practicum with ligaments pinned.
Objective:	Compare and contrast the midline and paramedian approaches. (Cell A2, intermediate level–cognitive domain)
Evaluation:	Multiple-choice question: Which approach is least affected by calcified ligaments?
Objective:	Demonstrate acceptable performance of a spinal block. (Cell B2, intermediate level–psychomotor domain)
Evaluation:	Use a skills checklist to evaluate if a student performed the block appropriately using a spinal injection simulator.

Objective:	Discriminate appropriate from inappropriate performance of a spinal block.
	(Cell C3, advanced level–affective domain)
Evaluation:	Oral or written critiques of instructional videos or mock anesthetic exercises.

By using Table 19.4 to evaluate these examples, the instructor can demonstrate that the objectives covered 4 different cells. To use a game analogy, when evaluating objectives for a course of instruction, there is an attempt to cover the grid like filling the rows and columns on a Bingo card. By "filling the card," the instructor is attempting to address as many levels and types of learning as possible. To further demonstrate the use of Table 19.4, the instructor should consider these objectives and methods of evaluation for a lecture on propofol.

Objective:	State the induction dose (mg/kg) for a healthy adult.
	(Cell A1, basic level–cognitive domain)
Evaluation:	Multiple-choice question: Identify the induction dose of propofol (mg/kg) for a healthy adult.
	Oral board examinations and quizzing of the students.
Objective:	Calculate the induction dose of propofol for a given patient.
	(Cell A2, intermediate level–cognitive domain)
Evaluation:	Multiple-choice question: How many milliliters of 10% propofol would you give to induce anesthesia in a healthy 75-kg adult man?

Table 19.4. Suggested Terminology for Writing Measurable Objectives for Various Categories and Levels of Learning

Domain of learning	Suggested level of performance		
	1. Basic	2. Intermediate	3. Advanced
A. Cognitive (knowledge base)	**A1** Cite/state Define Describe Discuss Draw Explain Identify Label List Name	**A2** Analyze Apply Calculate Categorize Compare Contrast Differentiate Interpret Solve	**A3** Assess/evaluate Compose Construct Create Design Formulate Manage Organize Rank
B. Psychomotor (technical skills)	**B1** Adjust Distinguish Duplicate Locate Prepare	**B2** Calibrate Demonstrate Illustrate Manipulate Operate	**B3** Adapt Construct Create Develop Design
C. Affective (behavior and attitude)	**C1** Accept Comply Recognize	**C2** Defend Influence Value	**C3** Discriminate Judge Relate

(Adapted from written communication with Ruth Patterson, EdD, professor emerita, Medical University of South Carolina, Charleston, South Carolina, 2008.)

Objective:	Develop an anesthetic plan for various patient populations and operative procedures. (Cell B3, advanced level–psychomotor domain)
Evaluation:	Present a case study for an elderly patient presenting for a colonoscopy. Proper management of patient simulation exercises.
Objective:	Defend your choice of induction drug and dose for a given patient. (Cell C2, intermediate level–affective domain)
Evaluation:	Oral boards and mock anesthetic exercises.

Getting Started: Lesson Planning

Although establishing measurable objectives is arguably the most important component of a lesson plan, preparation for a lecture begins with the instructor's knowledge of the subject matter. In addition to clinical experience and reviewing recently published materials, an instructor is able to determine the current level of understanding and to apply the latest research findings for a given topic. The review should begin with the required book list for the course being taught so that the presentation will correspond with student reading assignments. It is important to note common areas addressed in numerous references, including discrepancies found in various sources. To confirm adequate coverage of material, it is beneficial to consult the content outline for the Council on Certification of Nurse Anesthetists Certification Examination.

After establishing the prerequisite knowledge base, the instructor will be in a position to write the learner objectives. As described, it is important to determine content with clinical significance and relevance to practice. The instructor should recall that objectives should be written in measurable terms to provide the ability to confirm successful completion. Namely, it should be possible to restructure each objective into an examination question to be employed for evaluation. Recalling an earlier example, there might be an objective for the student to list the correct sequence of structures encountered with a midline subarachnoid block. An appropriate criterion-referenced examination question could then be constructed as follows: "Which is the most superficial ligament encountered with the midline approach to a spinal anesthetic?" This strategy allows the student and instructor to measure the success to which the objective was achieved. Clearly written objectives can also serve as a guide for prioritizing the volumes of assigned readings that typically accompany a lesson plan. Students should be able to use the set of objectives as a study guide that provides a source for follow-up questions and clarification.

It is also important to provide 2 versions of an outline of the subject matter. The draft for the students can be referred to as the lesson plan, and the instructor's copy is the teaching plan. Proper sequencing and transitions are important for an organized delivery of the material. The key is to provide enough detail on the students' lesson plan to guide instruction but still promote active learner participation by taking appropriate notes and contributing to class discussions. Specifically, some key points should be omitted from the students' lesson plan to allow the instructor to ask questions for which answers are not provided on the outline. This strategy is employed to help the students develop their critical thinking skills. It mimics the real-life situation in the operating room in which the anesthetist is given a set of patient variables and then must choose the proper course of action. Another suggestion for the outline is to include a second column for identifying media content or supporting materials. Excerpts from a sample outline for a lesson plan and teaching plan are shown in Table 19.5.

In addition to providing an appropriate outline, it is important to incorporate supporting materials into the lesson plan. For example, class handouts that include applicable tables and figures can provide a valuable extension to the written content. These graphic displays help provide visual reinforcement of key points. At the same time, the instructor must ensure consistency and sequencing of the visual aids to avoid distraction from the lecture. While preparing for a class, instructors might find it appropriate to adopt a philosophy that the presentation should only be minimally affected if the video projector or computer fails. Instructors should be cautious to avoid getting carried away with technology. They must ensure that the use of media supports the lecture but does not overwhelm the content. The Internet and electronic media have provided a vast supply of information and digital images, but it is the instructor's responsibility to tailor this to an appropriate amount for student consumption.

Before discussing the presentation of a lesson plan, it may be helpful to first consider some of the characteristics of an effective teacher. Lowman,[10] although acknowledging complicated methodology, conducted research in an attempt to describe what constitutes exemplary teaching. His work resulted in a model of effective college teaching that considers the quality of instruction in 2 dimensions. The first involves the instructor's skill at creating intellectual excitement in learners. Components of this dimension include the clarity of all of the instructor's presentations and his or her stimulating emotional impact on students. As

---

Table 19.5. Example of Lesson and Teaching Plan Outlines

Lesson plan (student copy)

A. Cardiovascular effects of ketamine	
1. Tachycardia	Figure X
2. Increases systolic blood pressure	Table Y
Leave space for notes on student copy.	

Teaching plan (instructor copy)

A. Cardiovascular effects of ketamine	
1. Tachycardia	Refer to Figure X in handouts Slide No.:
Why? Sympathetic stimulation.	
Have questions prepared to facilitate discussion of implications for coronary artery disease, etc.	
2. Increases systolic blood pressure	As shown on Table Y Slide No.:
Ask students to compare this with other induction agents.	

Lowman describes it, clarity is related to what material is presented, whereas the emotional impact is determined by the way in which material is presented. The second dimension concerns interpersonal rapport with the students. This refers to an instructor's skill at communicating with students to increase their motivation, enjoyment, and independent learning. Beneficial characteristics in this realm include being warm, open, predictable, and highly student centered. Lowman concluded that exemplary instructors excel in 1 or both of these dimensions, or are at least adequate in each one.

Presenting the Lesson Plan

With successful completion of these preliminary steps, all that remains is the execution of the lesson plan. For initial presentations, it is difficult to predict the appropriate time allotment and amount of material to cover. This is where a supportive spouse, colleague, or innocent bystander can assist by participating in a dry run through the material. With a new presentation, the instructor often covers the material faster than expected. As such, it may be helpful to have supplementary material or case discussions prepared that can provide a buffer at the end of the presentation. Subsequent lectures will then allow for fine-tuning, with expansion or contraction of content as needed for the class time allotment. It is important to allow time for student interaction during class. By having an instructor assign several readings ahead of time or having the class review case studies on the topic, the students will be able to prepare for active participation. For example, the allotted class time can be broken down as follows: lecture on the key elements and principles, review of case studies, discussion of anesthetic implications, and if available, employment of a simulator to demonstrate care for the patient in the operating room.

To begin the presentation, it is important for the instructor to gain the audience's attention with an appropriate introduction. This could include the clinical relevance of the topic, such as the expected impact on patient management. For example, the instructor might begin by relating the incidence of a disease or the frequency of a particular surgical procedure. Relating his or her own background and experience with the given topic can help establish credibility in presenting the material. It is also helpful for the instructor to specifically address the learning objectives that have been written. This will give the students a sense of priority and organization of the information to be discussed.

For the actual lecture content, it is paramount to ensure proper sequencing of the subject matter to ensure clarity. For the students to gain maximal benefit from the presentation, it is necessary for them to easily follow the outline. This is in contrast to students fumbling through their lesson plans trying to figure out what notes need to be taken vs what material has been provided. However, the presenter should omit some content to provide an opportunity for class discussion and problem solving. Again, it is helpful to have a teaching copy of the lesson plan that is congruent with the student draft and that also includes questions and cues for making key points.

Instructional aids should be considered supplemental to the lesson plan. Multimedia presentations should be applicable and entertaining, but should not distract from the fundamental information. Graphics programs such as PowerPoint (Microsoft Corp, Redmond, Washington) are simple tools that can be employed to augment a presentation. Search engines can provide access to a vast array of digital images that can be incorporated as visual aids (eg, Google Image Search; Google Inc, Mountain View, California; http://www.google.com/imghp). In addition, various resources are available in CD-ROM format that provide tables and figures for teaching purposes.

Formatting the Lesson Plan

A variety of formats can be employed for constructing a lesson plan. To begin, check with the program faculty to determine if there is a standard format that the parent institution requires. Although the sequence of information on a lesson plan may vary, the information required is typically consistent. This begins with an identification of the institution and instructor, including appropriate credentials. It is usually standard to provide information such as the targeted audience, course number, placement in the curriculum, class location, and type of instruction employed (eg, lecture, demonstration, and audiovisual aids). A helpful hint is to include some type of identification (ie, file name) that can be used for file storage and retrieval. It is essential to list the references that were used in preparation of the lecture, along with the reading/study assignment for which the students will be responsible.

The body of the lesson plan can begin with introductory comments and a list of objectives for the lecture. This will be followed by the ever-important outline of material that has been described. The specific style of the outline should not overwhelm the importance of the content. Thus, the use of bullets or outline tools in the various word-processing programs should not supercede the task of providing the appropriate amount and sequence of information. Appendix 19.1 provides a sample of a lesson plan format that instructors can adapt to their own needs.

With regard to supporting materials, one suggestion is to use a separate handout with figures and tables. This allows individual manipulation of the lesson plan text and visual aids as necessary for updates or corrections. Students are then able to view each simultaneously, thereby avoiding the distraction of shuffled pages. Except for figures or tables that have been incorporated from a required text, it may be better to avoid displaying excessive material that is not included in the handouts. This will save students from taking needless notes and facilitate their hearing of what is being said, rather than trying to reproduce a drawing or graph. Software such as PowerPoint can make this task simpler because it includes a print command that allows one to choose handout options (eg, sequence and number of slides per page). Before the actual lecture time, many facilities may be able to distribute lesson plans and presentations via the Internet (eg, Blackboard/WebCT; Blackboard Inc, Washington, DC) to allow for better class preparation by the students.

The lecturer should finalize the presentation with a thorough summary that includes repetition of the most relevant concepts. This last step is necessary to encourage retention of clinically significant issues. During the review of key points, it is essential to include ample time for questions from the students to promote their understanding of the subject matter. This also provides an opportunity to evaluate the lesson plan and determine the learner's level of understanding. This time might also be used to ensure clarity of the study assignments or to provide an example of possible test questions.

Another consideration about the format of a lesson plan is the content of the course syllabus. Most academic institutions require specific information on file for courses in order to comply with various accreditation standards. In addition to the items suggested for the cover page of a lesson plan, information on the syllabus should include course goals, required textbooks, contact information for instructors, prerequisite courses, and examination and grading policies.

It may be beneficial to review the syllabus to ensure that the lecture content is congruent with the overall goals of the course. Compared with the learner objectives written for an individual lesson plan, course goals are more generic statements of the expectations for students. For example, on the syllabus, a goal might be as follows: "The student will be able to perform an endotracheal intubation on an adult or pediatric patient." In comparison, an objective written for the lesson plan on airway management could read: "The student will demonstrate proper placement of a straight-bladed laryngoscope." A corresponding examination question could then be constructed in the following example. "Where is the tip of a straight blade placed when performing direct laryngoscopy?" A suggested format with typical inclusions for a course syllabus is provided in Appendix 19.2.

Summary

A lesson plan is a valuable tool for presenting subject matter that should incorporate the basic principles of teaching and learning. Although the format can vary, the content should be thoroughly covered with careful attention to the needs of the learner. The important components of a well-structured lesson plan include the following: a title page with appropriate references and course information, an introduction for gaining attention and establishing importance, measurable and appropriately defined learning objectives, and a properly sequenced outline that provides guidance for instruction. Many experienced teachers believe that giving a lecture boils down to telling the class what you are going to tell them, presenting the information, and then telling them what you told them. Of course, there should be considerably more learner participation to ensure successful execution of the lesson plan.

Despite the importance of teaching processes and lesson planning, there is another somewhat intangible item that may be of equal priority. The instructor must approach teaching with passion and enthusiasm. If the students sense that a subject is not important to the instructor, it is doubtful that they will give much effort toward learning it. Similar to anesthesia, effective instruction involves both the art and science of teaching. The most knowledgeable teacher will not be effective unless he or she presents the right material in the right way.

With the increased emphasis on distance education and virtual classrooms, this will be an especially challenging aspect of instruction. Knowles[11] made this statement more than 20 years ago: "Our great challenge now is to find ways to maintain the human touch as we learn to use the media in new ways."

Appendix 19.1. Sample Lesson Plan Format

Instructor's name/credentials

Lesson Plan: ABC-123 (file name)

Topic of Lecture

Presented to: First-year students, AFN-526: Principles of Anesthesia Practice

Location: Classroom number and building (as necessary)

References: Examples of frequently used texts

> Barash, chapter(s)
> Dorsch, chapter(s)
> Guyton, chapter(s)
> Longnecker, chapter(s)
> Miller, chapter(s)
> Morgan, chapter(s)
> Nagelhout, chapter(s)
> Stoelting (*Anesthesia and Co-Existing or Pharmacology and Physiology*), chapter(s)

Reading assignment:
From required booklist for course (includes references noted above)

Type of Instruction: Lecture (1 hour)
Others: video, demo/return demo, laboratory exercises, simulator training

Introduction: Used to gain attention and establish the format of the presentation

Objectives: The learner will be able to:
1. Describe . . .
2. Identify . . .

Outline: Proper sequencing and the correct amount of material are critical elements

Summary and Key Points: Emphasize the most important areas for retention

---

Appendix 19.2. Sample Course Syllabus

Course number

Credit allotment: Number of credit/semester hours

Course hours: Number of hours of lecture or lab per week

Placement: Term and year

Prerequisite and/or concurrent courses:

Faculty coordinators: Contact information for instructors in the course
(such as names, office hours, phone numbers, email addresses)

Description of course: In addition to a catalog excerpt, provide a rationale for the course and present a topical outline for the material to be covered.

Goals: At the conclusion of this course, students will be able to . . .

Format: Lectures, group discussions, video, laboratory exercises, and demonstrations.

Evaluation: Explanation of assignments and policies for exams and course grades

Required textbooks and supplies:

Meeting time and location:

Class schedule:

References

1. Gagne RM, Briggs LJ, Wager WW. *Principles of Instructional Design.* 4th ed. Fort Worth, TX: Harcourt Brace Jovanovich College Publishers; 1992.

2. Knowles M. *The Adult Learner: A Neglected Species.* 3rd ed. Houston, TX: Gulf Publishing; 1984.

3. Mager RF. *Preparing Instructional Objectives.* 2nd ed. Belmont, CA: Pitman Learning Inc.; 1984.

4. Rogers CR, Freiberg HJ. *Freedom to Learn.* 3rd ed. Columbus, OH: Merrill/Macmillan; 1994.

5. Hotchkiss MA, Biddle C, Fallacaro M. Assessing the authenticity of the human simulation experience in anesthesiology. *AANA J.* 2002;70(6):470-473.

6. Bloom BS. *Taxonomy of Educational Objectives: The Classification of Educational Goals.* New York, NY: Susan Fauer Co Inc; 1956.

7. Anderson LW, Krathwohl DR, Bloom BS, eds. *A Taxonomy for Learning, Teaching, and Assessing: A Revision of Bloom's Taxonomy of Educational Objectives.* New York, NY: Addison Wesley Longman Inc; 2001.

8. Pickard MJ. The new Bloom's taxonomy: an overview. *J Fam Consumer Sci Educ.* 2007;25(1):45-55.

9. Marzano RJ, Kendall JS. *The New Taxonomy of Educational Objectives.* 2nd ed. Thousand Oaks, CA: Corwin Press; 2007.

10. Lowman J. *Mastering the Techniques of Teaching.* 2nd ed. San Francisco, CA: Jossey-Bass Publishers; 1995.

11. Knowles MS. *Andragogy in Action: Applying Modern Principles of Adult Learning.* San Francisco, CA: Jossey Bass Publishers; 1984.

Chapter 20

Simulation-Based Education: Practical Approaches to Curriculum Integration

Celeste G. Villanueva, CRNA, MS

Key Points

- Advancing patient safety and the quality of patient care is a fundamental driving force for simulation-based education.

- Anesthesia crisis resource management is a high-fidelity manikin-based simulation methodology based on aviation crew resource management team training principles that is widely accepted as an essential strategy to improve patient safety.

- Nurse anesthesia programs should strive to incorporate an anesthesia crisis resource management component into the curriculum, emphasizing development of anesthesia nontechnical skills.

- Standards and guidelines for endorsement of simulation programs and centers have been established by some professional healthcare organizations (eg, the American Society of Anesthesiologists and the American College of Surgeons). Accreditation standards and processes for simulation programs are in development by the Society for Simulation in Healthcare, a broad-based, multidisciplinary, international organization.

- Curriculum designs for simulation integration that are longitudinal (extending the full length of the program) and integral to other curricular components will enhance the effectiveness of simulation-based education. An evidence-based set of 10 ideal educational conditions leads to more effective learning while using high-fidelity simulation.

Key points continue on page 340.

- Designating and providing resources for a simulation champion in each nurse anesthesia program faculty is an important first step in full curricular integration of simulation. Collaboration with other programs will accelerate the development and maintenance of standardized curricular components and centralized resources for effective simulation programs.

- High-fidelity manikin-based simulation, if well incorporated into a curriculum, can provide evidence of an institution's educational effectiveness. The key is to establish explicit linkages between learning objectives of a simulation-based learning activity and the desired competencies.

Introduction

A provocative statement regarding simulation was published several years ago in 1992: ". . . no industry in which human lives depend on the skilled performance of responsible operators has waited for unequivocal proof of the benefits of simulation before embracing it . . . Neither should anesthesiology."[1] That call to action spawned volumes of literature, countless hours of education and training using simulation, and many well-designed studies seeking the ultimate proof of its benefit. Yet in 2004, the same author continued musing whether or not the year 2025 would see simulation-based education inextricably woven into the fabric of our healthcare system.[2] The message of simulation must be promulgated, and more collaborative work needs to be done if, by 2025, the question of benefit will no longer be asked.

Alfred Lupien's chapter (chapter 14) on simulation in this book provides fundamental definitions, a conceptual framework, and a general plan for using simulation in a nurse anesthesia educational curriculum. This chapter is intended to complement Lupien's chapter by providing information and resources to enhance effective integration of simulation-based education (SBE) into the nurse anesthetist's practice, whether that practice has an educational or clinical focus. That said, most of the information is applicable primarily for educators. Turcato[3] describes the results of a 2008 national survey related to the use of simulation technology in nurse anesthesia educational programs, which indicate that the majority of programs do not incorporate high-fidelity manikin-based (HFMB) simulation into their curricula. A robust body of evidence supports this specific type of simulation methodology in the education of healthcare providers,[4,5] and in particular, anesthesia providers.[6] Some of the earliest adaptors of HFMB simulation were nurse anesthetists.[7,8] Given these facts, there is clearly a need to bridge the gaps in communication and resources between colleagues who actively use simulation and those who do not. Turcato also delineates what program administrators identify as barriers to incorporation of HFMB simulation into their curricula and proposes strategies to overcome these barriers.[3] Those strategies aim to achieve the following goals: to disseminate the benefits of simulation to decision makers, to generate enthusiasm among colleagues, and to pool resources among colleagues. The information provided here is intended to facilitate the attainment of these goals.

As is often the case with an emerging knowledge domain, the use of terms related to healthcare simulation can be inconsistent among authors, which can lead to decreased clarity for the reader. A glossary is included at the end of this chapter in an attempt to transfer knowledge more effectively. The definitions represent a synthesis of information from the literature on healthcare simulation.

Current Driving Forces For Simulation-Based Education

During the past decade, there has been an explosion of interest in patient simulation, which is the result of several highly influential forces. The simulation phenomenon has moved quickly—propelled by these forces—from a topic of academic interest to a catalyst for major expenditures of healthcare education dollars, research grant funding, time, and intellectual energy. Educators, especially the program administrators who interact with institutional decision makers, should be conversant in the origins and evolution of these forces in preparation for making a case—business, strategic planning, or curricular—for a simulation-related project.

Patient Safety and Quality of Care

Improvement in patient safety and quality of care is universally acknowledged by the simulation community as the driving force for using immersive simulation techniques for professional education, performance assessment, preparation for clinical work, remediation of provider skills, or research.[2] The landmark publication by the US Institute of Medicine,[9] which set the national agenda for reducing human error and formulating a comprehensive approach to patient safety, identifies simulation team training patterned after the aviation industry's crew resource management (CRM) training as a way to prevent and mitigate harm to patients. The same report designated the Agency for Healthcare Research and Quality (AHRQ) as the federal government entity that would essentially serve as a clearinghouse for patient safety matters. The AHRQ published a report in 2001 containing a critical analysis of patient safety practices, which included a review of the evidence supporting the impact of CRM training (using HFMB simulation) on reduction of medical errors. Although no direct evidence existed then or exists to date that unequivocally supports this relationship, in large part because a study design and measurement of outcomes is difficult at best, the report implied that healthcare decision makers should accept the irrefutable validity of CRM, as the aviation industry has for the equivalent type of training.[10] Another compelling indicator that patient safety is a driving force for simulation is the fact that, in 2006, the AHRQ awarded more than $5 million in grants for 19 projects that focus on assessing and evaluating the roles that simulation can play in improving the safety and quality of healthcare delivery.[11]

Simulation Activities of Healthcare's Stakeholders

Gaba[2] identifies the driving forces for full integration of simulation into the US healthcare system and submits his notion of the strategies various influential simulation stakeholders might employ to forward a simulation agenda. Table 20.1 lists specific examples of the strategies and mechanisms currently in place that are especially relevant to anesthesia education and practice. These examples should provide powerful motivation for leaders of our profession to enhance the work nurse anesthetists are currently doing to promulgate simulation-based education. More importantly, they should facilitate the development of processes and guidelines for simulation integration into the curricula of educational programs and continuing education programs.

Professional Organizations That Advance Simulation

The Society for Simulation in Healthcare (SSH) is a rapidly growing organization that is broad based, multidisciplinary, international in membership and focus, and has a clear mission to advance patient safety initiatives. Since 2003, the leadership

Table 20.1. Key Influences for the Integration of Simulation into Healthcare

Name of organization	Mechanisms to implement forces	Driving forces
Society for Simulation in Healthcare (SSH)	*Simulation in Healthcare: Journal of the SSH* Simulation Alliance[a] SSH Simulation Program Accreditation[b]	Promulgate simulation.
Advanced Initiatives in Medical Simulation	Building a National Agenda for Simulation-Based Medical Education (2004 report)[12] Political advocacy for the Enhancing SIMULATION[c] Act of 2009 (H.R. 855)	Improve patient care and safety.
American Association of Nurse Anesthetists	Simulation user group[d]	Improve performance.
American Society of Anesthesiologists	ASA Committee on Simulation Education ASA Simulation Education Program[e]	Avoid government regulation.
National Board on Certification and Recertification of Nurse Anesthetists	No simulation-based education requirement to date	Improve performance. Ensure maintenance of competency.
American Board of Anesthesiology	MOCA components include PPAI,[f] which entails simulation-based education for recertification.	Respond to public pressure.

[a] A coalition of stakeholders in simulation, the think tank for simulation initiatives. This group establishes standards for simulation-based education and training.

[b] Process for accreditation of simulation program development under the auspices of the SSH.

[c] Indicates Safety In Medicine Utilizing Leading Advanced Simulation Technologies to Improve Outcomes Now.

[d] Special interest group with informal meetings scheduled during the Assembly of School Faculty (AANA Education Committee).

[e] Advocates the promotion of learning through simulation; specifically approves programs of quality in anesthesiology simulation training.

[f] MOCA indicates Maintenance of Certification in Anesthesiology (recertification process); PPAI, Practice Performance Assessment and Improvement, phased in January 2008.

of this highly motivated group established (1) an annual international conference featuring world-class speakers, interactive workshops, and roundtable discussions; (2) a specialty journal that includes articles from all disciplines and all focus areas, such as education, assessment, research, clinical practice; and (3) Internet-based resources such as an active listserv and access to key resources for all simulation users, from novice to expert. Among its many activities is the establishment of the Credentialing, Accreditation, Technology, and Standards Committee, charged with developing standards and processes for accreditation of simulation programs and centers. The launch of this pilot program in July 2009 was announced during the SSH International Meeting on Simulation in Healthcare in January 2009. The move toward establishing standards for the field of simulation-based education indicates industry growth and the increasing value that stakeholders place in its products.

From a more practical point of view, the availability of processes and standards makes the creation of simulation programs (ie, curricula) less of a daunting task for those with a developing level of expertise.

Also established in 2003, the Advanced Initiative for Medical Simulation is an organization with a purpose complementary to the SSH in that its members seek to positively influence national healthcare policy and long-term federal economic investment to support simulation development.[13] Nurse anesthetists are active participants in current key task forces and committees of the SSH; however, a continued and much larger engagement of our professional community would serve to advance the mission of both of these simulation-focused organizations and would accelerate the much-needed integration of simulation into all areas of nurse anesthesia practice.

Simulation and Certification

The provocative topic of incorporating HFMB simulation into high-stakes assessment for anesthesiologists and nurse anesthetists is often raised during discussions of simulation-based education. This is a complex issue that is of intense interest, largely driven by the many forces, both internal and external to our discipline, that demand the demonstration and documentation of professional competence throughout a provider's practice lifetime. Many challenges to incorporating simulation into professional certification processes exist. To date, the only reports of HFMB simulation-based performance assessments incorporated into anesthesiology board examinations relate to the Israeli Board of Anesthesiology Examination Committee processes, active since 2003.[14,15]

Most simulation experts concur on the notion that simulation-based methodologies, specifically the HFMB type, will almost certainly be a requirement for certification, recertification, and continuing education across all medical subspecialties, and possibly across all healthcare disciplines.[16] Thus, it will be essential that nurse anesthetists as a group be well informed, be credible in the delivery of simulation-based learning, and be engaged in collaborative efforts in preparation for making critical decisions about simulation as it relates to certification and recertification.

Malpractice Premium Incentives

Another compelling fact that should be part of a case for aggressive simulation integration is the growing number of medical specialties that use CRM training as a risk-management strategy.[17,18] The Controlled Risk Insurance Company (CRICO) Risk Management Foundation of the Harvard Medical Institutions, in collaboration with the Center for Medical Simulation of Cambridge, Massachusetts, set the prototype for a program that provides discounted malpractice insurance premiums to physicians who complete an 8-hour CRM training course provided by Center for Medical Simulation. Discounted premiums began in 2001 at 6% below the usual rate. An actuarial analysis CRICO completed 5 years after initiating the program compared the malpractice claims numbers of anesthesiologists who had undergone the CRM with those who had not completed the program. The decreased number of claims of those who had completed the program was significant enough for CRICO to increase the discount to 19% in 2007.

A similar premium incentive program has not yet been established for Certified Registered Nurse Anesthetists because the malpractice insurance for nurse anesthetists at the Harvard Medical Institutions is covered by the hospitals' policy.[19] By 2002, CRICO had launched a similar premium incentive program for obstetricians and gynecologists with similar success patterns; this proven model as a safety initiative is certain to be repeated by other risk-management companies and across multiple clinical specialties.

Trends in Higher Education

A final category of current driving forces for SBE is related to the current climate and realities of higher education. Most students enrolled in nurse anesthesia educational programs come from the generations dubbed Generation X and Generation Y (also known as the Millennials; see chapter 8). Interestingly, these 2 generations, despite having age ranges less than 2 decades apart, have notably different sets of collective values and characteristics, and both generations have different value sets from the Baby Boomer generation, which comprises most of the nurse anesthetists in practice.[20] Members of Generation X and Generation Y have commonalities when it comes to technology and how it affects every aspect of their lives. Frand,[21] in describing their set of attitudes and aptitudes, refers to the "information-age mindset," developed as a result of growing up in a culture described as globally connected, service and information intense, and digitally based. The pedagogical implications of this mindset are further outlined, an important one being that students prefer—and learn more effectively—via experiential, interactive, and authentic learning methodologies.[22]

The simulation-based learning techniques and curricular characteristics described in the following section are ways to meet a distinct need—indeed, an expectation—of the students that enter our programs. Contemporary nurse anesthesia students not only tend to have a mindset as previously described, they also often have backgrounds that include the use of simulation-based education, either during their prelicensure nursing programs or via hospital-based, point-of-care simulations in which they have participated. Based on surveys and evaluations completed by potential applicants and enrolled students at Samuel Merritt University, Oakland, California, it is crystal clear that having a simulation facility available for learning opportunities is an important marketing tool. Even more compelling for potential students is the knowledge that their education will have an effective simulation component, which brings us to the core topic of this chapter: curriculum integration.

Curricular Integration of Simulation-Based Education

A common message simulation experts repeatedly deliver when providing advice on the appropriate use of simulation technologies is "it's all about the curriculum."

Glavin[23] describes a curriculum as "a statement of how learners can achieve a prescribed set of abilities that will equip them to identify and solve the problems they will face after they complete their program of study." The value of any simulation technology purchased does not depend on how much it costs or even how well the user can operate it. It depends on how well the technology user understands the content and the logic of an educational program's curriculum and how it leverages the interactive nature of a simulator to accomplish the curricular goals. A simulation program that is well integrated into a curriculum optimally matches the functionality of a type of simulator and the design of a simulation to a specific set of learning objectives. Furthermore, those learning objectives should be aligned with the designated learning outcomes and competencies upon which a program curriculum is constructed. In this section, an exemplar of simulation integration into a nurse anesthesia educational curriculum is used as a practical point of reference for discussion of relevant concepts.

Where and how does one begin to infuse simulation-based methodologies into an established nurse anesthesia program curriculum? Much of the answer to this question depends on the range of the program's inventory of (or access to) simulators; the availability of facilities (eg, a simulation center or a dedicated laboratory space for simulation) and infrastructure (eg, trained simulation staff and information technology and audiovisual support staff); the number of nurse anesthesia faculty trained in simulation methodologies; and the level of philosophical and fiscal support provided by institutional administrators from the program level through the higher administrative echelons of an academic or hospital institution. An essential first step is to identify and empower a designated simulation champion, well described by Medley[24] as "a faculty member who believes in the technology, is informed and excited about its use, and has a "contagious" effect on other faculty members." Program administrators would be wise to designate resources for such an individual.

The Samuel Merritt University (SMU) simulation curriculum presented in Appendix 20.1 at the end of the chapter represents a dynamic work in progress. Deliberate integration of HFMB simulation began approximately 8 years ago. Our faculty began incorporating simple manikin-based simulation techniques in 2001 in a small teaching space that was inconsistently accessible and was equipped with rudimentary audiovisual technology. In 2006, the approval of capital funding by our university (a private institution) and the garnering of philanthropic donations for the construction of our state-of-the-art simulation center was largely predicated on our program's success with curricular integration of simulation. I raise this point to state emphatically that an effective simulation curriculum can be delivered in a wide range of physical facilities with varying levels of technological sophistication. Key elements of success are clear and deliberate curricular planning by faculty and taking incremental steps in the implementation of set plans. Such a plan begins with understanding educational concepts that provide a good foundation for a simulation curriculum.

Learning Theories and Simulation

Just as clinicians seek a strong evidence base for their practice, current higher education standards dictate that strong theoretical constructs should form the basis of how educators approach teaching clinicians to practice. Most textbooks related to SBE in healthcare contain a chapter in which the author discusses conceptual frameworks that provide structure and rationale for immersive-type educational strategies.[25-28] The theoretical underpinnings of simulation-based education, generally attributed to the experiential learning theories of Kolb[29] and Lewin,[30] can be graphically described as a circular model linking the 4 major concepts of concrete experience, observation and reflection, forming abstract concepts, and experimenting in new situations. Figure 20.1 illustrates how this model integrates with elements of simulation, especially HFMB simulation, standardized patients, and to some extent, computer-based simulation.

Brain-Based Learning

New and exciting advances in brain-related sciences have prompted the emergence during the past 2 decades of a biologically driven educational framework referred to as brain-based learning (BBL).[30-33] This framework is an evidence-based metaconcept that encompasses many educational strategies, including practical simulations and experiential learning. What makes BBL particularly revolutionary is the notion that placing its concepts at the core of one's teaching leads to the development of the prefrontal cortex of the brain. Executive functions

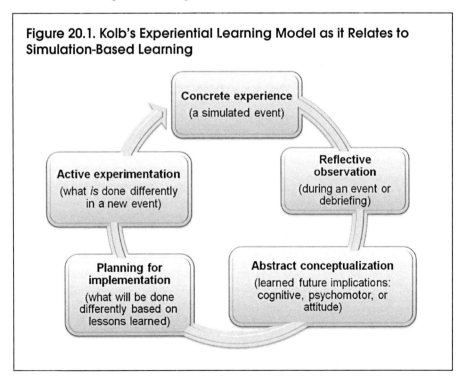

Figure 20.1. Kolb's Experiential Learning Model as it Relates to Simulation-Based Learning

Concrete experience
(a simulated event)

Reflective observation
(during an event or debriefing)

Abstract conceptualization
(learned future implications: cognitive, psychomotor, or attitude)

Planning for implementation
(what will be done differently based on lessons learned)

Active experimentation
(what *is* done differently in a new event)

(Adapted with permission from Dunn.[25(p17)])

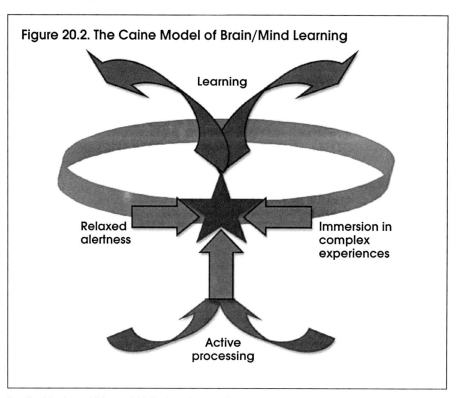

Figure 20.2. The Caine Model of Brain/Mind Learning

Learning

Relaxed alertness

Immersion in complex experiences

Active processing

A critical feature of this model is that each of the 3 elements has a profound effect on the other 2 and is never separate.

are housed primarily in that front area of the brain. "Individuals with highly developed executive functions have mastered the ability to plan and organize their thinking, use reason, engage in risk assessment, make sense of ideas and behavior, multitask, moderate emotions, work with longer time horizons, think critically, access working memory, and reflect on their own strengths and weaknesses."[30] This skill set is one that all patients and fellow healthcare providers would certainly seek in an anesthetist, indeed, in all individuals responsible for human lives. Thus, we educators who are responsible for the development of future generations of nurse anesthetists have a duty to ensure that the teaching methodologies we employ and the curricula that we deliver keep apace with what sound science demonstrates as effective in developing higher-order thinkers.

Figure 20.2 illustrates the 3 essential elements of the Caine model of BBL and the accompanying Table 20.2 summarizes the model's basic elements, offering examples of how those elements apply to SBE for nurse anesthetists. Brain-based learning is a teaching paradigm that is not only applicable in the setting of a simulated patient care environment, but also applies to the classroom and to the operating room, the ultimate immersive experience for our students.

A Plan for Simulation Infusion Into a Curriculum

Please refer to Appendix 20.1 while considering the following curriculum features.

Table 20.2. Application of the 3 Elements of the Caine Brain-Based Learning Model

Element	Description and application to simulation-based education
Relaxed alertness (emotional climate)	The optimal state of mind and atmosphere for learning consists of low threat, high expectations, and high challenge. The desired state of mind of the learner combines confidence, competence, and intrinsic motivation. *Application:* A philosophy that fosters this type of learning environment in the classroom and simulation setting facilitates successful integration of a simulation program into a curriculum. Faculty responsible for debriefing simulation scenarios should understand that less fear on the part of the learner translates (via encoding of memory) to better long-term learning. Also, simulation training has been shown to increase the confidence of students and residents before entering a clinical setting.[34-37] Thus, we can infer that decreased fear and increased confidence of learners in the real clinical setting will lead to a state of relaxed alertness and more effective learning.
Orchestrated immersion in complex experience (instruction)	The only way to simultaneously engage the many processes and capacities reflected in the natural (ie, brain) learning system is through complex experience. The brain learns by making connections between what is experienced and what that experience means to the learner. *Application:* The classic design and orchestration of a HFMB simulation scenario involves prompting learners to make links between the new (simulated) experience and what they already know; place new knowledge within the "big picture"; frame their own, learner-centered, adaptive questions; use new knowledge in spontaneous situations, and receive feedback on their work. Because the real experience of providing anesthesia care is context rich and complex by nature, replicating this during simulation-based learning activities is not difficult to conceive (Although it may be challenging to suspend the disbelief of the learner.)
Active processing (consolidation)	Continuous and personal engagement by the learner is considered active processing. Learners should have "in the moment," ongoing, instant feedback as well as continuous reflection that solidifies and expands knowledge. They should be challenged to think more deeply, identify specific characteristics and see relationships, analyze situations, think on their feet, make critical decisions, and communicate their understanding. *Application:* High-fidelity manikin-based scenarios reinforce concepts of pathophysiology and pharmacology and are examples of the active processing element present in SBE. Such scenarios usually incorporate common clinical care controversies or conflicting patient issues related to comorbidities that force the learner to engage in the type of thinking (deep, analytical, on your feet) described above. Debriefing, whether it occurs as reflection in action, or in a separate room with a group of learners, provides the opportunity for analysis and ongoing reflection.

The 3 essential elements of the Caine brain-based learning model can be directly applied to simulation-based learning strategies. These elements emerge out of a set of 12 brain/mind learning principles, from which the definitions and descriptions presented here are adapted.[30] Examples specific to anesthesia education are provided.

Distributed Curricular Design

Kozmenko[38] describes 2 major formats of a simulation-based curriculum: a brief, intensive course that spans a few weeks with daily sessions that last 6 to 8 hours, or a longitudinal curriculum that provides for a distributed learning interval. The SMU simulation curriculum is based on a longitudinal format that spans the length of the 27-month program. Positive features of this "infusion" (vs bolus) type of format are: (1) It allows for a synchronized combination of didactic teaching and simulator based activities, (2) Each activity builds on the foundation of internalized experiences from previous learning activities, and (3) It allows for multiple repetitions of key themes in a curriculum. An example of a key recurring theme throughout simulation activities is patient safety. Most of our simulation scenarios, irrespective of complexity, contain some element reinforcing current safety practices expected of all anesthesia providers, for example, the Joint Commission Universal Protocol for Hospitals (preprocedure verification process, mark the procedure site, and time-out performance)[39] or the Institute for Healthcare Improvement's situation-background-assessment-recommendation communication model.[40]

Somewhat related to the longitudinal nature of the curriculum is the fact that the simulation-based learning (SBL) activities (see Appendix 20.1, left column) are constructed as a continuum where experiences from preceding activities are considered prerequisites for subsequent activities, the activities increase incrementally in complexity and challenge, and all activities are mandatory for proceeding from one to the next.

Simulation is Defined Broadly

The curricular plan is based on the use of all simulation modalities. Refer to chapter 14 for a description of simulator categories and the type of learning best suited for each category. That information should be consistent with the SBL activity description (see Appendix 20.1, middle column) and its correlating primary goal (see Appendix 20.1, right column) Note that the conceptual strategy for simulation Lupien describes in chapter 14 invokes Vygotsky's Zone of Proximal Development. The SBL activities listed for semesters 1 and 2 generally follow the 4 stages of this zone of proximal development learning process.

Figure 20.3 represents the principle of using multiple modalities of SBL within a simulation curriculum. It is a graphic representation of our program's interpretation of a framework for developing competence in healthcare provider skills, referred to as the circle of learning (COL).

A full description of the components of the COL can be found on the website of the Laerdal Medical Corporation[41]; the framework is based on the concept of using ongoing, interrelated methodologies to engage learners in the process of gaining competence. The activities listed on the wedges of the circular figure correlate to SBL activities listed in Table 20.2. This pattern of using a variety of modalities to engage the various parts of the learner's brain is a common theme in the SMU curriculum. Interestingly, components of the COL framework are consistent with some of the basic precepts of the Caine model[29] of experiential and brain-based learning, which include a set of 12 brain/mind learning principles.

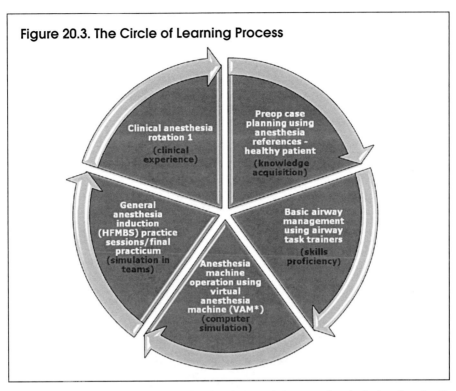

Figure 20.3. The Circle of Learning Process

Preop case planning using anesthesia references – healthy patient
(knowledge acquisition)

Clinical anesthesia rotation 1
(clinical experience)

General anesthesia induction (HFMBS) practice sessions/final practicum
(simulation in teams)

Anesthesia machine operation using virtual anesthesia machine (VAM*)
(computer simulation)

Basic airway management using airway task trainers
(skills proficiency)

A critical feature of this model is that each of the 3 elements has a profound effect on the other 2 and is never separate.

*VAM is an online computer simulation program that serves to reinforce concepts/skills gained in hands-on anesthesia machine training sessions.

The following examples illustrate how 3 of these 12 principles correlate with components of the COL.

Brain/Mind Learning Principle 9: There are at least 2 approaches to memory: archiving isolated facts and skills or making sense of experience.
COL: Knowledge acquisition combined with computer-based simulation (focus on problem-solving)
Brain/Mind Learning Principle 10: Learning is developmental.
COL: Skills proficiency development is fundamental to moving toward competency with complex tasks
Brain/Mind Learning Principle 11: Complex learning is enhanced by challenge.
COL: Simulation in teams using HFMB simulation methodology

As a result of the simulation revolution, many textbooks and other types of publications are readily available as resources for simulation curriculum developers. The references cited here are recommended specifically to increase awareness of the various teaching strategies that best leverage the features of various simulation modalities.[27,28,42-44]

Focus on Nontechnical Skills

The SBL activities scheduled in the latter part of the SMU curriculum (activities 12 through 15) are designed for a strong focus on the development of anesthesia nontechnical skills (ANTS). The definition and conceptual framework of ANTS adopted for use in our curriculum are those established via a collaborative effort of anesthesiologists and industrial psychologists.[45] This partnership between professionals in 2 seemingly unrelated disciplines evolved because of the parallels that exist between high-risk industries (eg, aviation or air traffic control) and anesthesia. Both domains have a safety-focused culture, and in both domains, it has been clearly demonstrated that applying the requisite book knowledge and procedural expertise to a situation, especially a crisis situation, is not sufficient to consistently result in competent practice and positive outcomes. There is another skill set that, when used in a complementary fashion to the more knowledge-based or technical skills, is more likely to yield a smooth and effective implementation of an action plan. The concept of nontechnical skills is not yet part of the common lexicon of most healthcare disciplines, but there is widespread agreement in the patient safety literature that providing nontechnical skill training to all personnel involved in acute patient care is a critical step in what has been called "the war against error."[46-48]

Another term used synonymously with nontechnical skills is human factors, defined as "the way people think and feel, and interact with each other and with their environment."[48] Human factors are not to be construed as risk factors. The important concept to grasp is that human factors can lie at the core of a major critical event that may cascade into a bona fide crisis, but they are also the factors that often lie at the core of averting crises. For the purposes of this chapter, the term nontechnical skills will be used, but the synonymous term mentioned is widely used in the parlance of patient safety and simulation.

The anesthesia nontechnical skills (ANTS) system is currently the only peer-reviewed, empirically derived, quantitative tool available in the anesthesia domain for assessing an individual's ability to demonstrate nontechnical skills.[45] The ANTS system has 3 levels of descriptions of nontechnical skills: categories, elements, and behavioral markers that are specifically defined. See Table 20.3 for a summary of the major levels. A numerical rating scale is part of the system that, when used by trained individuals, has the potential to provide a metric that reflects the individual's nontechnical skills. The ANTS system is incorporated into the SMU simulation curriculum in the manner suggested by its authors, primarily as a tool for teaching or for structuring feedback to learners during debriefing, because of the absence of data indicating reliability and validity of the tool as a formal summative assessment instrument. The terminology and concepts in the ANTS system may be applied easily to any other clinical specialty.

Anesthesia Crisis Resource Management

Recent data indicate that principles of anesthesia crisis resource management (ACRM) are not formally integrated into most nurse anesthesia educational

Table 20.3. Categories and Elements of the Anesthetists' Nontechnical Skills System

Category	Elements
Task management	Planning and preparing Prioritizing Providing and maintaining standards
Team working	Identifying and using resources Coordinating activities with team members Exchanging information Using authority and assertiveness Assessing capabilities Supporting others
Situation awareness	Gathering information Recognizing and understanding Anticipating
Decision making	Identifying options Balancing risks and selecting options Reevaluating

(Adapted with permission from Fletcher.[40])

curricula; moreover, many of the programs that do have an ACRM curricular component do not use high-fidelity manikin-based simulation as a teaching methodology specifically for ACRM.[3] The Institute of Medicine's strong endorsement in 1999 of the aviation industry's crew resource management training was not a passing trend. A recently published and critically acclaimed book on patient safety and quality care states that, despite the substantial work done to reduce human errors during the past decade, "The United States healthcare industry still has not established a culture of safety."[47] The compelling message is for all healthcare professions to use the safety-building strategies of the aviation industry's CRM, the model upon which ACRM was developed.

As indicated in SBL activities 12 to 15 (see Appendix 20.1), the SMU curriculum integrates ACRM concepts across several simulation modules. The SMU faculty incorporates discussions of ACRM principles (including the concepts fundamental to ANTS) into all their didactic courses where appropriate, as precursory to the formal ACRM sessions.

Several nurse anesthesia programs have a strong ACRM element integrated into their curricula. A wealth of resources is available in our professional community that can be tapped by educators seeking to incorporate or expand the ACRM component of their programs using HFMB simulation. Anecdotally and based on discussions during nurse anesthesia educator forums, there is a desire and need to establish mechanisms to share and access such resources. As indicated in the introductory paragraphs of this chapter, an important goal in including the topic of simulation into this book is to initiate more aggressive actions to meet that need.

Future Integration Focused on Simulation-Based Assessment

Appendix 20.2 lists the SBL exercises under active consideration for incorporation into the SMU curriculum. They have 1 common goal: to assess a student's level of proficiency with the cognitive and technical skills required for advanced cardiac life support, pediatric advanced life support, difficult airway management, and common, acute intraoperative events. At SMU, the primary focus of our HFMB simulation sessions has been on formative teaching with a clear emphasis on concept reinforcement, clinical reasoning, and the development of nontechnical skills. To date, the literature that provides sufficiently strong evidence for the use of simulation-based assessment, particularly for high-stakes assessment, has been inconsistent. Although recent studies indicate that the field is closer to having reliable and valid measurement tools and processes,[49-57] most simulation users await further research before adopting simulation-based assessment for high-stakes purposes.

With that caveat in mind, the SMU strategy is to construct HFMB simulation scenarios that would accomplish the purposes described in Appendix 20.2 for the 4 activities listed, to follow the literature regarding the establishment of robust assessment tools, and to plan and implement the new curricular elements incrementally as appropriate and as logistics (time and personnel) allow.

Quantity of Simulation-Based Learning

A question sometimes posed by educators developing a simulation program is: "How much simulation should be used in a curriculum?" There are no published standards or guidelines relative to the number of hours or percentage of curricular content that should incorporate simulation-based methodologies. McGaghie and colleagues[52] report the results of an analysis of 31 quantitative studies that sought to correlate the number of practice hours using simulation techniques to achievement of learning outcomes. Although the study results primarily bring to light the need for more rigorous methodology in this area of research, a notable principal finding is that, across all learner levels and clinical specialties (eg, medicine, nursing, and allied health) there is clear evidence that repetitive practice involving simulation techniques is associated with improved learner outcomes in a dose-response curve relationship.

An interesting and not surprising trend evident in the SMU program is that the paradigm for classroom teaching is changing as a result of the aggressive growth of our simulation program. Once faculty members experience the overwhelmingly positive feedback of students (and faculty) to learner-centered, experiential activities incorporating simulation methodology, they become highly motivated to invest the time and energy to revise old lesson plans to include innovative teaching strategies. One consequence of this change is a steady increase in hours using simulation-based and other experiential methodologies with a concomitant decrease in the traditional didactic lecture style. This resonates well with our students, who personify the information-age mindset. To date, this has not resulted in a downturn in metrics used to assess student performance in classroom activities.

On the contrary, the impact of using HFMB simulation has significantly improved the first-year student nurse anesthetists' level of skill, competence, and confidence before entering clinical residency. Activities 1 through 9 listed in Appendix 20.1 describe an intense use of simulation methodologies, particularly HFMB, during semester 1. The impact on knowledge, skills, attitude, and ability for safe practice has been similar, if not more effective, than that recently brought to light in 2 studies on first-year anesthesiology residents who experienced simulation-based learning. In one study,[34] the first-year clinical anesthesiology residents were given an intense, 3-day preparation course featuring basic airway management and operating room preparation, preparation for and completion of a general anesthesia/endotracheal tube induction, and transfer care of the patient to the postoperative care unit, all on relatively healthy patients. In the second study,[35] the first-year clinical anesthesiology residents received HFMB simulation training during the first 6 weeks of their residency training in the basic management of intraoperative hypoxemia and hypotensive events.

The purpose of each study was to evaluate the knowledge and confidence level of the residents (first study) and the level of competence and safe practice (second study). Both study results showed improvement over baseline and, by inference, improvement over groups that did not receive simulation-based preparation. If the simulation-intense preparation extends to a 16-week period and includes significantly more content (eg, semester 1 activities in our program), increased competence and confidence seem to be reasonable results. Our course evaluations bear this out, as do the informal reports that we receive from the clinical faculty on the level of preparedness of first-year student nurse anesthetists. Anecdotally, clinical faculty have consistently indicated that our HFMB simulation curriculum has resulted in students who are much more prepared during first rotations, which allows them to focus earlier and more effectively on subjects not normally broached until well into that first rotation.

Effectiveness of Simulation-Based Learning

Is there evidence to support the statement that high-fidelity patient simulation actually results in learning? A landmark article by Issenberg[53] reported on a review of the simulation literature spanning 34 years. This was a study done through the Best Evidence Medication Education Collaboration, and attempted to answer the question: "What are the features and uses of high-fidelity medical simulations that lead to most effective learning?" There was evidence to support the claim that optimal learning occurs if as many as possible of 10 conditions are present in the educational environment. It seems reasonable that in the course of developing a plan for simulation integration into a curriculum, we would aspire to achieve all 10 conditions, listed in Table 20.4. At SMU, these criteria are applied when performing an annual assessment of our simulation curriculum.

Aligning a Simulation Curriculum With Other Curriculum Components

Simulation-based education is not touted to replace all other teaching methodologies incorporated into a curricular plan. Rather, it serves as an excellent adjunct

(Adapted from Issenberg,[50] with permission.)

to what already exists in most program blueprints. It cannot replace actual clinical experience as the ultimate teaching methodology, assuming the experience meets accreditation and practice standards. Simulation is not only applicable to teaching students; it is another technique for assessing if a student has accomplished educational objectives. The use of simulation as an assessment strategy (formative or summative) is full of challenges,[54] and a comprehensive discussion of simulation as an assessment method is well beyond the scope of this book.

Simulation's Position in Miller's Pyramid

In the medical education literature, any discussion of curriculum components unfailingly calls up the framework for clinical assessment proposed by Miller[55] in 1990, often referred to as Miller's pyramid of assessment levels, which is built from the bottom up:

- *Knows* (knowledge) is the broad base of the pyramid and pertains to the recall of facts, principles, and theories. Traditionally it is assessed via written examinations, usually multiple-choice questions.
- *Knows how* (competence) refers to the ability of a practitioner to acquire information from a variety of sources, analyze the information, and then make rational judgments in the form of a diagnosis or a management plan; this is primarily assessed via case-based, problem-oriented essay examinations or oral examinations.
- *Shows how* (performance) was the innovative concept when Miller proposed his performance pyramid. Miller was a strong advocate of simulation via standardized patients in an objective structured clinical examination. He opined that research should focus on providing concrete evidence in support of this educational and assessment methodology. Miller's original discourse includes an observation about the "astonishing array of physical abnormalities [that]

can be simulated"[55] and discusses how students' performance in such realistic situations is invaluable to assessing competency. Thus, it is reasonable to infer that Miller would have wholeheartedly supported the use of HFMB simulation to assess the *Shows how* level of competency.

- *Does* (action) is the top level of the pyramid and refers to assessment of a clinical practitioner when functioning independently (ie, without the presence of supervisory personnel); assessment at this level is currently approached via different techniques (eg, provider case records, or multirater feedback), which usually are not (but may be) simulation based.

Simulation's Role in Assessment of Core Competencies

High-fidelity manikin-based simulation learning activities fit well into a schema for assessing a student's attainment of an anesthesia program's educational outcomes, or at least their progress toward outcome attainment. Samuel Merritt University, like all institutions of higher education, requires each academic department to delineate a plan indicating how they measure and document students' attainment of both the department's and the institution's established core competencies. A substantial component of the SMU Program of Nurse Anesthesia "Core Competency Assessment Plan" involves our SBL activities, which address the *Shows how* level of assessment. Figure 20.4 illustrates some of our assessment mechanisms for key program and

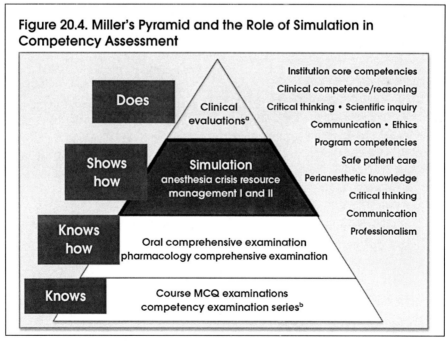

Figure 20.4. Miller's Pyramid and the Role of Simulation in Competency Assessment

Does	Clinical evaluations[a]
Shows how	**Simulation** anesthesia crisis resource management I and II
Knows how	Oral comprehensive examination pharmacology comprehensive examination
Knows	Course MCQ examinations competency examination series[b]

Institution core competencies
Clinical competence/reasoning
Critical thinking • Scientific inquiry
Communication • Ethics
Program competencies
Safe patient care
Perianesthetic knowledge
Critical thinking
Communication
Professionalism

(Adapted from Samuel Merritt University assessment mechanisms.)
[a] Clinical evaluations refer to assessment of graduates. The does level represents performance in the professional practice environment.
[b] This series comprises multiple-choice questions, randomly presented and grouped in the categories of the CCNA National Certification Examination, administered via the e-learning platform Blackboard.

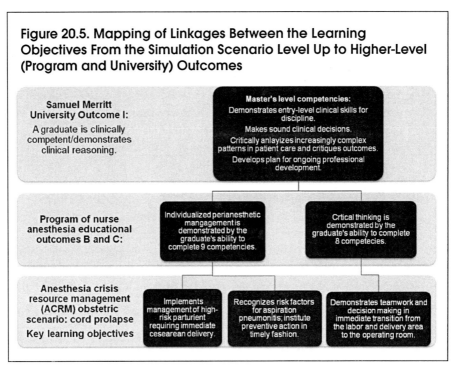

Figure 20.5. Mapping of Linkages Between the Learning Objectives From the Simulation Scenario Level Up to Higher-Level (Program and University) Outcomes

(Adapted with permission from Samuel Merritt University, Oakland, California.)

institutional competencies, represented in the context of Miller's assessment pyramid. Specific metrics for each student are recorded for each of the assessment activities (eg, multiple-choice question examinations, the competency examination series, pharmacology comprehensive and oral comprehensive examinations, and the ACRM sessions in which the student was an active participant in the scenario). Additionally, an electronic portfolio is compiled for each student, consisting of digitized recordings of key SBL activities throughout the curriculum (items 4, 9, 10, 12, 14, and 15 in Appendix 20.1). This provides a visual record of progress made throughout the course of the curriculum, especially since each recording is associated with a completed activity-specific assessment instrument.

One final aspect of using simulation as an assessment strategy is the concept of linking learning objectives for an SBL activity to outcomes and competencies upward through the curriculum. Ideally each objective of an activity (eg, an ACRM scenario) will logically link to a program outcome, which will subsequently link to a core university competency. Figure 20.5 illustrates 1 set of many linkages that would exist throughout a simulation-based curriculum, and the snapshots from a digitized recording of a simulation (Figure 20.6) provide examples of the physical evidence of the learning and assessment session. Simulation methodologies are powerful mechanisms in the academic setting, and they have the potential to provide compelling evidence of a program curriculum's effectiveness.

Figure 20.6. CRNA Simulation-Based Education

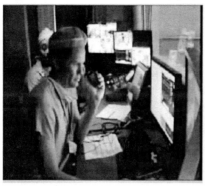 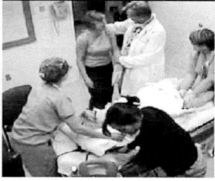

Nurse Anesthesia simulation faculty controlling a patient simulator via computer and observing an ACRM scenario while completing the assessment instrument (left); screenshot from the digitized recording of the cord prolapse scenario showing transition from the labor and delivery department to the operating room (right). This section of the recording demonstrates the teamwork and decision-making learning objective noted in the graphic in Figure 20.5. The student is wearing the scrub cap.

Summary

The undeniable connections between simulation in healthcare and patient safety initiatives make it imperative that nurse anesthesia education programs have strong simulation-based curricular components. Although the evidence is not unequivocal that patient outcomes are improved by simulation training, the indirect evidence is compelling and the face validity of the methodologies is high. The case for effective learning with the use of high-fidelity simulation has been made. Thus, simulation, especially high-fidelity manikin-based simulation, should no longer be viewed by educators as technology that is simply nice to have. It should be perceived as an innovative technique to incorporate with other strategies for learning and part of an ongoing plan for program growth and curriculum development. Most experts agree that it is only a matter of time before simulation-based education becomes the norm, and eventually, the standard for nursing (all levels) and physician (medical school and postgraduate) education.

Fortunately for us in the field of anesthesiology, from whence the true pioneers of medical simulation came (including some very innovative nurse anesthetists), there are volumes of scientific studies about all aspects of simulation that are directly relevant to our practice. The technology is almost tailor-made for our training and educational requirements. A generation of experienced simulation experts and enthusiasts are available as resources. The simulation literature is growing richer by the day with contributions from all facets of the healthcare disciplines, often with collaborative, multidisciplinary themes. Contemporary, neuroscience-based educational theory (brain-based learning) is enhancing the strong social psychology-based framework of experiential learning that is fundamental to simulation-based learning.

A successful simulation program has a carefully constructed, adaptable curriculum that uses the various simulators in ways that maximize the simulators' functionality. Simulation-based learning activities must be focused on clear learning objectives and considered integral to the rest of the curriculum. This encourages collaboration among faculty members and can help spread the contagious enthusiasm that simulation often causes. I hope the examples in this chapter have piqued the interest of those whose programs have not yet started a simulation curriculum, have raised more questions for those who engage in simulation-based education, and have encouraged those who passionately advocate for this methodology to network and collaborate.

Glossary

Anesthesia crisis resource management (ACRM): A training course that uses high-fidelity manikin-based simulation, structured around learning objectives specifically focused on principles of complex problem solving, decision making, resource management, and teamwork behaviors. A course generally entails learners actively engaging in a series of simulated clinical situations that are constructed to facilitate their abilities to prevent, ameliorate, and resolve critical incidents and crisis situations. A key feature of ACRM-type courses is the opportunity for learners to interact intensely and realistically with each other and to reflect on their experiences through debriefing sessions.

Debriefing: Universally considered to be the crucial component of simulation-based, immersive learning, healthcare simulation debriefings are facilitated conversations among learners involved in a particular simulation exercise. These conversations generally (but not always) occur immediately after a simulation scenario, and they are guided to allow participants to explore, analyze, and make sense of their actions, thought processes, and emotional responses during the particular simulation. Debriefing facilitators should be individuals trained to ensure that the conversations between learners meet established criteria for optimal learning.

High-fidelity manikin-based simulation: An educational technique that employs the use of a full-scale human patient (manikin) simulator, capable of manifesting realistic physiologic responses, either via computer-generated responses observed on the manikin or its associated vital sign monitor. High fidelity refers to a high degree of accuracy not only in the simulation of a human patient but also in the reproduction of the environment in which the patient/manikin is placed. Accurate reproductions of environments include physical, environmental, and psychological levels of reality.

Human factors: The spectrum of factors that results in the way people think and feel and interact with each other and their environment and thus influence, positively and negatively, decisions made and actions taken. Human factors influence behavior at an individual, team, and organizational level.

Objective structured clinical examination: A method used in healthcare professional education programs to assess the competence level of learners in certain clinical skills. The term *objective* refers to the fact that (1) the performance assessment is criterion-based and results in quantifiable metrics, and (2) trained, standardized patients (a form of simulators) are involved instead of real patients. The term *structured* is used because the OSCEs are formatted as a series of interactive, objective-focused stations that the learner experiences in a preplanned, systematic manner, and each station has an associated assessment checklist that is completed by the individuals evaluating the learner (eg, the standardized patient and/or a faculty member/instructor). The OSCE was initially introduced in 1975 as a method for assessing medical student competency. This type of simulation-based methodology is now commonly used in medical, nursing, allied health, and basic science curricula.

Point-of-care simulation: High-fidelity manikin-based simulation that is implemented in actual patient care settings—points of care. The term is used synonymously with *in situ* simulation. This type of simulation-based methodology has the potential advantages of (1) reduced cost of implementation (as compared to simulations implemented in a simulation center), (2) opportunities for individuals and teams who normally work together to undergo simulation training together, and (3) opportunities to identify system or organizational issues that may exist as barriers to safe patient care.

Scenario: A structured learning activity that uses some type of simulator (usually a manikin-based simulator) as the teaching tool. A clinical simulation scenario is essentially a scripted vignette in which learners are engaged. Scenarios are based on specific learning objectives and a few key lessons. All components of the scenario should serve to accomplish the set objectives.

Session: Learning activities consisting of a series of simulation scenarios that together meet an established objective of an educational curriculum. The purpose of distinguishing between a scenario and a session is that the logistics of planning and implementing a single scenario vs multiple scenarios entails different, but related skill sets, both scenarios and sessions are important for educators to understand and master when implementing a simulation-based curriculum.

Simulation: Simulation is a technique—not a technology—to replace or amplify real experiences with guided experiences that evoke or replicate substantial aspects of the real world in a fully interactive manner.[2]

Standardized patient (SP): An SP is a person who has been specifically trained to simulate a patient so accurately that the simulation cannot be detected by a skilled clinician. In performing as the simulator, the SP presents the gestalt of the patient being simulated, not just the history, but the body language, the physical findings, and the emotional and personality characteristics as well. Standardized patients can contribute to the performance evaluation of clinicians by completing a validated assessment tool after each simulation encounter.

References

1. Gaba DM. Improving anesthesiologists' performance by simulating reality. *Anesthesiology.* 1992;76(4):494.

2. Gaba DM. The future vision of simulation in health care. *Qual Saf Health Care.* 2004;13(suppl 1):i2-i10.

3. Turcato N, Robertson C, Covert K. Simulation-based education: what's in it for the nurse anesthesia educators? *AANA J.* August 2008;76(4):257-262.

4. Hamman WR. The complexity of team training: what we have learned from aviation and its applications to medicine. *Qual Saf Health Care.* 2004;13(suppl 1):i72-i79.

5. Hunt EA, Shilkofski NA, Stavroudis TA, Nelson KL. Simulation: translation to improved team performance. *Anesthesiology Clinics.* June 2007;25(2):301-319.

6. Gaba DM, Howard SK, Fish KJ, Smith BE, Sowb YA. Simulation-based training in anesthesia crisis resource management (ACRM): a decade of experience. *Simulation and Gaming.* 2001;32(2):175-193.

7. O'Donnell J, Fletcher J, Dixon B, Palmer L. Planning and implementing an anesthesia crisis resource management course for student nurse anesthetists. *CRNA.* 1998;9(2):50-58.

8. Fletcher J. ERR WATCH: Anesthesia crisis resource management from the nurse anesthetist's perspective. *AANA J.* 1998;66(6):595-602.

9. Kohn LT, Corrigan JM, Donaldson MS. *To Err Is Human: Building a Safer Health System.* Washington, DC: National Academy Press; 1999.

10. Wachter RM, Shojania KG, Duncan BW, McDonald KM. Making health care safer: a critical analysis of patient safety practices. Evidence Report/ Technology Assessment No. 43. Rockville, MD: Agency for Healthcare Research and Quality; July 2001.

11. AHRQ awards more than $5 million to study the safe delivery of health care through medical simulation. [press release]. Rockville, MD: Agency for Health Care Research and Quality; November 13, 2006.

12. Eder-Van Hook J. Building a national agenda for simulation-based medical education. [Report]. Telemedicine and Advanced Technology Research Center, US Army Medical Research and Materiel Command. July 30 2004. Medical Simulation Organization website. www.medsim.org/articles/ AIMS_2004_Report_Simulation-based_Medical_Training.pdf. Accessed May 20, 2009.

13. Dawson S, Alverson D, Bowyer M, Eder-Van Hook J, Waters RJ. The complementary roles of the advanced initiative in medical simulation and the society for simulation in healthcare. *Simul Healthc.* 2007;2(1):30-32.

14. Ziv A, Rubin O, Sidi A, Berkenstadt H. Credentialing and certifying with simulation. *Anesthesiol Clin.* 2007;25(2):261-269.

15. Berkenstadt H, Ziv A, Sidi A. Incorporated simulation-based objective structured clinical examination into the Israeli National Board Examination in Anesthesiology. *Anesth Analg.* 2006;102(3):853-858.

16. Sinz E. Simulation-based education for cardiac, thoracic, and vascular anesthesiology. *Semin Cardiothorac Vasc Anesth.* 2005;9(4):291-307.

17. Blum RH, Raemer DB, Carroll JS, Neelakantan S, Felstein DL, Cooper JB. Crisis resource management training for anesthesia faculty: a new approach to continuing education. *Med Educ.* 2004;38(1):45-55.

18. Gardner R, Walzer TB, Simon R, Raemer DB. Obstetric simulation as a risk control strategy: course design and evaluation. *Simul Healthc.* 2008;3(2):119-127.

19. McCarthy J, Cooper JB. Malpractice insurance carrier provides premium incentive for simulation-based training and believes it has made a difference. *Anesth Patient Saf Found Newsletter.* 2007;22(1):489.

20. Merwin E, Stern S, Jordan LM. Supply, demand, and equilibrium in the market for CRNAs. *AANA J.* 2006;74(4):287-293.

21. Frand J. The information-age mindset: changes in students and implications for higher education. *EDUCAUSE Review.* 2000;35(5):15-24.

22. Oblinger DG. Boomers, Gen-Xers, and Millennials: understanding the "new students." *EDUCAUSE Review.* 2003;38(4):37-47.

23. Glavin RJ. When simulation should and should not be in the curriculum. In: Kyle RR, Murray WB, eds. *Clinical Simulation:Operations, Engineering and Management.* Amsterdam, The Netherlands: Elsevier; 2008:71-75.

24. Medley CF, Horne C. Using simulation technology for undergraduate nursing education. *J Nurs Educ.* 2005;44(1):31-34.

25. Dunn WF. *Simulators in Critical Care and Beyond.* Des Plaines, IL: Society of Critical Care Medicine; 2004:15-23.

26. Henson LC, Lee AC. *Simulators in Anesthesiology Education.* Rochester, NY: Springer; 1998:1-8,23-28,29-37.

27. Loyd GE, Lake CL, Greenberg RB. *Practical Health Care Simulations:* Louisville, KY, Elsevier Mosby; 2004:205-244,245-281.

28. Kyle RR, Murray WB. *Clinical Simulation:Operations, Engineering and Management.* Amsterdam, The Netherlands: Elsevier; 2008:71-75, 77-84,135-151.

29. Kolb DA. *Experiential Learning: Experience as the Source of Learning and Development.* Englewood Cliffs, NJ: Prentice Hall; 1984:21-37.

30. Nummela-Caine R, Caine G, McClintic C, Klimek KJ. *12 Brain/Mind Learning Principles in Action: Developing Executive Functions of the Human Brain.* 2nd ed. Thousand Oaks, CA: Corwin Press; 2009:1-18,21-37.

31. Jensen E. *Brain-Based Learning: The New Paradigm of Teaching.* 2nd ed. Thousand Oaks, CA: Corwin Press; 2008:1-17,141-153,200-233.

32. Zull JE. *The Art of Changing the Brain: Enriching the Practice of Teaching By Exploring the Biology of Learning.* Sterling, VA: Stylus; 2002:13-88.

33. Sousa DA. *How the Brain Learns.* 3rd ed. Thousand Oaks, CA: Corwin Press; 2006:248-260.

34. Oravitz TM, Metro DG, McIvor WR. The benefits of a human simulator training course for initial first-year anesthesia residency education. *Open Anesthesiol J.* 2008;2:13-19. http://www.bentham.org/open/toatj/index.htm. Accessed May 20, 2009.

35. Park CS, Rochlen LR, Yaghmour EA, Deleon AM, McCarthy R. Assessing performance for safety and competence in novice residents using high-fidelity simulation. ASA Abstracts. *Anesthesiology.* 2008;109(A760-).

36. Cooke JM, Larsen J, Hamstra SJ, Andreatta PB. Simulation enhances resident confidence in critical care and procedural skills. *Fam Med.* 2008;40(3):165-167.

37. Vandrey C, Whitman M. Simulator training for novice critical care nurses. *Am J Nurs.* 2001;101(9):24GG-24LL.

38. Kozmenko V, Kaye AD, Morgan B, Hilton CW. Theory and practice of developing an effective simulation-based clinical curriculum. In: Kyle RR, Murray WB, eds. *Clinical Simulation:Operations, Engineering, and Management.* Amsterdam, The Netherlands: Elsevier; 2008:135-151.

39. The Joint Commission Universal Protocol: Hospitals. 2008. Joint commission website. http://www.jointcommission.org/NR/rdonlyres/AEA17A06-BB67-4C4E-B0FC-DD195FE6BF2A/0/UP_HAP_20080616.pdf. Accessed March 26, 2009.

40. SBAR technique for communication: a situational briefing model. Institute for Healthcare Improvement website. 2005. www.ihi.org/IHI/Topics/PatientSafety/SafetyGeneral/Tools/SBARTechniqueforCommunicationA SituationalBriefingModel.htm. Accessed 26 March 2009.

41. The circle of learning. Laerdal Medical Corporation website. www.laerdal.info/document.asp?docID=6681900. Accessed May 13, 2009.

42. Jeffries PR, ed. *Simulation in Nursing Education: From Conceptualization to Evaluation:* New York, NY: National League for Nursing; 2007:22-23.

43. Gallagher CJ, Issenberg SB. *Simulation in Anesthesia.* Philadelphia, PA: Saunders Elsevier; 2007:277-341.

44. Seropian MA. General concepts in full-scale simulation: getting started. *Anesth Analg.* 2003;97(6):1695–1705.

45. Fletcher GCL, Flin RH, McGeorge P, Glavin RJ, Maran NJ, Patey R. Anaesthetists' non-technical skills (ANTS): evaluation of a behavioural marker system. *Br J Anaesth.* 2003;90(5):580-588.

46. Fletcher GCL, McGeorge P, Flin RH, Gavin RJ, Maran NJ. The role of non-technical skills in anaesthesia: a review of current literature. *Br J Anaesth.* 2002;88(3):418-429.

47. Nance JJ. *Why Hospitals Should Fly: The Ultimate Flight Plan to Patient Safety and Quality Care.* Bozeman, MT: Second River Healthcare Press; 2009:vii-ix,11-32.

48. St. Pierre M, Hofinger G, Buerschaper C. *Crisis Management in Acute Care Settings—Human Factors and Team Psychology in a High Stakes Environment.* Berlin, Germany: Springer-Verlag; 2008:4-15.

49. Boulet JR, Murray D, Kras J, Woodhouse J. Setting performance standards for mannequin-based acute-care scenarios: an examinee-centered approach. *Simul Healthc.* 2008;3(2):72-81.

50. Henrichs BM, Avidan MS, Murray DJ, et al. Performance of Certified Registered Nurse Anesthetists and anesthesiologists in a simulation-based skills assessment. *Anesth Analg.* 2009;108(1):255-262.

51. McIntosh CA. Lake Wobegon for anesthesia . . . where everyone is above average except those who aren't: variability in the management of simulated intraoperative critical incidents. *Anesth Analg.* 2009;108(1):6-9.

52. McGaghie SC, Issenberg SB, Petrussa ER, Scalese RJ. Effect of practice on standardised learning outcomes in simulation-based medical education. *Med Educ.* 2006;40(8):792-797.

53. Issenberg SB, McGaghie WC, Petrussa ER, Gordon DL, Scalese RJ. Features and uses of high-fidelity medical simulations that lead to effective learning: a BEME systematic review. *Med Teach.* 2005;27(1):10-28.

54. Glavin RJ, Gaba DM. Challenges and opportunities in simulation and assessment. *Simul Healthc.* 2008;3(2):69-71.

55. Miller GE. The assessment of clinical skills/competence/performance. *Acad Med.* 1990;65(9 suppl):S63-S67.

Appendix 20.1. Exemplar of Simulation-Based Learning Integrated Into a Curriculum

Simulation-based learning (SBL) activity	Methodology: brief description	Curriculum placement (Integrated nurse anesthesia curriculum format) — Semester, clinical phase / Title of course / Primary goal of activity	Hours per student
1. Introduction to simulation concepts	Lecture/discussion: Orientation of new students to the conceptual foundations of simulation, tour of simulation facility	Semester 1, preclinical / Basic Principles I / Establish ground rules for SBL sessions, explain program philosophy, establish relaxed alertness environment.[a]	4
2. Orientation to operating room (OR) environment	Experiential activity: Orientation to OR work environment (all aspects)	Semester 1, preclinical / Basic Principles I / Establish sensory familiarity with the environment and general overview of team roles early in training.	2
3. Introduction to Induction: general endotracheal anesthesia (GETA)	Demonstration with HFMBS[b]; Modeling by various faculty of proper sequencing, technique, decision-making	Semester 1, preclinical / Basic Principles I / Provide exemplars for psychomotor, cognitive, and affective skills for basic induction.	3
4. Preoperative planning sessions, supervised practice of GETA, or general anesthesia with Laryngeal Mask Airway (LMA)	Lecture/discussion/group work/role playing, experiential activity with HFMBS; 3 case-based lectures, each followed by mock preoperative assessment exercise (fellow student plays role of patient). Student develops anesthetic plan, presents plan to faculty (preceptor), Implements Induction under supervision; Incrementally complex patients.	Semester 1, preclinical / Basic Principles I / Develop assessment and clinical reasoning skills; early bridging of theory to practice (actual implementation of a plan). Note: Students are also provided frequent opportunities to practice induction-emergence sequences for GETA or GA-LMA with faculty assistance available outside course hours.	12
5. Technical skills workshops (not a comprehensive listing of sessions)	Lecture/discussion, experiential activity: Didactic instruction followed by repetitive, supervised practice utilizing an array of task trainers/simulators Including: • Airway trainers (basic and difficult) • Back simulators • Central venous access/peripheral nerve block trainer (ultrasound capability) • SimSuite (central venous access simulator for cardiology, which is housed in a simulation center at a clinical affiliate site) • Task trainers for fiberoptic intubation skills development (including dexterity trainer) • Arterial line insertion task trainer	Semester 1, preclinical / Basic Principles I / Basic airway management Semester 1, preclinical / Basic Principles I / Advanced airway management I (includes basic fiberoptic intubation skills) Semester 1, preclinical / Basic Principles I / Subarachnoid block (SAB)/epidural Insertion/management (basics) Semester 2, clinical phase I / Basic Principles II / SAB/epidural insertion/management Semester 2, clinical phase I / Basic Principles II / Peripheral nerve block insertion/management	8 7 8 4 12

#	Activity	Method	Details	No.
			Semester 3 or 4, clinical phase II — Advanced Principles I or II — Advanced airway management II (difficult airway management and neonatal resuscitation program)	8
			Semester 3, clinical phase I — Advanced Principles I — Thoracic anesthesia airway management	3
			Semester 3, 4, or 5, clinical phase II — Advanced Principles I or II — Central venous line and pulmonary artery catheter insertion using the SimSuite (via arrangements with University of California, Davis Medical Center Simulation Center)	4
6.	Anesthesia machine seminars	Lecture/demonstration, experiential activity: Hands-on practice with machine check, troubleshooting during manikin-based simulation scenarios; Computer based simulation (in process)[c]	Semester 1, Preclinical — Basic Principles I — Focus of initial seminars is on basic competence and safety; all subsequent HFMBS scenarios include opportunities to reinforce competencies related to anesthesia machine operation and troubleshooting.	14
7.	Advanced health assessment skills workshops	Lecture/demonstration, experiential activity using: Harvey cardiopulmonary simulator (IP); Standardized patients culminating in objective structured clinical examination (OSCE)[c]	Semester 1, preclinical — Advanced health assessment (curricular revision in progress to meet anticipated 2009 Council on Accreditation of Nurse Anesthesia Educational Programs requirement); Refinement of assessment skills (for both preoperative and postoperative patients)	8 anticipated
8.	Clinical Orientation Workshop	Demonstration, experiential: Series of hands-on workshops comprising teaching stations (with preceptors) dedicated to essential anesthetic tasks and skills: Drug and equipment set-up; Positioning and monitoring; Documentation; Sterile technique for neuraxial block placement; Malignant hyperthermia protocol; Basic pediatric drug and equipment set-up	Semester 1, preclinical — Basic Principles I — Reinforce concepts from lectures and previous laboratory sessions, foster students' confidence and ability to practice safely during initiation to clinical residency. Note: These station-based workshops entail a substantial use of the teaching services of selected senior nurse anesthesia students as preceptors (with faculty supervision) In appropriate stations. This strategy transforms the activity into an experiential learning session for the senior students as well as those they are teaching.	8
9.	Assessment of preparedness to enter clinical residency	Experiential activity with HFMBS: Student completes a basic case from preoperative assessment (of standardized patient) including presentation of plan to preceptor, presurgical briefings (Joint Commission protocols), induction, emergence, and postanesthesia care unit.	Semester 1, preclinical — Basic Principles I (end of semester) — Assess basic competency with essential knowledge, skills, and behaviors related to a basic induction of general anesthesia associated with a common postinduction/postemergence anesthetic complication; foster student confidence and ability to practice safely during initiation to clinical residency. Note: Students must attain a threshold numerical score on the assessment checklist used for this mock induction - emergence session in order to progress into the clinical curriculum. Remediation opportunities are available if the student does not succeed on first attempt.	4

Appendix 20.1. Exemplar of Simulation-Based Learning Integrated Into a Curriculum (continued)

10. Pathophysiology integrative simulation sessions	Experiential with mid-fidelity MBS: Two, 4-hour sessions in triads who are presented with scenarios related to a pathophysiologic state recently studied. Students required to plan for and implement preoperative preparation of the patient followed by induction, maintenance, and emergence; common complications (mild-severe degrees) are included as part of the scenario; described as mid-fidelity because full-scale intraoperative setting is not simulated during maintenance and intermittent teaching occurs during scenario. Experiential activity with computer-based simulation.	Semester 2, clinical phase I Pathophysiology and Basic Principles II Reinforce physiology and pathophysiology concepts gained via reading, lecture/discussions, and clinical experience; clinical reasoning and decision making also a focus. Example: scenario involving airway and other pulmonary issues follows the pulmonary pathophysiology lectures. MicroSim[d] computer simulation course assignments include completion of certain case studies that complement learning by other described modalities.	8
11. Pediatric GETA mock induction sessions	Lecture/discussion, experiential activity with HFMBS: Each student is required to prepare for and implement a GETA induction on an infant.	Semester 2, clinical phase I Basic Principles II Application of principles of pediatric anesthetic management to practice; foster student confidence and safe practice before first encounter with pediatric patient during clinical experience.	4
12. High-risk obstetric anesthesia simulation sessions	Experiential activity with HFMBS and standardized patients: Seminar in ACRM-type° format with all scenarios related to high-risk obstetrical patients. These are multidisciplinary learner sessions with both nurse anesthesia and maternal-child health nursing students participating.	Semester 4, clinical phase II Advanced Principles I Reinforcement of obstetrical anesthesia management principles obtained via reading, lecture/discussions, and clinical experience, with emphasis on clinical reasoning and decision making; major concepts of anesthesia nontechnical skills (ANTS) are introduced.	8
13. Neuroanesthesia and trauma anesthesia simulation sessions	Experiential activity with HFMBS and standardized patients: Seminar in ACRM-like format with all scenarios related either to neurosurgical or trauma patients. Multidisciplinary learners will likely be present.	Semester 4, clinical phase II Advanced Principles II Reinforce neuroanesthesia and trauma anesthesia management principles obtained via reading, lecture/discussions, and clinical experience, with emphasis on clinical reasoning, decision making, and continued development of ANTS.	8
14. Anesthesia crisis resource management I (ACRM)	Lecture/discussion, experiential activity with HFMBS: Sessions using the ACRM format described by Gaba Six, complex, full-scale scenarios (both adult and pediatric) situated in a variety of anesthetizing locations (operating room, post operative patient room, interventional radiology suite) are presented to groups of 6 learners.	Semester 6, clinical phase III Master of Science in Nursing Synthesis requirement[f]. Build upon the goals delineated for activities 12 and 13, and refine ANTS. Nonanesthesia healthcare personnel are often members of the faculty/staff that present the scenarios to the students, thus providing an interprofessional component to the learning.	10

15. Anesthesia crisis resource management II	Experiential activity with HFMBS: ACRM session as described above. Scenarios are more complex and include 2 obstetric situations.	Semester 7, clinical phase III Master of Science in Nursing Synthesis requirement. Further refine all skills described above and conduct emphatic discussion with learners during debriefings to bring the team training lessons into their clinical practice as CRNAs	8
16. Interdisciplinary simulation sessions with podiatric medicine students (Selected students are provided this optional opportunity.)	Experiential activity with HFMBS: Nurse anesthesia students take the role of instructor for second-year podiatric medical students who are enrolled in a clinical rotation run entirely in the simulation center to prepare them for hospital and clinic rotations.	Semester 6 or 7, clinical phase III Clinical Anesthesia V or VI Primary goal of nurse anesthesia students: Instruct podiatric peers in the proper execution of presurgical briefings, and facilitate the development of interpersonal and communication skills between anesthetists and surgeons during a conscious sedation/local anesthetic case, and during an intraoperative crisis (eg, anaphylaxis).	4

(Adapted with permission from Samuel Merritt University (SMU) Program of Nurse Anesthesia)

[a] The optimal emotional state for learning as defined by Caine;[29] see Table 3 for definition and reference.

[b] HFMBS: High-fidelity, manikin-based simulation. The SMU inventory of full-body patient simulators includes: multiple SimMan and SimBaby simulators (Laerdal Medical Corporation, Wappinger Falls, NY); Noelle with Newborn Hal (Gaumard Scientific, Miami, FL); multiple mid-level manikins: Vital Sim family and ALS simulator (Laerdal).

[c] See glossary.

[d] MicroSim (Laerdal Medical Corporation, Wappinger Falls, NY): self-directed, computer screen-based simulator provides learner with realistic, interactive case scenarios.

[e] ACRM indicates anesthesia crisis resource management. "ACRM-type" refers to the fact that the debriefing periods for these sessions have more of an instructional teaching component (relative to the clinical topic of the scenarios) vs true ACRM sessions.

[f] The SMU Master of Science in Nursing Synthesis is a master's thesis equivalent. Nurse anesthesia students meet this requirement via completion of comprehensive exams (written and oral) and completion of ACRM I and II, as described in the table.

Appendix 20.2. Additional Simulation-Based Learning Activities Under Consideration for Integration Into Samuel Merritt University Curriculum

Simulation based learning (SBL) activity	Methodology: brief description	Curriculum placement - integrated curriculum Proposed semester, clinical phase in program Title of course Primary goal of activity	Hours per student
1. Advanced cardiac life support (ACLS) algorithm competency assessment	Experiential activity with mannequin-based simulation (without full, high-fidelity context): Student is presented with a series of short scenarios that would require proficiency with ACLS, PALS and DAA algorithms or common protocols for managing common intraoperative critical events. Performance is observed, using standardized checklist /evaluation tool (to be determined). **Assessments will be low stakes, due to continued need for reliable and valid tool for simulation-based assessments.**	Semester 1, clinical phase I Clinical Anesthesia II Assess proficiency with ACLS skill set in perioperative setting.	8
2. Pediatric advanced life support (PALS) algorithm competency assessment		Semester 2, clinical phase I Clinical Anesthesia III Assess proficiency with PALS skill set in perioperative setting.	8
3. Difficult airway algorithm (DAA) competency assessment		Semester 5, clinical phase II Clinical Anesthesia IV Assess knowledge of difficult airway algorithm and proficiency with adjunct airway equipment used during difficult airway situations.	8
4. Acute intraoperative critical event management skills assessment		Semester 6 and 7, clinical phase III Clinical Anesthesia V and VI Assess proficiency with skills required to recognize and manage common and serious acute intraoperative events.	8

(Adapted with permission from Samuel Merritt University, Oakland, California.)

Chapter 21

Testing the Student's Knowledge

Vicki Coopmans, CRNA, PhD

Key Points

- Effective teaching and testing are based on clearly defined student learning objectives.

- Good test questions address important content and are well-constructed.

- The instructor should provide clear examination instructions and expectations to the student.

- The instructor should develop scoring and grading methods in advance.

Introduction

There are a variety of ways to assess student knowledge in the didactic setting; however, developing effective measures can be quite challenging. Anyone who has ever been responsible for writing examination questions can appreciate that it is easier said than done as evidenced by the following concerns often voiced by students:

1. The content on the examination was not covered in class.
2. The questions were:
    a. too vague.
    b. confusing.
    c. poorly worded.
    d. tricky.
    e. too complicated.
    f. overly time consuming.
3. The "book" says something different.

The intention of this chapter is to provide guidance on selecting and developing testing modalities that will appropriately reflect mastery of content and generate little or no protest from those being evaluated.

Purpose

This chapter will provide an overview of testing methods in the didactic setting with particular attention to multiple-choice questions (MCQs). The National Certification Examination (NCE) and Self-Evaluation Examination (SEE) have traditionally been administered using MCQs using the single-best-answer format, although alternative item formats are currently being considered to supplement the MCQ format. Both are computerized adaptive tests (CATs), in which the questions are selected and administered dynamically, such that the difficulty of the questions is targeted to the estimated ability level of the examinee. The difficulty of the test questions is calibrated using item response theory (IRT). Item response theory is a type of mathematical model that determines the difficulty of questions based on responses from a pilot sample of examinees. Once the questions have been calibrated according to their difficulty, IRT can also be used to estimate the examinee's ability.

The development of valid test questions is a rigorous process, and it is necessary to calibrate a large bank of test questions in order to administer a CAT. New questions must be analyzed and evaluated before being added to the test bank. There are several statistical software platforms that include IRT item analysis. The use of CATs and IRT generally exceeds the resources of individual nurse anesthesia programs, but many do use MCQ format throughout their curricula to prepare students for the types of questions they will see on the SEE and NCE. For this reason, most of this chapter will be devoted to the use and development of MCQs. Essay testing will also be reviewed and some creative assessment techniques will be introduced.

Teaching and Testing

Before I address the process of test construction, I will present a discussion of the relationship between teaching and testing and other general testing concepts. Teaching has been defined as the act of imparting knowledge.[1] Testing has been described as a method for determining the "skill, knowledge, intelligence, capacities, or aptitudes of an individual or group."[2] The work of imparting knowledge and then measuring that knowledge in the student are inextricably wedded and challenging to accomplish. For instruction to be successful, the learner must be informed of the expected outcomes. Effective teaching is based on clearly identifying and defining these outcomes, which are generally expressed as learning objectives. It is upon these learning objectives that tests should be developed. Thus, both teaching and testing methods are designed and carried out based on the student learning objectives developed by the instructor.

There are 2 basic types of assessment: norm-referenced and criterion-referenced. The purpose of norm-referenced testing is to determine how well learners perform in relation to one another. Norm-referenced testing can be used to distinguish between low and high achievers. This type of assessment ranks how the examinee performs within the group, and it is sometimes referred to as "grading on a curve." This means that a certain small proportion of students will receive an A or an F and the rest will fall somewhere in between. Norm-referenced testing has been said to interfere with student learning and to suborn unhealthy competition for grades.[3]

Criterion-referenced assessment is used to determine mastery of a specific set of skills and/or concepts. The NCE is based on criterion-referenced principles with the purpose of establishing the level of knowledge and skills necessary to perform as an entry-level practitioner.[4] The National Council Licensure Examination for Registered Nurses is also criterion-referenced.[5] It is generally agreed that criterion-referenced testing is preferable because it is intended to ensure the level of competency necessary for safe practice.[3,6-8] Theoretically, all examinees could either pass or fail, depending on whether the established benchmark has been met. With norm-referenced testing, an individual could still pass without meeting minimum standards if the rest of the learners performed poorly. The primary goal of nurse anesthesia educational programs is to prepare competent anesthesia practitioners; it is important to consider this when selecting the type of assessment to be used.

Testing Methods

There are various methods available for measuring student knowledge in the didactic setting, such as MCQs; short answer questions, essay tests, written assignments, and oral examinations. Some more creative assessment techniques include concept mapping, journal assignments, and portfolio development.

Multiple Choice Items

Multiple choice items can be divided into 2 basic groups: true or false questions and single-best-answer questions. True or false questions require the examinee to select all responses that are correct. The single-best-answer questions, (also referred to as 1-best-answer questions) require selection of the correct or most appropriate response.

Single-Best-Answer Questions

The classic 1-best-answer MCQ model includes a single stem (an introductory question or statement), a correct response, and 3 or 4 distractors. Other single-best-answer questions include matching and extended-matching questions (R-type questions[9]).

Regardless of the type of question used, the choice should be based on content addressed by predetermined learning objectives and should be well constructed. Poorly-worded items can have the unintended consequence of either unfairly assisting or penalizing examinees.[10,11] Well-accepted item-writing guidelines and many examples of flawed item construction have been presented in numerous publications.[9,12-14] Recommendations for the development of each component and various types of the MCQ will be reviewed.

As describe earlier, all MCQ begin with a stem. The stem can take the form of a question (closed stem), an incomplete statement (open stem), or a description of a situation or issue, and should be developed with the factors listed in Table 21.1.

All examination items should measure a specific, important learning objective. The stem should be clear and grammatically correct both alone and in combination with the responses. The examinee should not have to read through the responses to discern the central concept of the question. Extraneous information not relevant to the purpose of the question should be avoided to minimize examinee confusion; however, the stem should have the necessary information and be focused so that all responses fall within a single subject area. Stems with negative wording should be used sparingly, if at all, because they add unnecessary difficulty to the question. When used, the negative word should be capitalized, bolded, and/or underlined. Some examples of stem format include:

Table 21.1. Recommendations for Multiple Choice Questions

The content should be based on well-defined learning objectives.

The content should be focused on 1 theme or problem.

The stem should be grammatically correct and concisely presented.

The stem should be phrased positively.

The stem should not include personal pronouns.

Closed stem: Where is the stellate ganglion?

Open stem: The stellate ganglion is located near the:

Description: During administration of a stellate ganglion block, an intervascular injection occurs. The most appropriate action is to:

The stem is followed by a number of responses or branches. The correct response should be absolutely correct or clearly the best choice. The distractors should be incorrect but plausible alternatives to the correct response. Recommendations for response construction are listed in Table 21.2.

Table 21.2. Recommendations for Multiple Choice Question Response Construction

The correct answer should be clearly the best choice.

Distractors should be plausible alternatives, but clearly incorrect.

Responses should be homogeneous (conceptually and structurally similar).

Repetitive words should be included in the stem.

Keywords from the stem should not be repeated in the responses.

Responses should be presented in a logical or numerical order.

Absolute terms (such as "always" or "never") should be avoided.

Responses should be of equal complexity and length.

Responses should be grammatically consistent with the stem.

Overlapping and "double barrel" options should be avoided.

"All of the above" and "none of the above" options should be avoided.

One of the pitfalls of question development is cueing, or providing clues within an item that unintentionally direct the examinee to the correct response for that or another item. For example, the correct response is given more attention because it is longer, more detailed, or more complete than the distractors. The examinee is also given an unintentional advantage if some of the distractors do not flow logically from the stem, but the correct answer does.

Cueing also may occur when the correct response has the most in common with the other options. This has been described as "convergence" and can take many forms. For instance, with numeric options, the correct response tends to be in the middle rather than at either extreme. It also can happen when the item writer makes slight variations to the correct answer to form the distractors, resulting in the "double barrel" question, for which the correct response contains more common elements from all of the options and is less likely to be an outlier.

Similar wording or phrasing in the stem and correct response is another source of cueing. Absolute terms such as "always," "never," "completely," and "totally" should be avoided because they are frequently associated with false statements. "Throw away" distractors such as "all of the above" and "none of the above" are generally not recommended. If an examinee has partial knowledge (for instance, that at least 2 of the 3 responses are correct), this may clue students to select "all of the above," relying more on test-taking strategy than on their own knowledge. Using "none of the above" can be problematic, particularly when judgment is involved and the options are not absolutely true or false. The more knowledgeable student may select "none of the above," believing an option that is not available may be more correct than the instructor's intended correct response.

The common concern of students regarding trick questions deserves some attention, if for no other reason than to provide the item writer with some insight on student perception. A study by Roberts[15] revealed that students believed trick items were deliberately used on examinations to deceive them. Students and faculty were asked to describe the characteristics of trick items. Results are listed in order of prevalence:

1. Intention
2. Trivial content
3. Too fine answer discrimination
4. Window dressing
5. Multiple correct answers
6. Content presented opposite from instruction
7. High ambiguity

Because there may be a fine line between the fair, challenging item and one that may be perceived as tricky and overly difficult, the item writer can minimize complaints by taking recommended guidelines into consideration. In some cases, what was thought to be an excellent question does not perform well for reasons that surface after its use. On the other hand, student allegations of trick questions also may be an excuse for poor test performance due to lack of knowledge. It is important to maintain objectivity in reevaluating test items. Questions that consistently exhibit poor performance by examinees probably need to be revised.

The following are examples of flawed items, along with suggestions for revision. **For clarity, flawed examples will be in gray boxes and corrected examples will be in white boxes.**

The question in example 1 has an unfocused stem and provides no information of the problem to be solved. The examinee should be able to read the question and construct the answer without looking at the responses. This type of question can be referred to as a hidden true or false question (with 1 true and 3 false statements).

Example 1

The stellate ganglion:

- a. is named for its neatly compact appearance.
- b. comprises the superior thoracic and inferior cervical ganglion.
- c. typically lies over the first thoracic vertebrae near the 2nd rib.
- d. can also be referred to as the thoracolumbar ganglion.

The stem in example 2 contains extraneous material, or "window dressing," not relevant to the problem or concept to be tested. The stem should only contain the information necessary to arrive at the correct response.

> **Example 2**
>
> You will be performing a stellate ganglion block for a 55-year-old man who is 62″ tall, and weighs 81kg, with well-controlled hypertension and gout in his right great toe. His wife of 30 years just left the room and he is very anxious about the procedure. During administration, an intravascular injection occurs. What should you do?

A more concise presentation of the question is presented in example 3.

> **Example 3**
>
> During administration of a stellate ganglion block, an intravascular injection occurs. The most appropriate initial intervention is to:

The distractors of the question in example 4 contain overlapping numeric data. It is preferable to avoid overlapping options or discrimination that is too fine. The item may have 2 correct answers and can be confusing to the examinee.

> **Example 4**
>
> The duration of intravenous succinylcholine after an induction dose is approximately:
>
>   a.   1 to 5 minutes.
>   b.   4 to 8 minutes.
>   c.   8 to 15 minutes.
>   d.   10 to 20 minutes.

Example 5 is a representation of a "double-barrel" question. With limited knowledge, examinees can easily rule out half the options, significantly improving their guessing odds. The savvy test taker may further deduce the correct answer based on the fact that "acetylcholine" is used in a majority of the responses.

> **Example 5**
>
> Nondepolarizing neuromuscular blockers act as:
>
>   a.   reversible competitive agonists for dopamine receptors.
>   b.   irreversible competitive antagonists for acetylcholine receptors.
>   c.   reversible competitive antagonists for acetylcholine receptors.
>   d.   irreversible competitive agonists for acetylcholine receptors.

Extended Matching Questions

While the single-best-answer MCQ is the only accepted format for the NCE, other single-best-answer item types are useful and well supported in the literature.[11-13,16,17]

The National Board of Medical Examiners also uses extended matching questions (EMQs), and only recently stopped using the traditional matching question (MQ) in favor of the EMQ.[11]

The conventional MQ is characterized by a set of options at the top or the right, and a set of stems (sometimes referred to as stimuli) underneath or at the left. Instructions for the examinee on how to respond are provided at the beginning. Typically, matching items are limited to 4 to 5 options and to 2 to 5 stems. Advantages of MQs include relative ease of construction and concise scoring and relatively short reading and response times; however, it can sometimes be challenging to develop homogeneous options and stem sets, and MQs typically only measure simple recall and association. While MQs can be used to test higher cognitive processes, these types of MQs are more challenging to construct. Recommendations for development of MQs are listed in Table 21.3.

Table 21.3. Recommendations for Matching Question Development

Provide clear instructions.

Address a single theme with each question.

Ensure homogeneity of stems and options.

Arrange stems and options in a random manner.

Use positive phrasing and consistent grammar in stems and options.

To avoid cueing, consider presenting an uneven number of stems and options. While each stem has only 1 correct response, allowing options to be used once, more than once, or not at all eliminates guessing by the process of elimination. Example 6 shows a poorly designed item and example 7 has suggestions for revision. The question in example 6 demonstrates several flaws. The directions are inadequate. The stems and options are heterogeneous and there is no central theme. Ordering of the options and stimuli are not random and are even in number. There is an obvious clue to the matching of Alice Magaw as the mother of anesthesia.

Example 6

Match the following:

___ 1.	The mother of anesthesia	A.	Alice Magaw
___ 2.	The first ether anesthetic	B.	William T. G. Morton
___ 3.	A theory of anesthetic action	C.	Meyer-Overton Rule
___ 4.	First used by Griffith and Johnson	D.	Curare
___ 5.	Year the AANA was founded	E.	1931

In example 7, the question has been revised. A central theme of the history of anesthesia is evident, and the stimuli and options are homogenous. The directions are more specific, the options are listed in random order, and cueing has been minimized.

Example 7

Match the response choices (right) with the stimuli (left). Responses may be used once, more than once, or not at all.

_____ 1. First use of N_2O in anesthesia	A.	Harold Griffith
_____ 2. The first ether anesthetic	B.	August Bier
_____ 3. The first spinal anesthetic	C.	Horace Wells
_____ 4. First used curare in anesthesia	D.	William T. G. Morton
_____ 5. First described IV regional anesthesia		

A variation of the conventional MQ, EMQs are theme-based, 1-best-answer type questions that typically include a set of 10 to 26 options, a lead-in statement, and at least 2 stem questions. For each stem, the examinee must select a single answer from the list of options. Research supports the use of EMQs for testing higher-order cognitive processes, such as application and analysis.[8,16,18] Like traditional MQs, advantages of EMQs include ease of construction, concise scoring, reasonable reading and response times (although this does increase proportionally with the number of options), and appropriateness for large-scale examinations. In addition, EMQs may be more resistant to cueing and guessing strategies.

It has been suggested that the theme, options, and lead-in statement be developed first and the stems be written last.[11] Recommendations for development of EMQs are provided in Table 21.4.

Table 21.4. Extended Matching Questions

Provide clear instructions.

Address a single theme with each set.

Establish the relationship between the options and stems with a lead-in statement.

Make the options short and the stems long.

Ensure homogeneity of options.

Avoid the use of verbs in the options.

Use positive phrasing and consistent grammar in stems and options.

Example 8 shows a poorly designed item, and the suggestions for revision appear in example 9. Although this item set appears to have a central theme of regional anesthesia, it is too broad. The options are not homogeneous and include the use of verbs. The instructions are not clear and there is no lead-in statement to establish the relationship between the options and stems. The stems cannot be answered without looking at the options, and rank-ordering to select the best option for each stem is nearly impossible.

In example 9, a more homogeneous set of options and stems are based on the more focused theme of interscalene block complications. The directions are clear, and a lead-in statement linking the options to the stems is present.

Example 8

Match the following:

A. Cardiopulmonary arrest

B. History of coagulopathy

C. Risk of postoperative nausea and vomiting

D. Decreased extremity movement

E. Potential for congestive heart failure

F. Interference with potassium channels

G. Postoperative pain management

H. "Nothing-by-mouth" status

I. Increased headache sensitivity

J. Seizure disorder

1. An important factor to consider prior to performing a regional block

2. A principle effect of local anesthetics during regional anesthesia

3. Possible adverse effect of regional anesthesia

Example 9

Directions: Match the appropriate option (top) to the stem (below). Each option may be used once, more than once, or not at all.

Theme: Interscalene block complications

Options:

A. Hemidiaphragmatic paresis

B. Pneumothorax

C. Intravenous injection

D. Bronchospasm

E. Intrathecal injection

F. Cervical sympathetic block

G. Intra-arterial injection

H. Tracheal perforation

I. Recurrent laryngeal nerve block

J. Intraneural injection

Lead-in: For each of the following patients undergoing an interscalene block, select the most likely adverse effect.

Stems:

1. During administration of an interscalene block, the patient begins to complain of dyspnea and difficulty swallowing and then loses consciousness.

2. During administration of an interscalene block, the patient complains of sudden, severe pain in the block site.

3. During administration of an interscalene block, the patient's speech begins to slur. The patient quickly loses consciousness and exhibits uncoordinated muscle movement.

True or False Questions

True or false questions require the examinee to select all responses that are true. True or false item formats can be divided into 2 groups: simple true or false items and multiple true or false (MTF) items. The simple true or false item is presented as a statement the examinee must determine as true or false. Multiple true or false (MTF) items include the "A/B/both/neither" format, sometimes referred to as C-type[11] questions, and the complex MTF item, also known as the K-type[11] question.

The true or false format tends to be used in the classroom setting, but not on standardized examinations. The NCE does not use true or false questions, and the National Board of Medical Examiners discourages their use.[11] The item writer may have something in mind while developing the question that upon further scrutiny is not apparent to the examinee, making the item difficult to qualify as clearly true or false. True or false questions can be confusing or perceived as tricky, particularly when a single word in the stem changes the statement from true to false. It is often difficult to develop clear, unambiguous true or false items that are not reduced to the task of simple recall of isolated facts. Assessing higher-order thought processes with true or false questions can be done, but they are more difficult to develop. The simple true or false format also is more susceptible to guessing.

Reported advantages of the simple true or false format include ease of construction for testing knowledge and recall of facts, straightforward scoring, reasonable reading and response time, and suitability for large-scale examinations. Disadvantages include difficulty assessing higher-level cognitive domains, tendency of testing trivial content, and vulnerability for guessing. Complex MTF questions are generally not recommended for use because they tend to be more difficult and take longer to answer, but are no more discriminating than traditional MCQs.[9,19] Suggestions for writing true or false questions are listed in Table 21.5.

Table 21.5. Recommendations for True or False Question Development

Focus on a single concept or problem.

Use clear, concise, positive phrasing.

Make the items obviously true or false.

Avoid absolute terms.

Example 10 is an example of a flawed simple true or false item. This item is problematic for several reasons. The statement is negatively phrased and the absolute term "always" is used. The intent of the question is not clear; is it true because the writer intended that the procedure be delayed because of the full stomach, or is it false because patients with a full stomach should be intubated?

Example 10

It is always best to avoid intubating a patient with a full stomach.

    a.   True

    b.   False

Example 11 presents an improved question. The intent of this question is clear and phrased in a positive manner. It focuses on a single concept and the statement is defensibly true.

Example 11

Endotracheal intubation should be performed on the patient presenting with a full stomach for emergency abdominal surgery.

    a.   True

    b.   False

Completion Items

Completion testing items are constructed questions that require the examinee to either provide a short answer or fill-in-the-blank response with a single word or a few words. It is important to develop questions that elicit a short response; the longer the response, the more difficult it can be to score the item. Well-designed completion items have been shown to have high reliability and discriminate more effectively.[20,21] Advantages include the ability to test a broad range of content and the reduced impact of guessing. Completion items work particularly well for questions requiring math calculations. Noncalculation questions can be challenging to develop because there can be only 1 correct response for completion items. Other disadvantages may include difficulty reading the student's handwriting and more time required for grading due to unanticipated answers. Suggestions for creating completion items are presented in Table 21.6.

Table 21.6. Recommendations for Completion Item Development

Develop items that can be completed with 1 word or short phrase.

Ensure there is only 1 correct response.

Do not take direct statements from assigned readings.

When using blanks, place toward the end of the sentence and use a consistent length.

For math calculations, specify how precise the answer should be (nearest tenth).

Example 12 is ambiguous with many possible correct answers shown in parentheses.

Example 12

Succinylcholine acts at the _____ (neuromuscular junction, motor end plate, skeletal muscle, nicotinic cholinergic receptor).

The question has been revised in example 13 to ask for a single, correct response.

> **Example 13**
>
> Succinylcholine acts at _____ cholinergic receptor sites (nicotinic).

Essay Questions

Essay questions can range from short-answer questions to extended-response questions. An advantage of the essay question is the opportunity to assess higher-level cognitive processes of analysis, synthesis, and evaluation.[13,22] Questions can be designed to address a specific, narrowly defined area in a broader, open-ended manner to allow the examinee more flexibility in generating a response.

Although the essay question may be easy to construct, it can be challenging to develop a clear scoring rubric for grading. Developing the rubric in advance is critical for both the examinee and the instructor. Some of the disadvantages of essay tests are the amount of time required for grading, reduced objectivity and test reliability, increased response time requirement, and language or legibility issues. Extended-response items with broad, open-ended questions tend to be more challenging to grade objectively. Even with a predetermined scoring rubric, the examinee may respond in a way unanticipated by the instructor. Recommendations for essay questions are included in Table 21.7.

> **Table 21.7. Recommendations for Essay Question Development**
>
> Items should be based on a specific (complex) learning objective.
>
> A scoring rubric should be established in advance.
>
> Clear instructions and scoring criteria should be provided to the examinee.
>
> Issues related to spelling, grammar, and penmanship should be addressed in advance.
>
> Avoid questions that are too broad.
>
> A time limit should be established.
>
> If using multiple essay questions, all examinees should answer all questions (no optional or "select-2-out-of-3" formats).
>
> Score/grade the exams anonymously.
>
> All responses to 1 question should be scored before moving on to the next question.

The question in Example 14 is too broad and does not provide clear instructions or expectations.

> **Example 14**
>
> Describe the induction process for anesthesia.

Example 15 provides a more precise task but still allows for some creativity on the part of the examinee. A possible grading rubric for example 15 is presented in Table 21.8.

Example 15

Develop a care plan for general endotracheal anesthesia for an 80-kg patient with gastroesophageal reflux disease who also has asthma (assume that the patient needs neuromuscular blockade). Provide medication and dosing information in the following areas:

    a.   Premedication (5 points)

    b.   Induction (8 points)

    c.   Maintenance (6 points)

    d.   Emergence (3 points)

Also, list 2 medications you would consider avoiding in this patient (2 points each; must be from different drug classes) and explain why (2 points each).

Table 21.8. Scoring Rubric for Example 15

Premedication (5 points)	Name 0.5 points	Dose 0.5 points	Induction (8 points)	Name 1 point	Dose 1 point
Benzodiazepine			Opioid		
Beta agonist			Lidocaine		
H$_2$ antagonist			Sedative/hypnotic		
Prokinetic			Neuromuscular blocker		
Nonparticulate antacid					

Maintenance (6 points)	Name 1 point	Dose 1 point	Emergence (3 points)	Name 0.5 points	Dose 0.5 points
Inhalation/TIVA			Anticholinesterase		
Neuromuscular blocker			Anticholinergic		
Opioid/NSAID			Antiemetic		
			Subtotals		

Meds to avoid (8 points)	Name 2 points	Reason 2 points			
Beta blocker					
Histamine releaser					
Subtotals			Total (30 points possible)		

In addition to facilitating the process of grading essay questions, another benefit of developing a scoring rubric in advance is that it often leads to positive changes in the essay question itself. It may lead the writer to refine or narrow the question, or assign different point values to reflect more accurately the importance of certain aspects of the content the question is designed to cover. Providing information the examinee needs to organize and prioritize the response is critical in enabling the efficient use of the allowed testing time.

Other Techniques

This section is devoted to some creative assessment techniques the reader may or may not currently be using. For those interested in trying something different or as a complement to the more traditional didactic testing strategies, this section provides descriptions of and some general guidance on the use of these alternative evaluation methods. For those interested in more detailed information, sources for reference are provided.

Laboratory Practical

The laboratory practical is a series of stations where dissected anatomical parts are marked with a pin, or various cell structures are indicated by an arrow on a slide under a microscope to be identified by the examinee. This allows the instructor to assess precisely whether the learner can name a particular organ or structure. Although labor intensive and time consuming to set up, the traditional laboratory practical is a useful tool for straightforward assessment of knowledge. What if assessment of higher-order thinking is desired? Evolution of the laboratory practical into a more participatory experience can allow for this type of measurement. Instead of having the examinees look through microscopes and identify particular structures, they might be asked to focus the microscope and locate a particular structure. The creative laboratory practical might also take the form of a skills assessment in which students are evaluated on essential skills. Winnett-Murray[23] describes this approach in a department of biology, where students participate in laboratory practical examinations to assess proficiency in microscopy, animal handling, making serial dilutions, and other skills considered essential for biology majors.

The counterpart of this expanded laboratory practical in the training and assessment of healthcare practitioners has been termed the "Objective Structured Clinical Examination" (OSCE). The OSCE has been described as a tool for evaluation of didactic knowledge and clinical skills and has been used within the fields of nursing, medicine, occupational therapy, and radiation therapy.[24-26] The OSCE is a performance-based evaluation designed around a specific clinical skill or task to be completed within a certain time frame. An objective scoring tool is used to rate the examinee. In addition to evaluation, the OSCE can be used to provide feedback and ensure minimal competencies. Some specific examples of OSCEs include evaluations of neonatal resuscitation by neonatal nurse practitioner students,[27] the ability of medical students to share information and decisions with patients,[28] and physical examination and multidisciplinary management plan development by rheumatology clinical nurse specialist students.[26] The Israeli Board of Anesthesiology has implemented the use of the OSCE format into the Israeli National Board Examination in several areas, including trauma management, resuscitation, crisis management, regional anesthesia, and mechanical ventilation.[29]

Some nurse anesthesia programs continue to use the laboratory practical for the anatomy component. With the current variety and improved quality of simulation technology, the laboratory practical can also be implemented for skills assessment as another means to evaluate didactic knowledge. A search of the literature did not reveal any publications related to the use of OSCEs in nurse anesthesia education, although it is likely the OSCE format is currently being used by some nurse anesthesia educational programs. The practice of nurse anesthesia includes many essential skills that may be evaluated in a laboratory practical setting using the OSCE format, such as spinal and epidural anesthesia, central and arterial line placement, or laryngoscopy and intubation. Performance-based OSCEs in the areas mentioned earlier, such as resuscitation and crisis management, would also be appropriate within a nurse anesthesia program. The following is a brief example of a resuscitation scenario in Berkenstadt et al.[29]

Background: The examiner is a junior intern in the emergency room who calls on the anesthesiologists for help. The patient is a 70-year-old man with known heart failure admitted to the emergency room with shortness of breath.

The simulator: Sim-Man simulator, in the sitting position, is connected to a monitor that features noninvasive arterial blood pressure, an electrocardiogram, and a pulse oximeter. One intravenous line is inserted; no oxygen is given.

Scenario: Upon the anesthesiologist's (the examinee's) arrival at the emergency room, the examiner takes the role of a junior intern and the other examiner acts as an ER nurse. One of the examiners gives the anesthesiologist the patient's medical history and refers to the monitor. On the monitor, the heart rate is 120/min, oxygen saturation is 90%, and arterial blood pressure, measured 10 minutes previously, is 150/100 mm Hg. Respiratory rate is 26/min.

Expected Performance and Examiner Response:
1. Address the patient: the patient responds with a concern of shortness of breath.
2. Perform a physical examination: the examiner provides the information that the neck veins are dilated and rales are present on both lung fields, in accordance with the anesthesiologist's performance.
3. Give oxygen: The examiner posing as the nurse gives oxygen and sets up the oxygen flow on request.
4. Ask for 12-lead electrocardiogram and chest radiograph: One of the examiners gives the anesthesiologist both items on request and asks for an interpretation.

The checklist items (address the patient, perform a physical examination, administer oxygen, and ask for 12-lead electrocardiogram and chest radiograph) are scored in a binary fashion as "performed" or "not performed."

The OSCE can be used to evaluate a variety of clinical skills and scenarios in a way that written examinations cannot. However, the OSCE does not come without some disadvantages. Like the traditional laboratory practical, it can be labor intensive and time consuming to develop and implement. The financial resources needed to invest in the necessary equipment and physical environment can be substantial. The component of objectivity in the scoring process is essential, so developing a valid, reliable scoring tool and establishing minimal competency levels is critical.

Concept Mapping

A concept map is an organized visual representation of interrelated concepts of a central theme or major idea. Concept mapping has been widely reported as an instructional and assessment tool to teach and evaluate critical thinking in undergraduate nursing education.[30-34] Although not as numerous, there are reports of the use of concept maps in graduate and postgraduate nursing programs.[35,36] Concept maps can be used early in the semester as a formative evaluation tool, during the semester to evaluate progress, and at the end as a summative, final examination. In addition to using the concept map for themes or ideas, it can also be applied to a particular type of case or individual patient.[30-34] In general, feedback regarding concept mapping has been positive from both students and instructors.[30,31]

Using the concept map as a means of assessment requires careful planning and implementation. Students accustomed to and successful at objective style assessments may initially resist the idea of concept mapping as a testing tool. Clear instructions as to the process and expectations must be provided to the student well in advance, and it is helpful to provide examples and allow for draft submission and feedback.[33,37] It is important for both the student and the instructor to keep an open mind during this experience. Some students will excel at the more creative, individualized ability to express their ideas of interrelationships, while others will struggle with the somewhat abstract method of establishing and justifying these connections. Some concept maps will display thoughtful, profound representations while others will seem to exhibit superficial expression of basic content.

Schuster[38] provides a useful framework for patient care plan concept map development. Mezeske[37] presents detailed guidelines for concept mapping of themes and ideas in the field of education. General suggestions for use of concept maps include the following:

1. Provide clear instructions and expectations.
2. Establish a timeline.
3. Develop a grading/scoring rubric.

Instructions and expectations should include the format (computer generated or hard copy) and parameters on the size and type of materials that may be used. A timeline with multiple checkpoints and dates for draft and final submission can help facilitate progress, maintain the scope of the project, and emphasize its importance. Benefits of using concept maps include stimulation of critical and reflective thinking and reduced risk of plagiarism. The time required for development and evaluation is an obvious drawback but, with experience (on the part of the instructor and student), the time can be reduced to a reasonable length.[38]

Written Assignments

The written assignment is a long-standing tool for evaluating student learning and development. There are many formats available. This section will review reflective writing exercises and portfolio development as assessment tools. Reflective writing assignments can be described as a process whereby students learn from their own experience. Examples of reflective writing formats include case reports and journaling. Reflective writing is well supported in nursing education as a means to encourage critical thinking, increase engagement in the learning process, and improve self-awareness.[39-41] The use of portfolios, both at the undergraduate and graduate level, is also described in nursing education and other health-related programs.[42-45] The portfolio has been used as a means to facilitate and document achievement of learning objectives and clinical competencies, stimulate critical thinking, and enhance professional development.[42,43]

When using these forms of assessment, it is critical to provide clear guidelines to the student. Precise instructions and expectations save time and energy for both the student and instructor. Reflective writing assignments are not simply reports of observation and action. Students should also be making a connection between what occurred and their own reasoning and thought processes both during and after the experience. General suggestions for instructors interested in implementing reflective writing assignments include:

1. Define reflective writing for the student.
2. Facilitate the process (do not focus on the product).
3. Emphasize the importance of quality (not quantity).
4. Provide a safe environment that encourages freedom of expression.
5. Give constructive, supportive feedback.
6. Maintain confidentiality.

The student may not understand what reflective writing is, so providing an explanation and examples are helpful. Set guidelines for content and length, with emphasis on the quality of the work instead of the quantity. Establish a routine for submission and feedback that is timely and constructive. Students who feel intimidated by the instructor or the process will be hesitant to express their thoughts and feelings fully and thus will not experience the full benefit of the exercise.

The portfolio has been defined as "a collection of personal work or materials that demonstrates growth over time."[44] When used as a means of assessment, a written component is often added as a means for stimulating reflection and self-awareness of the growth process. This can take the form of reflective commentary on specific learning outcomes.[42,43] A variety of documents may be submitted as supportive evidence such as grade transcripts, standardized examination reports, assignments, meeting agendas, certificates of completion, licenses, certifications, resumes, job descriptions, performance evaluations, letters of reference, awards, clinical case tracking reports, and records of professional activities (to name a few). As with other writing assignments, explicit instructions and expectations should be given up front, and periodic, prompt, constructive feedback should be provided throughout the process. The individual nature of the portfolio does not lend itself well to precise comparison with other portfolios. Scoring a portfolio requires careful advance planning to minimize bias.[42,43,46] Some institutions have developed specific guidelines for portfolio development.[46] Basic recommendations for portfolio assignments include the following:

1. Divide the portfolio into manageable sections.
2. Establish set parameters for length and supporting documentation.
3. Identify the learning objectives to be evaluated.
4. Establish standards for spelling, grammar, and format.
5. Develop a precise scoring rubric.
6. Implement a process for random verification of supporting documentation.
7. Provide periodic, constructive feedback.

Possible sections of the portfolio could include a resume, learning objective commentaries or statements, a case report, and supportive evidence. Limiting the length of the commentary and number of supportive documents will result in a more compact, reflective portfolio. In order to maintain legitimacy of the assignment, random verification of supportive documents has been suggested.[46]

Oral Examination

Oral examinations are another tool for evaluating student knowledge. They are used in a variety of health-related disciplines periodically throughout the educational curriculum and as final, cumulative assessments. Many medical specialties include an oral examination component in their certification process, including the American Board of Anesthesiology (ABA). The degree to which nurse anesthesia programs use oral examinations has not been quantified in the literature, and there are few published reports of their use within the field of nursing.[47-49] A study comparing written and oral examinations in an undergraduate medical-surgical nursing course demonstrated effective evaluation of comprehension of content and clinical application with both techniques.[49] In Canada, a cohort of neonatal nurse practitioner graduates performed similarly to a group of pediatric residents on a comprehensive examination that included an oral examination component.[48] The use of oral examinations for certification by the ABA and Royal College of Physicians and Surgeons of Canada has been reported in the literature as reliable and valid.[50-53] In preparation for the board certification oral examination and as a method to ensure core competencies, many anesthesiology residency programs have incorporated oral practice examinations into their assessment plan.

Advantages to using oral examination are the ability to evaluate low-order and higher-order cognitive processes and problem-solving capability. Thorough evaluation of communication skills can be accomplished in a way not afforded by most other types of assessment. The exercise of organizing knowledge, ideas, and opinions and presenting responses in an effective, confident manner is invaluable. Some favor the face-to-face interaction with immediate ability to assess learner knowledge of the content area.

Disadvantages of oral examination include concerns regarding objectivity during the testing and grading process. The ABA oral examination is conducted with the examiners blinded to the candidate's training program, performance during residency, type or location of practice, or personality.[54] It would be difficult to achieve this level of objectivity for oral examinations administered during training. Associate examiners for the ABA are also required to attend training sessions each time they participate to ensure consistency in examination administration and grading techniques. Inter-rater and intra-rater reliability of examiners is a concern. One study of examiner reliability for oral practice examinations in 2 anesthesiology residency programs was reported as fair to good. The authors suggested using at least 2 examiners to improve reliability.[51] Conducting oral examinations can be labor intensive, particularly with large cohorts of students. Scheduling more than 6 students sequentially has been reported as being exhausting to the examiner.[47] Student feedback often includes complaints of stress and anxiety leading up to and during the examination.[47,49,52] In a study of anesthesiology residents participating in oral practice examinations, a higher self-assessed level of anxiety correlated with poorer performance than those who self-assessed at a lower level of anxiety.[52]

When using oral examination as a form of assessment, it is critical to prepare the examinee and provide clear instructions and guidelines as to how the examination will be administered, with particular attention to attenuating anxiety. Recommendations for instructors interested in administering oral examinations include the following:

1. Provide clear information as to how the oral examination will be conducted.
2. Develop a uniform list of questions in advance.
3. Provide a practice session with example questions during class.
4. Develop a standardized grading rubric in advance.
5. Audiotape or videotape the session if possible.
6. Provide a quiet testing environment free of distraction.
7. Use 2 simultaneous evaluators whenever possible.

Informing the examinee what to expect may alleviate the degree of stress and anxiety before and during the examination. Questions should be developed based on the learning objectives of the course and the cognitive processes the examiner wishes to evaluate. It is important to conduct the examination in a comfortable, quiet environment. Calls should be forwarded and a sign should be posted to prevent interruption. Permission to audiotape or videotape should be obtained in advance, and recording equipment should be placed in the periphery, if possible. It is also helpful for the examiner to set a predetermined time limit.

Summary

As nurse anesthesia educators, our goal is to prepare safe, competent, compassionate practitioners for the future. Although it is important to provide the student nurse anesthetist with the necessary tools, information, and experiences to be successful on the NCE, it is also vital to instill a commitment to periodic reflection and lifelong learning. How we evaluate our students in the classroom setting can inform their future behavior and self-awareness in these areas. Using a variety of testing methods, allowing for creativity, and stimulating engagement in the learning process can help achieve these goals.

References

1. Merriam-Webster Editorial Staff. Teach. *Merriam-Webster's Collegiate Dictionary.* 11th ed. http://www.merriam-webster.com/dictionary/teach. Accessed April 28, 2008.

2. Merriam-Webster Editorial Staff. Test. *Merriam-Webster's Collegiate Dictionary.* 11th ed. http://www.merriam-webster.com/dictionary/test. Accessed April 28, 2008.

3. Giordano PJ. Principles of effective grading. In: Buskist W, Davis SF, eds. *Handbook of the Teaching of Psychology.* Malden, MA: Blackwell Publishing; 2005:254-258.

4. Council on Certification of Nurse Anesthetists. 2008 candidate handbook: 115th certification examination for nurse anesthetists. http://www.aana.com/uploadedFiles/Credentialing/Certification/CCNA_Resources/ccna_candidate_handbook.pdf. Accessed May 7, 2008.

5. Wendt A, Kenny L. Setting the passing standard for the National Council Licensure Examination for registered nurses. *Nurse Educ.* 2007;32(3):104-108.

6. Maki P. *Assessing for Learning: Building a Sustainable Commitment Across the Institution.* Sterling, VA: Stylus Publishing; 2004:120-121.

7. De Champlain AF. Ensuring that the competent are truly competent: an overview of common methods and procedures used to set standards on high-stakes examinations. *J Vet Med Educ.* 2004;31(1):61-65.

8. McCoubrie P. Improving the fairness of multiple-choice questions: a literature review. *Med Teach.* 2004;26(8):709-712.

9. Case SM, Swanson DB. *Constructing Written Test Questions for the Basic and Clinical Sciences.* 3rd ed. Philadelphia, PA: National Board of Medical Examiners; 2002.

10. Downing SM. The effects of violating standard item writing principles on tests and students: the consequences of using flawed test items on achievement examinations in medical education. *Adv Health Sci Educ Theory Pract.* 2005;10(2):133-143.

11. Tarrant M, Ware J. Impact of item-writing flaws in multiple-choice questions on student achievement in high-stakes nursing assessments. *Med Educ.* 2008;42(2):198-206.

12. Haladyna TM. *Developing and Validating Multiple-Choice Test Items.* 3rd ed. Mahwah, NJ: Lawrence Erlbaum Associates; 2004.

13. Juve JA. Test construction. In: Buskist W, Davis SF, eds. *Handbook of the Teaching of Psychology.* Malden, MA: Blackwell Publishing; 2005:247-253.

14. Promissor, Inc. *Item Writing Guide.* Evanston, IL: Computer Adaptive Technologies; 1999.

15. Roberts DM. An empirical study on the nature of trick test questions. *J Educ Measurement.* 1993:30(4):331-344.

16. Beullens J, Van Damme B, Jaspaert H, Janssen PJ. Are extended-matching multiple-choice items appropriate for a final test in medical education? *Med Teach.* 2002;24(4):390-395.

17. Swanson DB, Holtzman KZ, Allbee K, Clauser BE. Psychometric characteristics and response times for content-parallel extended-matching and one-best-answer items in relation to number of options. *Acad Med.* 2006;81(10 suppl):S52-S55.

18. Coderre SP, Harasym P, Mandin H, Fick G. The impact of two multiple-choice question formats on the problem-solving strategies used by novices and experts. *BMC Med Educ.* 2004;4:23.

19. Haladyna TM, Downing SM, Rodriguez MC. A review of multiple-choice item-writing guidelines for classroom assessment. *Appl Meas Educ.* 2002;15(3):309-334.

20. Rademakers J, Ten Cate TJ, Bär PR. Progress testing with short answer questions. *Med Teach.* 2005;27(7):578-582.

21. Ramos KD, Schafer S, Tracz SM. Validation of the Fresno test of competence in evidence based medicine. *BMJ.* 2003;326(7384):319-321.

22. Tomey AM. Completion testing items. *Nurse Educ.* 1999;24(6):6-7.

23. Winnett-Murray K. Resurrecting the lab practical. In: Mezeske RJ, Mezeske BA, eds. *Beyond Tests and Quizzes: Creative Assessments in the College Classroom.* San Francisco, CA: Jossey-Bass; 2007:56-69.

24. Bromley LM. The Objective Structured Clinical Exam: practical aspects. *Curr Opin Anaesthesiol.* 2000;13(6):675-678.

25. Major DA. OSCEs: seven years on the bandwagon: the progress of an objective structured clinical evaluation programme. *Nurse Educ Today.* 2005;25(6):442-454.

26. Ryan S, Stevenson K, Hassell AB. Assessment of clinical nurse specialists in rheumatology using an OSCE. *Musculoskeletal Care.* 2007;5(3):119-129.

27. Brooks G. Assessment of student advanced neonatal nurse practitioners in resuscitation and stabilization of the newborn: the use of the objective structured clinical exam. *J Neonatal Nurs.* 2004;10(6):184-188.

28. Thistlethwaite JE. Developing an OSCE station to assess the ability of medical students to share information and decisions with patients: issues relating to interrater reliability and the use of simulated patients. *Educ Health.* 2002;15(2):170-179.

29. Berkenstadt H, Ziv A, Gafni N, Sidi A. Incorporating simulation-based objective structured clinical examination into the Israeli National Board Examination in anesthesiology. *Anesth Analg.* 2006;102(3):853-858.

30. Hicks-Moore SL. Clinical concept maps in nursing education: an effective way to link theory and practice. *Nurse Educ Pract.* 2005;5(6):348-352.

31. Hicks-Moore SL, Pastirik PJ. Evaluating critical thinking in clinical concept maps: a pilot study. *Int J Nurs Educ Scholarsh.* 2006;3:article 27.

32. Hsu LL. Developing concept maps from problem-based learning scenario discussions. *J Adv Nurs.* 2004;48(5):510-518.

33. Hsu LL, Hsieh SI. Concept maps as an assessment tool in a nursing course. *J Prof Nurs.* 2005;21(3):141-149.

34. King M, Shell R. Teaching and evaluating critical thinking with concept maps. *Nurse Educ.* 2002;27(5):214-216.

35. Giddens J. Concept mapping as a group learning activity in graduate nursing education. *J Nurs Educ.* 2006;45(1):45-46.

36. Hill CM. Integrating clinical experiences into the concept mapping process. *Nurse Educ.* 2006;31(1):36-39.

37. Mezeske RJ. Concept mapping: assessing pre-service teachers' understanding and knowledge. In: Mezeske RJ, Mezeske BA, eds. *Beyond Tests and Quizzes: Creative Assessments in the College Classroom.* San Francisco, CA: Jossey-Bass; 2007: 8-25.

38. Schuster PM. Concept mapping: reducing clinical care plan paperwork and increasing learning. *Nurse Educ.* 2000;25(2):76-81.

39. Harris M. Scaffolding reflective journal writing: Negotiating power, play, and position. *Nurse Educ Today.* 2008;28(3):314-326.

40. Kessler PD, Lund CH. Reflective journaling: developing an online journal for distance education. *Nurse Educ.* 2004;29(1):20-24.

41. Ruland JP, Ahern NR. Transforming student perspectives through reflective writing. *Nurse Educ.* 2007;32(2):81-88.

42. Schaffer MA, Nelson P, Litt E. Using portfolios to evaluate achievement of population-based public health nursing competencies in baccalaureate nursing students. *Nurs Educ Perspect.* 2005;26(2):104-112.

43. Jasper MA, Fulton J. Marking criteria for practice-based portfolios at masters' level. *Nurse Educ Today*. 2005;25(5):377-389.

44. Ray R. Tracking learning over time in health care education using clinical proficiency transcripts. In: Mezeske RJ, Mezeske BA, eds. *Beyond Tests and Quizzes: Creative Assessments in the College Classroom*. San Francisco, CA: Jossey-Bass; 2007: 139-151.

45. Kalet AL, Sanger J, Chase J, et al. Promoting professionalism through an online professional development portfolio: successes, joys, and frustrations. *Acad Med*. 2007;82(11):1065-1072.

46. Lettus MK, Moessner PH, Dooley L. The clinical portfolio as an assessment tool. *Nurs Adm Q*. 2001;25(2):74-79.

47. Bairan A, Farnsworth B. Oral exams: an alternative evaluation method. *Nurse Educ*. 1997;22(4):6-7.

48. Mitchell A, Watts J, Whyte R, et al. Evaluation of graduating neonatal nurse practitioners. *Pediatrics*. 1991;88(4):789-794.

49. Rushton P, Eggett D. Comparison of written and oral examinations in a baccalaureate medical-surgical nursing course. *J Prof Nurs*. 2003;19(3):142-148.

50. Eagle CJ, Martineau R, Hamilton K. The oral examination in anaesthetic resident evaluation. *Can J Anaesth*. 1993;40(10):947-953.

51. Kearney RA, Puchalski SA, Yang HY, Skakun EN. The inter-rater and intra-rater reliability of a new Canadian oral examination format in anesthesia is fair to good. *Can J Anaesth*. 2002;49(3):232-236.

52. Shubert A, Tetzlaff JE, Tan M, Ryckman JV, Mascha E. Consistency, inter-rater reliability, and validity of 441 consecutive mock oral examinations in anesthesiology: implications for use as a tool for assessment of residents. *Anesthesiology*. 1999;91(1):288-298.

53. Tetzlaff JE. Assessment of competency in anesthesiology. *Anesthesiology*. 2007;106(4):812-825.

54. James FM III. Oral practice examinations: are they worth it? *Anesthesiology*. 1999;91(1):4-6.

Chapter 22

Encouraging Scholarship Among Student Nurse Anesthetists: The Role of the Faculty Mentor

Chuck Biddle, CRNA, PhD

The amount of writings of a profession is a measure of its vitality and activity, whilst their quality is a rough indication of its intellectual state.

–Sir Robert Hutchinson

Key Points

- Scholarship assumes many forms but is defined broadly as the expansion and refinement of the scientific foundations for a specialty. Educators are heavily invested in supporting and promoting scholarly activity by our students.

- Students will often propose research questions or projects that are too broad in nature or ill defined. Rather than discourage their enthusiasm, faculty should redirect students' energy toward developing a highly relevant, focused, and researchable question or limited number of questions.

- In assuming the role of research mentor, one must be reasonably available to students, be prepared to help refer complex questions to appropriate domain experts, facilitate the development of a manageable timeline for students, and assist in clarifying the roles and responsibilities of students.

- Students should be educated about the purpose and responsibilities of the peer-review system and reminded that the process is an opportunity to have their work closely examined and critiqued by experts in the domain so that it can be presented in its most valid and useful form.

- Students must contend with barriers before engaging in a serious scholarly project, and they should seek out a faculty advisor who has demonstrated expertise and success in scholarly inquiry. Students should plan for things to go wrong and have contingencies in mind so that they are prepared to deal with setbacks. Intellectual curiosity, flexibility, patience, stamina, and perseverance are key attributes for success.

Introduction

Nurse anesthesia educators (NAEs) are heavily invested in supporting and promoting healthcare research in general and perioperative care in particular. In my view, research is a process by which we come to better understand the world around us, a process driven by asking important, relevant questions and seeking answers to them. Dissemination of the outcomes from that process is the essential next step. Research without dissemination is associated with a number of lost benefits (Table 22.1).

Scholarly activity in nurse anesthesia is a key component of our profession's activity, setting it apart from a merely technical enterprise performed by its members. One essential attribute of a profession is having a systematic body of knowledge that must be expanded by research and passed on to the next generation of its members.[1] Nurse anesthesia scholarship takes on many forms but can be viewed broadly as the expansion and refinement of our knowledge and skills, the sharing of ideas and expertise, the critical evaluation of existing and new approaches, and a commitment to growing the scientific foundations of our specialty. We also find ourselves at a critical evolutionary juncture given the national movement toward awarding the doctorate in nurse anesthesia practice. I am strongly of the view that NAEs have an obligation to promote scholarship among their students. The goals of this chapter are to advance this belief, and to offer some guidance in that quest.

It should be established at the outset that I have no intent to imply that all NAEs should be engaged in research, traditionally defined as engaging in the pursuit of new knowledge through rigorously controlled experiments. In fact, the definition, scope, and expectation of faculty scholarship have evolved considerably in university settings nationwide. Although the need for both basic science and clinical investigators is essential, there is also the clinical scholar role with which many of us may feel more comfortable. This role does not demand that we produce new knowledge; instead, our responsibility is to perfect and maintain our own clinical expertise and to impart that knowledge and skill set onto students and junior members of the profession.

Table 22.1. Benefits of Communicated Research

To the public:	Improvements and refinements in patient care
To the profession:	Enhancement of the image and stature of its members
To the institution:	Pride and reputation of its contributing staff
To ourselves:	Satisfaction, advancement, recognition among professional peers

Although Table 22.1 gives a broad overview of the benefits of engaging in and sharing the findings of research, I am also a pragmatist, and believe that, for the process to be truly embraced, we must help the student appreciate the associated rewards at the individual level. Table 22.2 gives an overview of these rewards and provides NAEs with talking points regarding the personal factors of engaging in scholarly activity. Faculty should not limit themselves to these points but should discuss, from the heart, what their personal views and passions are about engaging in scholarly activity.

> ## Table 22.2. The Personal Factors Associated With Scholarly Activity
>
> Personal satisfaction in executing a knowledge quest and sharing it with others
>
> Satisfying one's curiosity
>
> Helping to define and experience a potential career path
>
> Engaging in a personal passion for exploring, creating, or writing
>
> Potential monetary reward for created work
>
> Satisfaction in achieving recognition among professional peers

The Faculty Role in the Process of Scholarship

I am heartened by the number of recent graduates from programs of nurse anesthesia who actively seek careers in academia despite the barriers that may exist (eg, generally lower salary, exposure to vicarious liability, potential for not fully autonomous practice, and the often politically charged environment of a coexisting anesthesia residency program). I am also buoyed by the large number of papers submitted to the *AANA Journal* and other healthcare and biomedical journals by our students, faculty new to the profession, and established faculty. With respect to the student cohort, what can we do to further advance their contributions?

The research process can be simplified into 3 steps or stages: (1) planning, (2) execution of the plan, and (3) peer review of the outcome. It is vital for the faculty mentor to get to know something about the student's background, professional interests, and previous experience. To avoid this part of the process is naïve and will often result in a negative (ie, unpleasant, boring, frustrating) or disastrous (eg, giving up or otherwise failing to complete the project) experience. It is essential for the faculty mentor not to lose sight of the following: *students may feel an obligation to engage in a project that is of little personal interest because they do not want to disappoint the faculty member.* If a student is clearly unable to generate an idea, and the faculty member elects to "recommend" a topic or project, it is important to establish an open dialogue to assess the student's genuine interest and skill sets required to engage in the project.

A student may come to the faculty member with a preconceived question that is much too broad and lacks focus. For example, "I wish to study the autonomic response to our intravenous induction agents," "Is regional anesthesia preferable to general anesthesia?" or "What drug is best to prevent postoperative nausea and vomiting?" are questions that will overwhelm even the most passionate investigator and are sorely in need of focus. In this event, the best course is to encourage the student to take some time to come up with 3 to 5 focused questions that might fall under the umbrella of the initial broad question and then return to discuss which questions are of greatest interest and whether or not the questions can be addressed. Essential talking points at this stage are listed in Table 22.3 and will help the student and mentor to better assess the feasibility of the proposed enterprise.

Table 22.3. Assessing the Viability of the Student's Idea

The fundamental issue is whether or not the project can be completed. Issues to consider:

Do I (as faculty) have the expertise to advise the student or is a referral necessary?

Does the student have the knowledge and energy to complete the task?

Is the research question one that can be answered?

Can it be accomplished in the time that is available?

Can the student and faculty control the factors essential to the research?

Do the student and faculty have the space, equipment, research subject recruitment, funding, etc?

If applicable, what are the Institutional Review Board considerations?

Occasionally a student will come to a faculty member and profess the desire to do something substantial that will have immediate practice applications of such magnitude that major biomedical journals will clamor for the rights to publish it. Such unbridled enthusiasm should not be discouraged, but should be redirected constructively toward developing a relevant, focused question. Students should be reminded that what will ultimately yield a publication, poster, or invited presentation is not the question, but the answer generated by a well-conceived methodology. Because at this stage the answer is not yet known, it is better to focus on developing a question that is amenable to systematic inquiry with the resources that are available.

If you are willing to assume the role of mentor, what then are your responsibilities? This is a very complex question and only broad guidelines will be suggested. First, the faculty member must be available to the student to help with problem solving and counsel. Second, if the target of the research is not one amenable to your skill set, then assuming the role of referral agent is likely the best course of action. The ability to network professionally (ie, locally, regionally, or nationally) provides one with a powerful tool to assist students in their scholarly quest.

Third, recognize that it is the nature of the enterprise that far more projects are started than completed, and clearly, no unique algorithm, recipe, or approach works with all students. Just as teaching a student how to place an epidural catheter, or when to turn down the inhaled agent as the case ends, or how best to evaluate and treat new-onset bradycardia are all context-sensitive (requiring artful intervention and reminders), so is scholarly mentorship. Sometimes the faculty member will need to be more prescriptive than at other times. I do believe that if the project is truly a "student project" then it is vital for the student to be able to claim intellectual ownership. This means that the student can rightfully be listed as the first author on a resultant paper publication.

Fourth, an absolutely vital role is to assist the student in developing a reasonable and manageable timeline, one that ensures that the goals, roles, and milestones are clearly described and understood (by all!) from the outset. In virtually all situations, more time is required to complete a given project than is initially planned. Finally, it is essential that one facilitates clarification of the roles and responsibilities for the student, the faculty, and any others participating in the project. This is also the time to discuss the issue of authorship and the order of listed authors using established criteria (Table 22.4).

Table 22.4. Criteria for Authorship of a Published or Presented Work[2,3]

Authorship requires having made substantial input at all phases of the work. In the case of research, it implies substantial input at:

Study conception and design

Data analysis and interpretation

Drafting and critically revising the submitted and revised paper

Final approval of the published version

Figure 22.1. Submitting a Paper to a Peer-Reviewed Journal

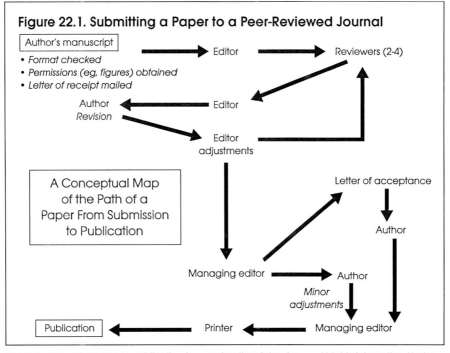

The path from submission to publication is complex, time intensive, and highly interactive. Under the guidance of a coordinating editor (usually the editor-in-chief), the paper is critically reviewed by domain experts and returned to the submitting author for revisions. There are a number of outcomes that might result from peer review that range from acceptance of the paper in its originally submitted form to outright rejection with no chance for reconsideration. The majority of papers fall somewhere between these extremes and with appropriate and timely revision can be published.

It comes as no surprise to experienced educators to learn of a situation in which the faculty mentor actually performed the project for the student. Watching a new student struggle with a clinical procedure or belabor a clinical decision can be frustrating. The desire (and sometimes the necessity) to intervene and simply do it yourself can be overwhelming. This can occur in the scholarship process as well. It is critical to maintain patience and judgment throughout, but, as in the process of clinical instruction, it is also important to know when to encourage and when to intervene directly.

Negotiating the Treacherous Waters of Peer Review

There are many dimensions to the peer review system. Perhaps the most common example involves presenting one's work for colleagues' critique. This can take the form of submitted manuscripts, abstracts, or book chapters. Other forms include poster presentations, oral presentations, grant applications, and even the traditional journal club, where published work is presented and evaluated by those in attendance. An overview of a rather typical process of submitting a paper to a peer-reviewed journal is found in Figure 22.1. A general set of guidelines to be considered when preparing a paper for submission to a peer-reviewed journal is found in Table 22.5, and is typical of what journal editors and reviewers will consider in their critique of a submitted paper.

Students should be informed that the process of peer review is an opportunity to have their work closely examined and critiqued by experts in the domain. The goal of peer review is to perform a collaborative gatekeeping, so that only the most meaningful, accurate, and rational information is formally disseminated. Too often, submitting authors experience anger or intense frustration when their work is criticized—it is not a process to be taken personally! When the submitting author receives the critique of the manuscript, it should be read and put away for a day or 2. Return to it only after a period of reflection with an open mind, free of emotional reactivity. Revise the paper based on reviewers' suggestions. If the student strongly disagrees with certain elements of the critique, emotively driven arguing should be avoided. Instead, the student should prepare a reasonable, scientifically based response to the editor, justifying the case in a well-constructed letter.

The Student Role in the Process of Scholarship

Students must make a substantial commitment to do a properly performed scholarly project. There are many barriers with which the student must contend and it is important to identify and reconcile (if possible) the barriers before moving forward with a serious scholarly project. Table 22.6 is a partial list of common barriers that students encounter in engaging in scholarly activities.

Students who are searching for a faculty advisor should "research the researcher," seeking the views of other students regarding the nature, quality, timeliness, and success of previous scholarly enterprises. The stages of research (from planning to dissemination) all have their inherent pitfalls. Students should be proactive; they

Table 22.5. Suggested Factors to Consider in Preparing a Manuscript for Submission

General considerations:

Adhere precisely to the guidelines and formatting instructions of the journal.

Avoid spelling and grammar errors, which indicate imprecision.

Consider the journal's audience, keeping them in mind as the paper is prepared.

Remain focused on the question(s) and objective(s) raised in the introduction.

Avoid generalizing beyond the scope of the project.

Make sure that the work is original and has relevance.

Avoid self-promotion; let the work stand on its own.

Do not overlook the relevant and important work of others.

Critically discuss cited work rather than simply regurgitating the findings.

Include appropriate references with precision.

Do not rely too heavily on secondary reference sources (textbooks).

Avoid the use of Internet references; these change and are often not peer reviewed.

Avoid editorialization of your personal views.

Discuss implications for practice and how the paper differs from previous work.

Have the paper proofread by a knowledgeable, critical party who is not associated with the paper.

Be as concise as possible.

Considerations specific to research projects:

If relevant, provide proof of Institutional Review Board approval.

Describe your methods in sufficient detail that the study could be replicated.

Carefully consider measurement reliability and validity issues.

If applicable, do a power analysis for appropriate sample size.

Explain how subjects were selected and discuss their representativeness.

Explain and justify the method of data analysis.

Consider the issue of clinical vs statistical significance.

Avoid cause-and-effect conclusions where associations among variables are appropriate.

Ensure that your conclusions are supported by the data.

Explain any conflicts with previous literature.

Suggest implications for practice and future research.

---

should plan for things to go wrong and have contingencies in mind so that they are prepared to deal with setbacks. For example, subject enrollment may not keep pace as anticipated, the database that was planned for the retrospective chart review may be temporarily unavailable, and the noninvasive cardiac output monitor promised for the duration of the study may be recalled.

The Unexpected Happens. Important characteristics of being a successful clinical anesthetist include the ability to solve problems and be resourceful. These attrib-

Table 22.6. Identifying Potential Barriers to Engaging in Scholarly Activity

The student should consider:

Do I have sufficient interest in the area to justify my involvement in this project?

Given my other personal and professional demands, do I have the time to do this project?

Do I have the confidence, experience, and skill set to do this project?

Am I doing this project simply because a faculty member asked me to participate?

Is my primary reason for doing this project because I don't want to offend the faculty?

Is the faculty advisor or mentor someone with whom I can work?

Does the faculty advisor or mentor have a history of success with other students?

If uncertain about your ability to engage in this project, consider choosing a smaller, less complex, less ambitious project.

utes are part of being a researcher. Students should, to the best of their ability, engage problems head-on and attempt to remedy them; however, as in the clinical area, having a successful and experienced mentor with whom the student regularly communicates pays dividends when particularly troublesome problems arise.

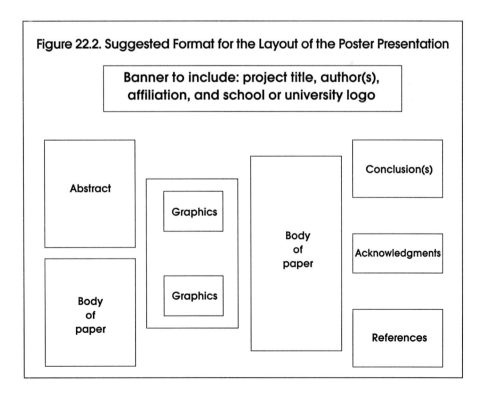

Figure 22.2. Suggested Format for the Layout of the Poster Presentation

Poster Presentations

A common form of scholarship is the poster presentation, which occurs at seminars, scholarly meetings, and clinical conferences. Posters provide the student researcher with the ability to display work visually and discuss research and findings with interested individuals or even small groups. Generally there is a designated location where posters are set up at meetings. For example, at the Annual Meeting of the American Association of Nurse Anesthetists, there is an extensive display of posters organized and located within the exhibit hall. This is a great opportunity for students to display and discuss their projects in a session specifically designed to promote scholarly discourse. Additional information regarding presenting a poster at the Annual Meeting can be found at the American Association of Nurse Anesthetists' website.[4]

There are many recipes for developing a poster, and the recommendations listed in Table 22.7 are provided to give the student some broad guidelines that I have

---

Table 22.7. Preparing a Poster for Presentation of a Scholarly Project

Aesthetic issues:

Keep the poster professional; avoid trying to be too trendy or unconventional.

Consider using contrasting colors for readability but limit your color use to 2 or 3 colors.

Mount your printed material on a colored background to create a border/frame.

Consider using relevant and interesting photographs or figures.

Avoid cramming your materials together even though space is limited.

Use a consistent spacing rule between the elements in your poster.

Consider aligning corners and vertical and horizontal lines (see Figure 22.2).

Organizational issues:

Use a consistent font style throughout the poster (sans serif fonts are easy to read).

The title should be easily read from 20 feet away.

The textual components of the poster should be easily read from 6 feet away.

Emphasize important textual components with bold typeface, color, or by underlining.

Avoid italics because they can be hard to read from a distance.

Organize layout in columns and counterclockwise starting in upper left (see Figure 22.2).

Make section headings distinct from the body of the text.

Graphics are good, but use only those that are relevant and necessary.

Related issues:

Remember you will be interacting with others about your work. Be prepared to discuss!

If the poster is a distillation of a full paper, have copies of the paper for distribution.

Alternatively, have a printed 1-page abstract for distribution.

Alternatively, have a printed 1-page handout of the key points of your research.

Dress professionally.

Have a dress rehearsal; invite others to quiz you before the formal poster session.

---

found to be successful in participating in and observing many poster sessions across a wide range of disciplines. Figure 22.2 offers a suggested format for the actual organization and layout of a poster, although it should be emphasized that many modifications are possible.

Summary

Nurse anesthesia educators find themselves in roles where significant and powerful professional influence occurs. The potential value of inculcation of scholarly activity can have immediate and long-term rewards for students. Think of your students as potential researchers and authors and do not hesitate to share that vision with them. Talk about other student and faculty publishing successes and help your students see that scholarly activities that culminate in poster presentations, oral presentations, and published papers are goals that they can realistically achieve.

Mentoring students by stimulating their interest in scholarly activity and facilitating their success is a deeply rewarding professional activity for NAEs. Ask students if they are considering a scholarly activity. Be supportive if initial enthusiasm wanes a bit as student priorities change. Don't become discouraged if a particularly promising student does not present or publish research. Your role should be defined as one that encourages and facilitates, rather than one that insists. To this end, don't be surprised if at a later time (sometimes even years later) former students send you a copy of their recently published paper or their invited presentation with a thank-you for giving them the inspiration and courage to try.

References

1. Greenwood E. Attributes of a profession. *Social Work.* 1957;2:45-55.

2. International Committee of Medical Journal Editors. Uniform requirements for manuscripts submitted to biomedical journals. *Ann Intern Med.* 1997;126(1):36-47.

3. Shapiro DW, Wenger NS, Shapiro MF. The contributions of authors to multiauthored biomedical research papers. *JAMA.* 1994;271(6):438-442.

4. Professional Development AANA Foundation. State of the science poster sessions guidelines. AANA website. http://www.aana.com/WorkArea/showcontent.aspx?id=18546. Accessed February 20, 2009.

Index